Principles and Methods of Explainable Artificial Intelligence in Healthcare

Victor Hugo C. de Albuquerque
Federal University of Ceará, Brazil

P. Naga Srinivasu
VNR Vignana Jyothi Institute of Engineering and Technology, India

Akash Kumar Bhoi
KIET Group of Institutions, India & Sikkim Manipal University, India

Alfonso González Briones
University of Salamanca, Spain

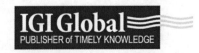

A volume in the Advances in Medical Technologies and Clinical Practice (AMTCP) Book Series

Published in the United States of America by
IGI Global
Medical Information Science Reference (an imprint of IGI Global)
701 E. Chocolate Avenue
Hershey PA, USA 17033
Tel: 717-533-8845
Fax: 717-533-8661
E-mail: cust@igi-global.com
Web site: http://www.igi-global.com

Library of Congress Cataloging-in-Publication Data

Names: De Albuquerque, Victor Hugo C., editor. | Srinivasu, Parvathaneni
   Naga, 1990- editor. | Bhoi, Akash Kumar, editor. | Gonzalez-Briones,
   Alfonso, 1985- editor.
Title: Principles and methods of explainable artificial intelligence in
   healthcare / Victor Albuquerque, Parvathaneni Naga Srinivasu, Akash
   Bhoi, and Alfonso Gonzalez-Briones, editors.
Description: Hershey, PA : Medical Information Science Reference, [2022] |
   Includes bibliographical references and index. | Summary: "This book
   focuses on the Explainable Artificial Intelligence (XAI) for healthcare,
   providing a broad overview of state-of-art approaches for accurate
   analysis and diagnosis, and encompassing computational vision processing
   techniques that handle complex data like physiological information,
   electronic healthcare records, medical imaging data that assist in
   earlier prediction"-- Provided by publisher.
Identifiers: LCCN 2022001647 (print) | LCCN 2022001648 (ebook) | ISBN
   9781668437919 (hardcover) | ISBN 9781668437926 (ebook)
Subjects: MESH: Artificial Intelligence | Diagnosis, Computer-Assisted
Classification: LCC RC78.7.D53 (print) | LCC RC78.7.D53 (ebook) | NLM W
   26.55.A7 | DDC 616.07/54--dc23/eng/20220131
LC record available at https://lccn.loc.gov/2022001647
LC ebook record available at https://lccn.loc.gov/2022001648

This book is published in the IGI Global book series Advances in Medical Technologies and Clinical Practice (AMTCP) (ISSN: 2327-9354; eISSN: 2327-9370)

British Cataloguing in Publication Data
A Cataloguing in Publication record for this book is available from the British Library.

All work contributed to this book is new, previously-unpublished material.
The views expressed in this book are those of the authors, but not necessarily of the publisher.

For electronic access to this publication, please contact: eresources@igi-global.com.

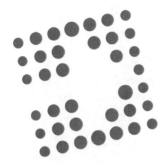

Advances in Medical Technologies and Clinical Practice (AMTCP) Book Series

ISSN:2327-9354
EISSN:2327-9370

Editor-in-Chief: Srikanta Patnaik SOA University, India Priti Das S.C.B. Medical College, India

MISSION

Medical technological innovation continues to provide avenues of research for faster and safer diagnosis and treatments for patients. Practitioners must stay up to date with these latest advancements to provide the best care for nursing and clinical practices.

The **Advances in Medical Technologies and Clinical Practice (AMTCP) Book Series** brings together the most recent research on the latest technology used in areas of nursing informatics, clinical technology, biomedicine, diagnostic technologies, and more. Researchers, students, and practitioners in this field will benefit from this fundamental coverage on the use of technology in clinical practices.

COVERAGE

- Nursing Informatics
- Clinical Data Mining
- Biomedical Applications
- Biometrics
- Clinical Studies
- Patient-Centered Care
- Clinical Nutrition
- Neural Engineering
- Telemedicine
- E-Health

IGI Global is currently accepting manuscripts for publication within this series. To submit a proposal for a volume in this series, please contact our Acquisition Editors at Acquisitions@igi-global.com or visit: http://www.igi-global.com/publish/.

Titles in this Series

For a list of additional titles in this series, please visit:
www.igi-global.com/book-series/advances-medical-technologies-clinical-practice/73682

Big Data Analytics and Artificial Intelligence in the Healthcare Industry
José Machado (Centro ALGORITMI, Universidade do Minho, Portugal) Hugo Peixoto (Centro ALGORITMI, Universidade do Minho, Portugal) and Regina Sousa (Centro ALGORITMI, Universidade do Minho, Portugal)
Medical Information Science Reference • © 2022 • 360pp • H/C (ISBN: 9781799891727) • US $395.00

Computational Intelligence and Applications for Pandemics and Healthcare
Sapna Singh Kshatri (Bharti Vishwavidyalaya, India) Kavita Thakur (Pt. Ravishankar Shukla University, India) Maleika Heenaye Mamode Khan (University of Mauritius, Mauritius) Deepak Singh (NIT, Raipur, India) and G. R. Sinha (Myanmar Institute of Information Technology, Mandalay, Myanmar)
Medical Information Science Reference • © 2022 • 357pp • H/C (ISBN: 9781799898313) • US $345.00

Quality Control Applications in the Pharmaceutical and Medical Device Manufacturing Industry
Eugenia Gabriela Carrillo-Cedillo (Universidad Autónoma de Baja California, Mexico) Karina Cecilia Arredondo-Soto (Universidad Autonóma de Baja California, Mexico) Kenia Palomino-Vizcaino (Universidad Autónoma de Baja California, Mexico) and Héctor Alfonso Magaña-Badilla (Universidad Autónoma de Baja California, Mexico)
Medical Information Science Reference • © 2022 • 298pp • H/C (ISBN: 9781799896135) • US $295.00

Bio-Inspired Algorithms and Devices for Treatment of Cognitive Diseases Using Future Technologies
Shweta Gupta (Jain University, Bengaluru, India)
Medical Information Science Reference • © 2022 • 309pp • H/C (ISBN: 9781799895343) • US $295.00

For an entire list of titles in this series, please visit:
www.igi-global.com/book-series/advances-medical-technologies-clinical-practice/73682

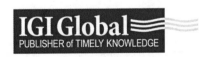

701 East Chocolate Avenue, Hershey, PA 17033, USA
Tel: 717-533-8845 x100 • Fax: 717-533-8661
E-Mail: cust@igi-global.com • www.igi-global.com

Table of Contents

Detailed Table of Contents

Chapter 1

Saravana Kumar N. M., M. Kumarasamy College of Engineering, India
Tamilselvi S., Bannari Amman Institute of Technology, India
Hariprasath K., Vivekanandha College of Engineering for Women, India
Kavinya A., Anna University, Chennai, India
Kaviyavarshini N., Anna University, Chennai, India

Diabetes is one of the most prevalent chronic diseases among all the age groups in developing nations like India. The work collates various machine learning techniques such as SVM, random forests, naive bayes and proposed MLP to perform better detection of diabetes in humans. The goal of this study is to predict the diabetes through neural network of multilayer perceptron. In this study, multilayer perceptron of deep learning algorithm is compared with different machine learning algorithms. The model for the different algorithm is validated with fivefold cross validation. The machine learning algorithms in this study are support vector machine, random forest, and naive bayes. The dataset used for this study is taken from UCI machine learning repository. This algorithm is trained and tested with all the features of the dataset. The algorithms are evaluated based on the accuracy measures. The result obtained shows that the multilayer perceptron of deep learning algorithm gives an accuracy of 98%.

Chapter 2

*Selvani Deepthi Kavila, Anil Neerukonda Institute of Technology and
Sciences (Autonomous), India*
Rajesh Bandaru, GITAM University (Deemed), India
*Tanishk Venkat Mahesh Babu Gali, Anil Neerukonda Institute of
Technology and Sciences (Autonomous), India*
Jana Shafi, Prince Sattam Bin Abdul University, Saudi Arabia

The heart is mainly responsible for supplying oxygen and nutrients and pumping blood to the entire body. The diseases that affect the heart or capillaries are known as cardiovascular diseases. In predicting cardiovascular diseases, machine learning and neural network models play a vital role and help in reducing human effort. Though the complex algorithms in machine learning and neural networks help in giving accurate results, the interpretability behind the prediction has become difficult. To understand the reason behind the prediction, explainable artificial intelligence (XAI) is introduced. This chapter aims to perform different machine learning and neural network models for predicting cardiovascular diseases. For the interpretation behind the prediction, the authors used explainable artificial intelligence model-agnostic approaches. Based on experimentation results, the artificial neural network (ANN) with multi-level model gives an accuracy of 87%, which is best compared to other models.

Chapter 3

*Wazir Muhammad, Balochistan University of Engineering and
Technology, Khuzdar, Pakistan*
Manoj Gupta, JECRC University, Jaipur, India
*Zuhaibuddin Bhutto, Balochistan University of Engineering and
Technology, Khuzdar, Pakistan*

Recently, deep learning-based convolutional neural networks method for image super-resolution has achieved remarkable performance in various fields including security surveillance, satellite imaging, and medical image enhancement. Although these approaches obtained improved performance in medical images, existing works only used a pre-processing step and hand-designed filter methods to improve the quality of medical images. Pre-processing step and hand-designed-based reconstructed medical image results are very blurry and introduce new noises in the images. Due to this, sometimes medical practitioners make wrong decisions, which are very dangerous for human beings. In this chapter, the authors explain that the hand-designed as well as deep learning-based approaches, including some image quality assessment metrics to open the gate to verify the images with different approaches, depend on the single image approach. Furthermore, they discuss some important types of medical images and their properties.

Chapter 4

S. Geetha, BNM Institute of Technology, India
M. Farida Begam, CMR Institute of Technology, India
Ayush Dubey, CMR Institute of Technology, India
Ayush Sengar, CMR Institute of Technology, India
Joshua Samuel Raj, CMR Institute of Technology, India

SARS-CoV-2 (n-coronavirus) is a global pandemic that has killed millions of people all over the world. In severe situations, it can induce pneumonia and severe acute respiratory syndrome (SARS), which can lead to death. It's an asymptomatic sickness that makes life and work more difficult for us. This research focused on the current state of the coronavirus pandemic and forecasted the global situation, as well as its impacts and future status. The authors used the FbProphet model to forecast new covid cases and deaths for the month of August utilizing various information representation and machine learning algorithms. They hope the findings will aid scientists, researchers, and laypeople in predicting and analyzing the effects of the epidemic. Finally, they conclude that the virus's second wave was around four times stronger than the first. They also looked at the trajectory of COVID-19 instances (monthly and weekly) and discovered that the number of cases rises more during the weekdays, which could be due to the weekend lockout.

Chapter 5

Jana Shafi, Prince Sattam bin Abdul Aziz University, Saudi Arabia
Shamayita Basu, University of Kalyani, India
Selvani Deepthi Kavila, Anil Neerukonda Institute of Technology and
*   Sciences, India*

Explainable artificial intelligence (XAI) concentrated on methods and models that simplify the comprehending and analysis of the ML models operation. Using XAI, systems deliver the essential facts to defend outcomes, mostly when unpredicted conclusions are made. It also certifies that there is an auditable and demonstrable way to guard algorithmic judgments including the factors of unbiased and being principled, which lead to building trust. Swift upsurge of non-communicable diseases (NCDs) turns out to be one of the severe health matters and one of the leading origins of death globally. In this chapter, the authors discussed XAI in healthcare, its benefits, and the deep Shapley additive explanations (DeepSHAP)-based deep neural network (DeepNN) framework provided with a feature selection method for prediction and explanation of non-communicable diseases followed by case study discussion about detection and progression of Alzheimer's disease (AD) with the help of XAI-based predictive models.

Chapter 6

Iswarya B., Sri G. V. G. Visalakshi College for Women, India
Manimekalai K., Sri G. V. G. Visalakshi College for Women, India

Deep learning has potential in the process of discovering drug, with enhanced method for analyzing image, structure of molecule and function prediction, along with preset synthesis based on the novel enzymatic structure along tailored features and its applications. Even with expanding quantity based on effective potential approaches, the statistical systems and Machine Learning algorithms that underpin them are sometimes difficult to grasp by the human mind. To meet the required recent paradigm for the automated structure of molecules, for the purpose of 'Explainable Artificial Intelligence' with deep learning approaches. In current era, there is a need for XAI with methods of deep learning to discourse the demand for a developed machine language of the molecular science. This review outlines the important concepts in XAI, possible approaches, and obstacles. It promotes to further development of XAI techniques.

Chapter 7

Hemaraju Pollayi, Department of Civil Engineering, GITAM University (Deemed), Hyderabad, India
Praveena Rao, Department of Civil Engineering, GITAM University (Deemed), Hyderabad, India

Machine learning (ML) has been slowly entering every aspect of our lives, and its positive impact has been astonishing. To accelerate embedding ML in more applications and incorporating it in real-world scenarios, automated machine learning (AutoML) is emerging. The main purpose of AutoML is to provide seamless integration of ML in various industries, which will facilitate better outcomes in everyday tasks. After a violent disaster, the supply of medical services may fall short of the rising demand, leading to overcrowding in hospitals and, consequently, a collapse in the healthcare system. In the chapter, the authors created learning models for COVID-19 to understand how to design a proper ML workflow, which results in an organized, efficient product that produces desired results in terms of diagnosis, prediction, and recommendations. Large amounts of labeled training data are processed and analyzed to identify correlations, patterns, and make predictions using these patterns about future trends.

Chapter 8

Topical Repute on Artificial Intelligence-Based Approaches in COVID-19
Supervision: Distinct Kingpin on Drug Re-Purposing Blueprint......................180
Shamayita Basu, University of Kalyani, India
Jana Shafi, Prince Sattam bin Abdul University, Saudi Arabia

The ongoing COVID-19 pandemic has led to a major oppression of worldwide healthcare infrastructure. In current times, artificial intelligence (AI) and network medicine provide groundbreaking implementation of information science in defining diseases, therapeutics, medicines, and in associating targets with the minimum fallacy. In this big data era, artificial intelligence (AI) has immensely reduced the time and investment of novel targeted drug discovery. As there is continual unfolding of the results of the possible drug combinations, exploitation of artificial intelligence is of utmost necessity so as to hone combination therapy plan. Drug repositioning or repurposing is a methodology by means of which subsisting drugs are being manipulated to handle challenging and emerging diseases, including COVID-19. In this chapter, the authors present the regulations on how to use AI to expedite drug repurposing or repositioning, for which AI propositions are not only intimidating but are also inevitable.

Chapter 9

An Efficient Multi-Layer Perceptron Neural Network-Based Breast Cancer
Prediction 211
Saravana Kumar N. M., M. Kumarasamy College of Engineering, India
Tamilselvi S., Bannari Amman Institute of Technology, India
Hariprasath K., Vivekanandha College of Engineering for Women, India
Kaviyavarshini N., Anna University, Chennai, India
Kavinya A., Anna University, Chennai, India

Cancer is the most deadly disease for human beings across the world due to the adoption of new food habits and pollution. Breast cancer is becoming a common disease for women. After years of research a better analysis and possessing a higher prediction of any kind of cancer, it is still a very imperative contribution in healthcare. In the literature, several attempts were made deploying machine learning methods yielding a significant prediction of cancer. The goal of this study is on machine learning techniques that can enable prediction of breast cancer from the attributes with more accuracy. In this study, Wisconsin Breast Cancer (WBC) dataset has been used to compute machine and deep learning algorithm. This research focuses on logistic regression, decision tree, and random forest and a novel deep learning adoption, multi-layer perceptron. The performances of these algorithms have been correlated with each other using accuracy percentage. Also, sensitivity and specificity are computed as evaluation metrics. The multi-layer perceptron (MLP) gives 97% accuracy.

Chapter 10

    Namana Murali Krishna, AVN Institute of Engineering and Technology,
        Hyderabad, India
    Harikrishna Kamatham, AVN Institute of Engineering and Technology,
        Hyderabad, India
    G. Raja Vikram, Vignan Institute of Technology and Science,
        Hyderabad, India
    J. Sirisha Devi, Institute of Aeronautical Engineering, Hyderabad, India

Human-computer interaction is a potential area of interest since the birth of the computer era. The chapter highlights the usage of electroencephalogram (EEG wave) signals to initiate a conveying medium for immobilized persons, who are not able to express their feelings, by the use of human brain waves or signals. In order to recognize the human feelings or expressions with some emotion by an disable persons, a classifier based on a gamma distribution is utilized. The characteristic of the human brain waves are extracted with the usage of cepstral coefficients. The extracted characteristic is classified into various emotion states using generalized gamma distribution. In order to experiment the proposed model, six healthy persons or subjects are taken aged between from 20 and 28, and a 64 electrode channel EEG system is considered to gather the EEG brain signals under audio as well as visual stimuli. In this chapter, the authors focused the study on four basic human emotions: boredom, sad, happy, and neutral.

Chapter 11

    Oladipo Idowu Dauda, University of Ilorin, Ilorin, Nigeria
    Joseph Bamidele Awotunde, University of Ilorin, Ilorin, Nigeria
    Muyideen AbdulRaheem, University of Ilorin, Ilorin, Nigeria
    Shakirat Aderonke Salihu, University of Ilorin, Ilorin, Nigeria

Artificial intelligence (AI) studies are progressing at a breakneck pace, with prospective programs in healthcare industries being established. In healthcare, there has been an extensive demonstration of the promise of AI through numerous applications like medical support systems and smart healthcare. Explainable artificial intelligence (XAI) development has been extremely beneficial in this direction. XAI models allow smart healthcare equipped with AI models so that the results generated by AI algorithms can be understood and trusted. Therefore, the goal of this chapter is to discuss the utility of XAI in systems used in healthcare. The issues, as well as difficulties related to the usage of XAI models in the healthcare system, were also discussed. The findings demonstrate some examples of XAI's effective medical practice implementation. The real-world application of XAI models in healthcare will significantly improve users' trust in AI algorithms in healthcare systems.

Chapter 12
Principles and Methods of Explainable Artificial Intelligence in Healthcare:
Framework for Classifying Alzheimer's Disease Using Machine Learning......272
Manimekalai K., Sri G. V. G. Visalakshi College for Women, India
Abirami D., Sri G. V. G. Visalakshi College for Women, India

Alzheimer's disease (AD) is a degenerative brain illness that primarily affects elderly adults. This sickness takes away people's capacity to think, read, and do many other things. Clinical trials investigating medications to treat this disease have a high failure rate, due to the difficulty in identifying the patients affected by this disease early on. It affects around 45 million people worldwide. Machine learning, a branch of artificial intelligence, incorporates a range of probabilistic methods. Several approaches showed potential prediction accuracies; however, they were tested using distinct pathologically untested data sets making a fair comparison difficult. Alzheimer's disease (AD) is a degenerative brain disease that mostly affects the elderly. Pre-processing, feature selection, and classification are just a few of the various factors that go into making the framework. This proposed approach directs researchers in the right direction for early Alzheimer's disease detection and can distinguish AD from other disorders.

Foreword

With the emergence of a new discipline, explainable artificial intelligence (XAI), artificial intelligence has witnessed a change in emphasis on implementing and evaluating intelligent systems that can be comprehended and explained. Because of its complexity and various parametric settings, XAI is an intriguing topic to investigate. Especially in healthcare engineering, there is a great demand for making the decision model evident for the audience to build a trustworthy environment. It's always helpful to know how a machine learning-centric healthcare system comes to a particular result. Explainability is crucial to ensure that the system is running as planned, satisfies regulatory requirements, and enables individuals impacted by a decision to question or alter that conclusion.

Explanation impacts on Artificial Intelligence and Machine learning model's acceptance and trustworthiness have also been studied empirically. Recently, XAI research has expanded its scope to include verbal explanations, explanations by prototype, and contrastive exposition, incorporating illustrations over the machine learning models, Iterative explanations, explanations in the training process, and other hybridizations of XAI approaches combining reasoning and learning. Increasingly dynamic features have been established in response to complaints about a lack of adaptability. Additionally, the issue of assessment goes beyond the primary appraisal of the decision model.

Explainability is a widely contested issue with consequences far beyond artificial intelligence features. When it comes to some analytical tasks in healthcare, machine intelligence algorithms have been shown to outperform humans. However, their lack of interpretability has been challenged in the medical decision-making system. Illegality and ethical ambiguity may hamper innovation and prevent breakthrough technologies from improving patient and public health. These technologies may reject critical ethical and professional norms, ignore regulatory problems and inflict significant damage if explainability is not thoroughly considered. However, the black-box nature of AI makes it hard for physicians and authorities to trust it, which is probably understandable in domains like healthcare, where errors may have deadly consequences. In this way, XAI technologies being developed for healthcare applications may justify their findings in a manner that people can comprehend. If you've ever tried to utilize an XAI algorithm, you'll know that it's confined to a handful of situations. However, as they develop, these algorithms will undoubtedly become the standard of care in the healthcare industry. It is in the best interest of health care technology businesses to invest in research and development. As a response to this problem, the notion of XAI has been presented. Rule-based and transparent methods such as Random Forest, Linear Regression, Decision Trees, Bayesian models, and Logistic Regression models are extensively utilized to create hybrid models with several explanation levels. This workshop intends to collect cutting-edge, newest advancements in healthcare applications and foster an open and broad conversation atmosphere for future research. XAI offers a wide range of issues to investigate and great scope for research in XAI-driven healthcare models.

Norita Md Norwawi
Centre for Graduate Studies, Universiti Sains Islam Malaysia, Nilai, Malaysia

Preface

Explainable Artificial Intelligence (XAI) techniques have been proven to record the effectiveness and interpretability of modern technologies featuring implementations over the text, audio, video processing, and predictive analysis in various domains. XAI approaches work with divergent techniques that include Machine Learning (Deep Learning, Artificial Neural Networks, etc.), Ecologically Inspired Computing, and Evolutionary approaches. The XAI would allow the individual to analyze and customize the underlying technology of the model, unlike traditional black-box models.

To ensure the reliability of data-driven AI models for computer-aided diagnostics and predictive analysis, novel Explainable Artificial Intelligence (XAI) techniques are required, effectively handling heterogeneous techniques, especially in fields like data analytics, image analytics, and signal processing. XAI is competent in operating and analyzing the unconstrained environment in fields such as robotic medicine, robotic therapy, and robotic surgery, all of which depend on computational vision to analyze complicated scenarios. AI data-driven models can acquire knowledge from previous experiences, making it possible to operate with divergent illnesses diagnosed through radiological imaging, pathological imaging, neural coding, and sensory data technologies. To obtain a sustainable level of performance in automated diagnosis and therapeutic planning, the designed models must be provided with a tremendous amount of training data. In some situations, the model must possess an excellent prior experience in decision making. In either case, the model must be capable of working with a large amount of healthcare data. XAI is a well-structured, situational, and adaptable technique that lets for promising impartial results. Virtual reality may aid in planning clinical procedures because of the model's capacity to handle diverse healthcare data and the depiction of biological structures. For example, clinical study screening, constant healthcare monitoring, probabilistic evolutions, and evidence-based procedures are all novel uses of XAI in the healthcare business.

The book is suitable for use as a reference guide in institutes with Artificial Intelligence and healthcare engineering specializations. It covers the most important research processes that will encourage new researchers to understand better the implementation methods and underlying issues of current methodologies. Individuals in academia, research, and business, particularly those working in healthcare, computer-aided diagnosis, and allied branches of computer science, would benefit from the suggested book. The proposed book's chapters are self-contained and autonomous of one another, and they include the whole issue formulation and consequent solution. The cutting-edge technology and context-specific approaches embodied in the book and its global scope of research will make this book attractive to the libraries of renowned universities. The healthcare industry can use the book to analyze the simulated results presented in the book.

Chapter 1 presents the deep learning model for diabetes prediction, which uses the XAI-driven model with various machine learning techniques such as SVM, Random forests, Naive Bayes, and Multi-Layer Perceptron over the UCI machine learning repository. The study has presented different classification models and their pros and cons to deal with diabetes prediction that assist in deciding the applicability of the model concerning the availability of the data. The results section has presented the performance analysis of the models mentioned above concerning Accuracy, sensitivity, and specificity. It is observed from the implementation outcome the Multi-Layer Perceptron has exhibited a better performance in the model.

Chapter 2 presents the cardiovascular disease prediction using the Model-Agnostic Explainable Artificial Intelligence technique using the Artificial Neural Network (ANN) approach. Authors have discussed various state-of-art methods for cardiovascular disease prediction in the literature. The study presents the different explainable techniques like SHAP and LIME in making the model interpretable. Multiple classifiers are discussed in the current research, including the K-Nearest Neighbors (KNN) classifier, Logistic Regression, Support Vector Machine with Normal Distribution Model (SVM-NDM), Single-Layered Artificial Neural Networks (SL-ANN), and Multi-Layered Artificial Neural Networks (ML-ANN). The models' performances mentioned above are compared in the results and discussion section of the study.

Chapter 3 presents the Role of Deep Learning in Medical Image Super-Resolution used in various fields, including security surveillance, satellite imaging, and medical image enhancement. The authors have proposed an image enhancement mechanism for improving the quality of the image and performed a statistical analysis of the model. In the current study, binary medical images, Grey Scale Medical images, and color medical images with real-time illuminations. Authors have discussed various image-related properties like bit depth, voxel, pixel, histogram, cross-correlation, natural scene statistics, and multiple noises like Gaussian noise, Salt and Pepper noise, and Mean, Median Filter. Different image formats are discussed in the current study for better comprehensibility.

In Chapter 4, the authors have presented a Tool for Analyzing and Forecasting the COVID-19 Situation using FbProphet Model Algorithms. The study includes the report's analysis over a period of time, and the impact of covid 19 is analyzed using the model's prediction. The weekly and monthly covid scenarios are discussed in line with deaths observed for a period of time. The authors have shown the predicted time series results concerning the plot for better comprehensibility of the study. The authors compare the obtained results with the ARIMA model, Exponential model, Deep Learning, Regression Methods, Compartmental methods, support vector machine, prophet algorithm, and Nature inspired models.

Chapter 5 presents the Role of Explainable Artificial Intelligence (XAI) in the Prediction of Non-Communicable Diseases (NCDs) using the Deep learning-based SHAP Additive Explanations named DeepSHAP over the Deep Neural Network (DeepNN) framework provided with a feature selection for detection and progression of Alzheimer's disease (AD) are discussed. The authors have discussed the benefits of XAI and its role in the healthcare domain. The results section presents the performances of the various prediction models like the KNN, Random Forest, and Support Vector Machine. The case study discussed in the current study would outline the implementation outcome of the XAI-driven prediction model.

Chapter 6 presents the Drug Discovery with XAI using the Deep Learning model for analyzing the image, the structure of the molecule, function prediction, present synthesis based on the novel enzymatic structure, tailored features, and applications presented in the study. The influence of XAI in the drug discovery process is discussed in the current study. Authors have presented the architecture of XAI in drug discovery and various deep learning models like Recurrent Neural Network, Convolutional Neural Network, Long Short-Term memory, and other approaches like Feature Attribute, Instance-based approaches, Graph Convolution method, and Uncertainty is discussed in the current study.

Chapter 7 presents the Learning Models for Healthcare Systems Using Python for COVID-19, the Susceptible-Exposed -Infected - Recovered-Death (SEIRD) model. Authors have discussed the mathematical model of the SEIRD for assessing the COVID 19 by partitioning the Susceptible (S), Exposed (E), Infections (I), Recovered (R), and Deceased (D). The authors have assessed the total death rate using the proposed model, and the model's performance has been evaluated against the actual deaths due to COVID-19. Authors have discussed the role of AutoML in dealing with unstructured and structured data. Few code snippets are placed in the manuscript, which could assist in building similar models for the smart analysis of the disease.

Chapter 8 presents the regulations on using AI to expedite drug repurposing or repositioning amid COVID-19. Authors have discussed various aspects like diagnosis, correlating ai with pharmaceutical studies, and the use of XAI in drug repurposing Blueprint. Authors have discussed the different existing state-of-art artificial intelligence-driven drug discovery techniques. They have briefly discussed XAI over deep learning architecture and graph representation learning in drug discovery.

Chapter 9 presents an Efficient Multi-Layer Perceptron Neural Network-Based Breast Cancer Prediction over the Wisconsin Breast Cancer (WBC) dataset. The study has focused on data collection, data pre-processing, implementation of classification algorithms, and corresponding activation functions. The authors have evaluated the performances of the proposed model with the Logistic Regression, Decision Tree, and Random Forest concerning the metrics like Accuracy, sensitivity, and specificity. The study has concluded that the multi-layer perceptron has exhibited better performance.

In Chapter 10, the authors have presented a model-based approach for Extracting emotional status from immobilized beings using EEG Signals. Authors have focused on four basic human emotions like boredom, sadness, Happy and neutral by analyzing the characteristic of the human brain waves, extracted with cepstral coefficients. The process of emotional recognition using the EEG signals and the Generalized Gamma Distribution are discussed, along with the methodology followed for acquiring the EEG signals. The results section compares the Double Truncated Gaussian mixture model and the generalized Gaussian distribution.

Chapter 11 presents the fundamental issues and challenges of Explainable Artificial Intelligence (XAI) in the Healthcare system. The authors have presented the framework for the XAI-driven healthcare system and the challenges associated with the XAI concerning the responsibilities of AI models. The other pivotal aspects like Bias, Data Learning, Fairness, Hardware dependencies, complexity, dealing with inadequate data, protection, and abstractions associated with the machine learning models in the healthcare domain are discussed. The future directions discussed in the current study would lay a road map for the XAI in the healthcare domain.

Chapter 12 shows the XAI-Framework for classifying Alzheimer's Disease using Machine Learning. The current study discusses various state-of-art techniques and their limitations in classifying Alzheimer's disease. Various feature selection approaches like the Best First Search (BFS), Greedy Stepwise over the Decision table, and ZeroR classifiers. Authors have compared the performance of the proposed XAI-driven classification model with Decision Tree, ZeroR, OneR, JRip, Naïve Bayes concerning execution time, Mean Square Error, Root Mean Square Error, and Kappa Statistics. The study would provide an insight into how the XAI would make the decision process of the classification model interpretable.

The proposed book focuses on Explainable Artificial Intelligence (XAI) for healthcare, offering a comprehensive review of cutting-edge technologies for accurate analysis and diagnosis of diseased. The book also includes computational vision processing approaches for dealing with complex data such as physiological information, discovery, and medical imaging data, which aid in providing appropriate medical treatment for the patients. The books currently on the market are limited to machine learning algorithms in healthcare to automate diagnosis and prediction models. In recent times, computer-aided diagnosis has shifted its focus toward a more adaptable algorithm and makes healthcare data management more effortless. XAI models make it feasible to alter them according to a context-specific demand that yields a better outcome.

Victor Hugo C. de Albuquerque
Federal University of Ceara, Brazil

P. Naga Srinivasu
GITAM University (Deemed), India

Akash Kumar Bhoi
KIET Group of Institutions, India, & Sikkim Manipal University, India

Alfonso Gonzalez Briones
University of Salamanca, Spain

Acknowledgment

The editors would like to appreciate the efforts of all those who were engaged in this project, especially the authors and reviewers who have contributed the best of their knowledge in formulating the chapters. We owe a debt of gratitude to each and every one of the editorial team for their consistent support throughout the process.

All the contributors in the book have obeyed the recommendations of the reviewers of reviewers in performing the necessary amendments in their chapter for better comprehensibility of the study. Timely responses of all the chapter contributors have assisted the editors in smooth handling of the project. We are thankful to those invited chapter reviewers who has examined the chapters to ensure that the publishing met the requisite level. The chapter reviews would not have been possible in a timely way without their critiques, helpful remarks, and suggestions.

We specially acknowledge the support of Editorial Advisory Board teams for their timely interactions on progress of the project and assistance in development phase. We thank Angelina Olivas and Elizabeth Barrantes, Assistant Development Editor, IGI Global for their unconditional support. The publisher, IGI Global, are most cordially appreciated.

Chapter 1
Deep Learning Model for Diagnosing Diabetes

Saravana Kumar N. M.
M. Kumarasamy College of Engineering, India

Tamilselvi S.
Bannari Amman Institute of Technology, India

Hariprasath K.
Vivekanandha College of Engineering for Women, India

Kavinya A.
Anna University, Chennai, India

Kaviyavarshini N.
Anna University, Chennai, India

ABSTRACT

Diabetes is one of the most prevalent chronic diseases among all the age groups in developing nations like India. The work collates various machine learning techniques such as SVM, random forests, naive bayes and proposed MLP to perform better detection of diabetes in humans. The goal of this study is to predict the diabetes through neural network of multilayer perceptron. In this study, multilayer perceptron of deep learning algorithm is compared with different machine learning algorithms. The model for the different algorithm is validated with fivefold cross validation. The machine learning algorithms in this study are support vector machine, random forest, and naive bayes. The dataset used for this study is taken from UCI machine learning repository. This algorithm is trained and tested with all the features of the dataset. The algorithms are evaluated based on the accuracy measures. The result obtained shows that the multilayer perceptron of deep learning algorithm gives an accuracy of 98%.

DOI: 10.4018/978-1-6684-3791-9.ch001

INTRODUCTION

Diabetes is a generic reference to a wide range of metabolic disorders caused by a high sugar level in the blood, which continues for a long duration. Diabetes can be cured only by predicting and identifying the diabetes in early stages and have an adaptive living pattern from person to person. They are two main reasons for the cause of diabetes in humans. The first reason is the insufficient supply of insulin in the pancreas, which may be of low insulin in the beta-cell. Thus, it requires sugar for the intensity of the body. The second reason is the resistance of insulin in the body and the reaction of the insulin, which is not sufficient for the cells in the body. By taking the food for the body, the carbohydrate will automatically be converted into a sugar called glucose. The then converted glucose will be dissolved in the human blood stream where it is stored as site. Zhu et al. (2019)

Insulin is a protein hormone utilized for the migration of glucose to handle energy. If the diabetes is not predicted at the starting stage, then the insulin cannot balance properly in the bloodstream. As a result, there is a significant increase in the sugar in the blood, which may severely affect either or give insistent damage to the parts of the body. Here numerous cells are required to build up a body which basically in demand to gain more energy. Parte et al. (2020) When consuming more liquid and solid foods, the body will split the whole particle into smaller blood glucose, giving energy for our regular activity. There is no direct delivery of glucose to the cells. For that, a bridge is generated that carries the glucose from the blood vessel to the liver, deposited in adipose tissue. When the glucose level is reduced, the sugar is withdrawn from the bloodstream. Insulin is an influential hormone that allows glucose from penetrating the body's cells for stamina. If the blood glucose level is reduced, then the sugar level in the blood is high, then it causes the disease called hyperglycemia. Ameena et al. (2020)

Types of Diabetes

Out of the wide spread types of diabetes, top three predominant types are referred to as Type I, Type II and Gestational diabetes.

- Type I - In Type I diabetes, the outcome is chosen from the pancreas's failure, which yields an adequate amount of insulin in procession for damage of beta cells. This damage of beta cells was formerly termed as insulin-dependent diabetes mellitus (IDDM) and is also commonly known as juvenile diabetes. The body responded with the immunity development against various diseases becomes the main cause for the damage of beta cells that are not identified in the past.

- Type II - In Type II diabetes, the outcome starts with the conflict of insulin. Conflict of insulin means the cells will not reply to the insulin properly. This case of disease developed will affect in deficiency of insulin. This insulin deficiency was formerly termed as non-insulin-dependent diabetes mellitus(NIDDM) and is also commonly referred to as an adult-onset diabetes across the globe. The main cause for the onset of the NIDDM is due to less physical activities like white collar jobs and irregular or no routine exercises which results in an undesirable and uncommon increase in body weight.
- Gestational diabetes – Gestational diabetes is mainly found during pregnancy in which the woman is not found diabetes in her history, which develops the blood glucose level to maximum.

The main step in healthcare is prevention and treatment. This step involves retaining a hale and better nutrition, regular physical workout, maintaining a normal weight, and avoiding tobacco which are the main health hazards. Blood pressure control foot and eye care maintenance are also more important for diabetes people. Type I diabetes, called IDDM which maintained with the help of insulin vaccination. Type II diabetes, called NIDDM, is maintained with treatment that may include insulin vaccination or may not include insulin vaccination. In some cases, the insulin vaccination or some treatment can also cause blood sugar levels to a minimum. Guttikonda et al. (2019) The surgery for weight loss for obese people will be an adequate treatment for Type II diabetes. Gestational diabetes, which is caused in pregnant ladies, will be resolved subsequently when the birth of a baby. The characteristic sign of diabetes, which is natural, is weight loss which happens without any intention. The sign may increase promptly in Type I diabetes within a week or month, which may not be present in type II diabetes. The other main sign may also be sleepiness frequently. In accumulation to the above case, many also have vision problems, blurred and headache, slow remedial of cut, and skin may be itching. Sarwar et al. (2018)

Data Science is one of the emerging scientific fields that may help in predicting the disease at starting stage. The patient's probability can be predicted with the help of the features available. Machine and deep learning can use for the accurate prediction of diabetes. They are classified into three types supervised, unsupervised, and reinforcement learning. Supervised learning helps to learn from the data available, and the result is predicted. In this study, various machine learning and deep learning algorithm like Random Forest, Naive Bayes, Support Vector Machine (SVM) are compared with deep learning named multi-layer perceptron, which gives more accuracy. In this paper, a model using Keras is built for more accuracy.

The chapter is organized as, In Section 2, the work related to the proposed work is discussed. In Section 3, the methodology of the work is provided, along with the dataset description and algorithms used. In Section 4, Evaluation metric used for analysis is discussed. In Section 5, the result produced for the entire algorithm is discussed. Finally, the study is concluded in Section 6 and future work. Rahman et al. (2020)

RELATED WORKS

Diabetes is widely regarded as one of the lethal diseases that caused due to imbalance in blood glucose levels. Dey et al. (2018) had proposed and tested a novel web application model that accurately predicts the onset of diabetes employing various machine learning approaches. The dataset used is PIMA Dataset. The preprocessing of the dataset would help for improving the accuracy. Data normalization plays a key role in boosting the accuracy and reducing the computational time significantly. In this paper, min-max scaling has been applied to improve accuracy. With the investigation done, the min-max scaling in ANN exhibits a better accuracy while the same scaling is applied with other machine learning approaches. The model can be used in future deep learning, and a location-based dataset can be collected.

Ayman et al. (2018) predicted diabetes using a machine learning algorithm. Healthcare is a rapid advancement technology in the field of research. The machine learning approach helps more diagnose diabetes and more in decision making. The classifier model is built using the weka tool. The experiment is done with the help of four classifier models like Naive Bayesian model, Support Vector Machine, conventional Random Forest and CART. From the experimentation results, the support vector machine outperforms well among the remaining algorithms.

Sneha et al. (2016) attempted to detect and predict diabetes by proposing a ML model built on a backpropagation neural network. The significant contribution made in the work is that they demonstrated the prediction by designing a light-weight artificial neural network with the help of backpropagation that is implemented with one input layer, fewer hidden layers and output layer. The input layer consists of 8 features, and the hidden layer has ten neurons for better performance. The backpropagation neural network outperforms well, with an accuracy of 81%.

Rahul et al. (2018) analyzed some classifiers to predict diabetes. Diabetes is very difficult to diagnose at the early stage. The significance of the work lies in the decision that the features were not chosen arbitrarily but from the probable features that carries information by analyzing the real-time health history of similar patients and then the analysis is carried out for early diagnosis and treatment. The experiment is done by training using PIMA India dataset. The classifier used here are as follows Support Vector Machine, Gradient Boosting, Decision Trees, Logistic Regression, Random Forest, Nearest Neighbors and Neural Network. For studying the performance of each classifier, optimization is carried out by tuning the parameters among various classifier Random Forest with a benchmarking 80% accuracy for real-time testing.

Saru et al. (2019) predicted diabetes with the help machine learning algorithm. The Healthcare industry has a huge amount of data that is sensitive. The growing fatal disease in the world is diabetes. A type of bioinformatics medical analysis is done with the help of a dataset collected from the UCI machine learning repository. In this paper, the resampling technique with the help of bootstrapping to enhance the accuracy is done for machine learning algorithms like Naive Bayes, Decision tree, and K Nearest Neighbor. Decision trees outperform with high accuracy of 94%. Faruque et al. (2019) has analyzed a machine learning algorithm to predict diabetes. Diabetes is common in humans who are caused due to increase in sugar levels. If diabetes is predicted early, it can be controlled and help save a life. Here, the machine learning algorithms are compared, such as Naive bays, Support Vector Machine, C4.5 decision tree, and K Nearest Neighbor. The decision tree algorithm performs well.

Yuvaraj et al. (2019) Predicted diabetes using machine learning algorithm on Hadoop Cluster. Diabetes is the major disease that causes blindness, failure in the kidney, and heart attack. Many healthcare monitoring systems are available around the world for diagnosing diseases. Hadoop cluster helps store the huge dataset and process it in a cloud environment. Random forest algorithm produces high accuracy in 4 node Hadoop environment. Verma et al. (2019) proposed a neural network system to predict diabetics. Diabetics are one of the silent metabolic disorders that affect a large number of humans worldwide. Diabetics damage the whole human body badly and have more complications in the body. This disease is difficult to identify in today's scenario lifestyle, which has less physical activity and more consumption of junk foods. In this paper, machine learning-based multi-layer perceptron is utilized to identify diabetics in patients. Here 5-fold cross-validation is also applied for a better result after training. The accuracy of the experiment is 82% for the prediction of diabetics. This result is compared with all other algorithms. They concluded by the future scope of using the ensemble technique for more accuracy.

Ashiquzzaman et al. (2017) introduced a prediction model by reducing the overfitting for predicting diabetic disease since overfitting minimizes the accuracy for prediction. This method is a dropout for the overfitting issue, and neural network in deep learning is combined with dropout by many layers. The proposed system has increased the prediction rate for the dataset. The process is started by introducing the entire dataset into the input layer, which is then pushed to the underlying connected layers thereby from each layer acts as a continual dropout layer. The fitted output which is the desired final result is found as a residue in the output layer and is also mapped with a single node. These layers are designed to form a multi-layer with perceptron. In the proposed system, the experimental results rate the accuracy of the NN models is 88.41% for the particular dataset. When the attempts to be made to address the overfitting, the accuracy of the system founds to be increased further.

Suresh et al. (2020) investigated various machine-learning based models to predict diabetes. Diabetes is a fatal disease globally, and it ends with complications like stroke, nerve disease, and damage in kidney and heart disease. They developed a system for predicting diabetics at a prior stage by utilizing different machine learning techniques. This paper has been analyzed using the statistical computing tool of R studio software. To perform the study and investigate the proposed models, the UCI machine learning dataset is used for training the model and testing. Initially, the data set is splitted for training and training 60-40 and then the model is trained to predict diabetics using R. Machine learning algorithms, namely Bayes, K Nearest Neighbor and Ensemble learning of Classification type and K-Means, Hierarchical agglomerative of cluster type and Logistic and multiple regression of regression type, are used to diagnose diabetics in early stage. The accuracy obtained in this model is 88% which is the maximum among all algorithms.

Tigga et al. (2020) performs a machine learning algorithm based approach for predicting more accuracy. In India, more than 30 million people are affected by diabetes. When this disease is identified early, then treatment can also be provided early to reduce the risk. Here different machine learning algorithm is applied for predicting diabetics with more accuracy. Early prediction of diabetics is more important in the field of healthcare. If the model is trained with better accuracy, the person can identify the risk of diabetics early. In this paper, they collected a dataset which has 952 instances that have been collected from questionnaires through online and offline mode, which includes 18 questions related to daily activity, background related to gene, and health-related. The data set is applied to some machine learning algorithms, and it is found that the random forest algorithm has more accuracy. They have also tested the dataset from the UCI repository, which shows the random forest has more accuracy.

Sahoo et al. (2020) suggested different machine learning and deep learning methods to identify diabetics. The dataset used for analysis is the diabetic dataset from the UCI machine learning repository. The different machine learning algorithms are compared with Convolutional Neural Network (CNN) based deep learning and found that the CNN based deep learning has more accuracy than all the machine learning algorithms. Parab et al. (2020) implemented the hybrid machine learning model to detect diabetics. Even though Bayes is used to detect diabetes, it is not detected with high accuracy and efficiency. So multi-layer hybrid machine learning is built for more efficiency. The Bayes model is combined with SVM for more accuracy in the hybrid model. They concluded that the hybrid system is in progress, and further research can improve the accuracy.

Table 1. Summary of some state-of-art works

Literature	Techniques used	Description	Limitation
Dey et al. (2018)	Supervised Machine Learning Approach SVM, KNN, Naive Bayes Algorithm, ANN	The proposed Artificial Neural Network model possess a higher accuracy of 82.35% than other supervised machine learning algorithms with Min-Max scaling on PIMA.	Other advanced NN models and Deep learning model shall be used for evaluation.
Ayman et al. (2018)	Supervised Machine Learning Approach Naive Bayes, Simple CART algorithm, Random Forest, SVM	High accuracy is achieved for SVM of 79%.	The machine learning models have been developed using a tool called WEKA.
Sneha et al. (2016)	Artificial Neural Network	Artificial Neural Network algorithm predicts whether the patients are diabetes or not diabetic within a few seconds with an accuracy of 81%.	For a medical aid, the model is not capable enough with lesser accuracy despite being faster.
Rahul et al. (2018)	Machine Learning algorithms like KNN, Gradient boosting, Decision trees, Logistic Regression, SVM Random Forest, and Neural network	Different parameters for better performance tune the algorithms. From all machine learning models, Random Forest performed well with an accuracy of 79.7% on the PIMA data set.	The ensemble method combines various base models to improve prediction accuracy.
Saru et al. (2019)	Machine Learning algorithms like Logistic regression with SVM, DT (J48), KNN (1,3)	The proposed method provides high accuracy with an accuracy value of 94% for the decision tree after bootstrapping.	Along with bootstrapping, min-max normalization can be applied.
Faruque et al. (2019)	Machine Learning algorithms like C4.5, Naive Bayes, Decision Tree, SVM, KNN	The decision tree C4.5 is significantly high in performance for classification with an accuracy of 73%.	The machine learning models have been developed using a tool called WEKA.
Yuvaraj et al. (2019)	Machine learning algorithms on Hadoop cluster	Random forest with 4 node Hadoop cluster environment has 94% of accuracy.	Metaheuristic algorithms can be accomplished with machine learning algorithms.
Verma et al. (2019)	Multilayer Perceptron Neural Network	The overall accuracy of the Multilayer Perceptron Neural Network model is 82%.	Time consuming for an average accuracy.

PROPOSED WORK

The proposed work attempts to investigate various machine learning approaches such

Figure 1. Workflow for Diagnosing Diabetes

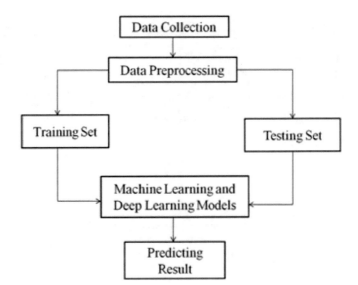

as Random Forest, Support Vector Machine, Naive Bayes, and a deep learning multi-layer perceptron model. The study is then carried out by the performance analysis of those algorithms is compared for the better prediction of diabetes. To perform the experimentation, the renowned UCI dataset is considered from the UCI machine learning repository. Since the dataset is incomplete for few entries, the dataset is initially preprocessed to find and address the missing values, thereby increasing the prediction capability of the models. The dataset, which is preprocessed, is then feed into the training model in which the model used grid search among various algorithms to predict the accuracy of the disease.

METHODOLOGY AND DATASET

Methodology

From figure 1, the workflow of the entire process has been demonstrated as various modules of the work. One of the contributions made here is the Preprocessing technique based on the median of mean range to fill the missing values. Then the dataset is split based on 10-fold approach for training and testing on the various machine learning and deep learning model. Then the result is compared among machine and deep learning algorithms.

Dataset Description

UCI Diabetes dataset is selected to carry out the research for two reasons. First being, most of the benchmarking literatures were carried out using the dataset, thereby to showcase our approach it would be easily comparable. The next important reason is the dataset is rich in terms of 9 attributes and 768 instances for the prediction which is huge and meaningful. It is to be note that all the records are female records. Naz et al. (2020) The attributes featuring in the corresponding dataset are glucose, skin thickness, blood pressure, pregnancies, insulin, diabetes pedigree function, BMI, age and outcome. In the dataset, the outcome attribute is a labelled dependent attribute which is based on the probability of having diabetes or not whereas all the other attributes such as glucose, blood pressure, skin thickness, pregnancies, insulin, BMI, diabetes pedigree function, age regarded as independent attributes. The attributes are described in table 1.

Table 2. Features of Dataset

Attribute	Description
Pregnancies	Total count of pregnant
Glucose	the concentration of Plasma glucose - 2 hours in the test of an oral glucose tolerance
blood pressure	Value of blood pressure (mm HG)
skin thickness	Skinfold thickness of triceps (mm)
Insulin	Level of insulin given in every 2 hours (mu U/ml)
BMI	Level of Body mass index BMI=weight/height (kg/m^2)
Diabetes Pedigree Function	The function whose scores likelihood of diabetes based on family history
Age	Age of individual in years
Outcome	Class variable (0 or 1) 0-No Diabetes 1-Diabetes

ALGORITHMS

10-Fold Cross-validation

Cross-Validation is used to train several models based on a subset of data. PIMA dataset split into 10 gatherings. The dataset is prepared for the prototype of 10-1 folds. The prototype is iterated form intervals. On every fold m data argumentation is utilized for validation.

$$CrossValidation\left(cv_{(m)}\right) = \frac{1}{m}\sum_{l=1}^{m}MSE_l \qquad (1)$$

Training Data

For training, 60% of data is utilized.

Validation Data

The data with more performance is selected and utilized to run the validation set. Commonly 10% to 30% of data is involved in the validation.

Test Data

For training, 5% to 20% of data is utilized to find unbiased values.

Pseudocode

Step 1:   Train Data: Split into 10 cohorts gathering.
Step 2:   Iteration l=1 to 10.
Step 3:   9 parts train model.
Step 4:   Calculate the accuracy with 1 part.
Step 5:   Typical accuracy is calculated with ten cohorts.

Support Vector Machine

Support vector machine (SVM) utilizes the theory of Vapnik Chervonenkis and the structural risk minimization principle. Soni et al. (2020) In SVM, the boundary possibilities are reduced on the train set. First, the sample group is introduced and implemented in the training model. Next, the kernel function is selected. With the help of feature selection, a minimum count of features is selected and utilized, improving the classifier's performance. Ladha et al. (2018)

The classification task is $\left\{i_x, j_x\right\}, x = 1....n, j_x \in \left\{-1,1\right\}, i_x \in R^d$, where i_x is spot-on data and j_x are labeled. The hyperplane is denoted by $v^t i + k = 0$ where v is the vector coefficient of d-dimension, k is an equalizer. Splitting linear Type is denoted as

$$\text{Maximum: } g\left(v, \xi\right) = \frac{1}{2}\left\|v\right\|^2 + c\sum_{x=1}^{w}\frac{3}{4}_x \qquad (2)$$

Figure 2. Support vector machine architecture

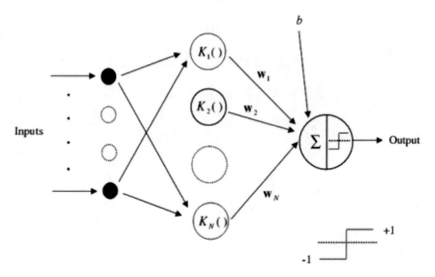

Focus to: $j_x\left(v^t i_x + k\right) \geq 1 - \xi_x \xi_x \geq 0$ (3)

After introducing Lagrangian multipliers as $\alpha_m\left(m = 1, 2, \ldots\ldots w\right)$,

Minimum: $\sum\limits_{x}^{w} \alpha_i - \dfrac{1}{2}\sum\limits_{x=1}^{w}\sum\limits_{y=1}^{m} \alpha_x \alpha_y j_x j_y i_x^t i_y$ (4)

Focus to: $0 \leq \alpha_x \leq C, \sum\limits_{x=1}^{w} \alpha_x j_{x=0}$ (5)

The Karush Kuhn–Tucker (KKT) states that,

$\alpha_x\left(j_x\left(v^t i_x + k\right) - 1\right) = 0$ (6)

11

If $\alpha_x > 0$, corresponding data is referred to as Support Vector and result receipts

are $v = \sum\limits_{x=0}^{w} \alpha_x y_x i_x$, where w is Count of SV. k *is* attained by $j_x \left(v^t i_x + k \right) - 1 = 0$,

where i_x is SV. When v and k are found. Linear Discriminant function is assumed as,

$$g\left(i\right) = sgn\left(\sum\limits_{x=1}^{w} \alpha_x j_x i_x^t i + k\right) \tag{7}$$

Mapped decision function is,

$$g\left(i\right) = sgn\left(\sum\limits_{x=1}^{w} \alpha_x j_x \varnothing(i_x)^t \varnothing\left(i\right) + k\right) \tag{8}$$

Where $i_x^t i$ *is* input space, referred to procedure $\varnothing(i_x)^t \varnothing\left(i\right)$ in the space parameter and elected kernel is known by $K\left(i_x, i_y\right) = \varnothing(i_x)^t \varnothing\left(i\right)$. This function is referred as,

$$g\left(i\right) = sgn\left(\sum\limits_{x=1}^{w} \alpha_x j_x K\left(i_x, i_y\right) + k\right) \tag{9}$$

In SVM, the parameter values are selected by a regularized parameter that decreases the error and gamma parameter that define the mapping of non-linear space, and finally, the kernel parameter.

Pseudocode
  Step 1: Read Dataset .
  Step 2: Set the kernel to linear.
  Step 3: Set random_state value, scaling value, and class value.
  Step 4: Test the dataset for accuracy.
  Step 5: Repeat from step 2 for maximum accuracy.

Advantages Ayman et al. (2018)

- Easy to deal with complex datasets.
- Overfitting risk is minimum in SVM.

- The accuracy value of the algorithm is more.

Disadvantage Ayman et al. (2018)

- More expensive for computational cost.
- Very difficult to train the kernel for more accuracy.
- Training time for the dataset takes more time.

Random Forest

Random Forest is one of the widely used supervised learning algorithms that carries a special tag of uniqueness than others. It is adaptable and equally convenient for decision-making for both regression and classification problems. It is also said as ensemble leaner, which creates a greater number of classifiers, and the classifier results are accumulated. Preetha et al. (2020) The random forest can create more number classification, and regression trees (CART) in which training is given based on the sample of bootstrap of the unique training data and search is based on the random method that is selected based on the subdivision of the input variables that is used for defining the split among them. Daghistani et al. (2020) Classification and regression trees are a binary decision trees built by the split of data in the node to the child node starting from the root node, which includes the whole sample node. Aliberti et al. (2019) The working process of random forest is selecting of samples, the decision is calculated based on tree and result is predicted, next the voting method is accomplished. Finally, the result is predicted based on the vote. Xu et al. (2019)

Pseudocode

Step 1:   Read the dataset.
Step 2:   Start with singe region.
Step 3:   Set number of iterations and splits.
Step 4:   Test the dataset for accuracy.
Step 5:   The average of voting combines prediction.
Step 6:   Repeat from step 2 for maximum accuracy.

Advantage Daghistani et al. (2020)

- The random forest has minimum variance.
- Random forest is more flexible.
- It gives accuracy even when the dataset is not scaled and has missing values.
- Combines the various decision tree for more accuracy.

Disadvantage Daghistani et al. (2020)

Figure 3. Random forest architecture

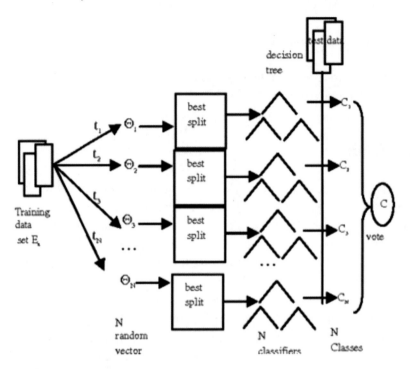

- Random forest is more complex for execution and construction.
- Random forest consumes more time.
- Random forest requires more computational resources.

Naïve Bayes

Naive Bayesian model is a classical probabilistic classification technique that utilizes the statistical method and supervises learning. Patil et al. (2020) It is also a learning algorithm of the inductive method and straight, straightforward probabilistic method of the Bayesian theorem with robust prospects. The performance goal is to test instances with the highest accuracy. The hypothesis probability is calculated. In this classifier, the class result does not depend on other parameters for the result. This classifier performs well in risk problems. Tyler et al. (2020)

The probability of the classifier is calculated through the instance $I_x,...., I_y$ as,

$$P(C = c \mid I_x = i_x,...., I_y = i_y) \tag{10}$$

Nondependent of the conditional class is given by,

$$P\left(C = c | I_x = i_x, \ldots, I_y = i_y\right) = P\left(C = c\right) * \prod_{I_z} P\left(I_z = i_z | C = c\right) \tag{11}$$

Finally, the more subsequent probability is given by,

$$max_c \prod_{I_z} P(I_z = i_z \mid A = a) \tag{12}$$

The four conditions of the Naive Bayes Classifier are,
Subsequent probability with Class A,

$$max_{c_x \in C} P(a_x \mid i) \tag{13}$$

Subsequent probabilities P(Axli) is calculated with help of,
$$P\left(a_x | i\right) = \frac{P\left(i | a_x\right) P\left(a_x\right)}{P\left(i\right)} \tag{14}$$
Probability P(ila$_x$) is evaluated by,

$$P\left(i | a_x\right) = \prod_{y=1}^{m} P(a_y \mid a_x) \tag{15}$$

Estimate the probabilities for P(A$_x$) and P(K$_y$la$_x$) with use train set,

$$P\left(k_y | a_x\right) = \frac{1}{\sqrt{2\pi}\sigma_{yx}} e^{\left[-\frac{\left(k - \mu_{yx}\right)^2}{2\sigma_{yx}^2}\right]} \tag{16}$$

Pseudocode
    Step 1:   Examine the train data.
    Step 2:   The mean and standard deviation of the different parameter is calculated in every class.
    Step 3:   Density equation used to calculate probability.

Step 4:   Class probability is calculated

Step 5:   Identify the class with the largest probability.

Advantage Saru et al. (2019)

Figure 4. Naïve Bayes flowchart

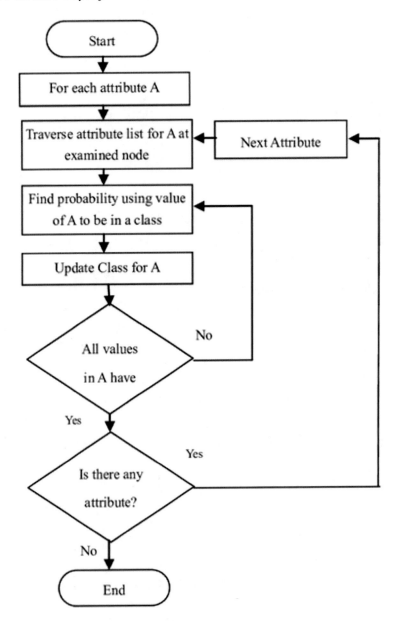

- The model of Naive Bayes is statistical.
- The efficiency of the training algorithm is more.
- It can be utilized in various problems and fields.
- Instance orders will not be affected.
- Novel Data can be predicted.

Disadvantage Saru et al. (2019)

- Assumptions for independent feature with not hold attribute.
- For large datasets, the precision value will be less.

Multilayer Perceptron

A Multi-layer perceptron (MLP) is a feed-forward artificial neural network. It exists of minimum nodes of 3 layers as input, hidden, and output layers. Other than the input node, every node is a neuron that utilizes a non-linearity activation function. MLP needs a supervised learning method (backpropagation) to train. Both the non-linear activation function and multiple layers categorize MLP from linear perceptron. It will categorize the data, which is separate in linear.

The concept of MLP is mainly used equivocally, almost to any feed-forward artificial neural network, also defined as the network which is combined of a multi-layer perceptron. These perceptions are commonly known as vanilla neural networks in colloquial, especially when we hold one hidden layer.

Activation Function

If multiple layer perceptron has activation function linearly in neurons, it means the linear function will sketch the inputs (weighted) to output in all neurons. Further linear algebra defines either layer could be modified to 2 layered input, output model. In Multilayer perceptron, few neurons are non-linear. It was evolved to the frequency model of biological neurons, which is action potentials. There are 2 accepted activation functions in sigmoids. They are,

$$y\left(v_i\right) = tanh\left(v_i\right) and y\left(v_i\right) = \left(1 + e^{-v_i}\right)^{-1} \tag{17}$$

Modern advancement in deep learning, Rectifier Linear Unit (ReLU) is high intermittently utilized as the potential method to overwhelm the problems in numerical relevant to sigmoid.

17

In this, the hyperbolic tangent sort from -1 to 1, also the remaining is the logistic function related to the shape but sort from 0 to 1. Now, y_i is the output of the ith neuron, and v_i is the input connections of the weighted sum. Here alter activation function is developed for both rectifier and soft plus activation functions. The most specific activation function comprises the radial basis function.

Learning

Learning arises in perceptron by adjusting the connection of the weights. Subsequently, all data is measured, depending on the number of errors during the execution (output) to the desired result. It illustrates supervised learning then achieves backpropagation, the proposal of the algorithm of least mean square to the linear perceptron. Verma et al. (2019)

Here we show the degree of the output node error j in the nth data point by $e_j(n) = d_h(n) - y_j(n)$, where d is a target variable, and y is a perceptron value. The weights of the node are further modified, which depends on the corrections that increase the error in the result that is given by

$$\in (n) = \frac{1}{2} \sum_j e_j^2 (n) \tag{18}$$

Now gradient descent is used to alter every weight is

$$\Delta w_{ji}(n) = -\cdot \frac{\partial \in (n)}{\partial v_j(n)} y_i(n) \tag{19}$$

Where y_i is output of preceding neuron and η is learning rate, has preferred to ensure that the weights suddenly converge to feedback excluding oscillations.

The derivation must be computed based on activated local field v_j, which changes. Also, it is simple to validate for an output node. This derivation can be made simple to

$$\frac{\partial \in (n)}{\partial v_j(n)} y_i(n) = e_j(n) \varnothing'(v_j(n)) \tag{20}$$

Where $\varnothing'$ is the derivation of the activation function mentioned above, which did not change. The study is complicated for the adjustment of weights in hidden node, yet it can program that known derivation is

$$-\frac{\partial \in (n)}{\partial v_j (n)} = \varnothing'\left(v_j (n)\right)\sum_k -\frac{\partial \in (n)}{\partial v_k (n)}\, w_{kj}(n) \tag{21}$$

This is dependent on the variation in weights of kth nodes, which means the output layer. So to modify the weights of the hidden layer, the weights of the output layer may vary according to the derivation of the activation function. Thus, this algorithm performs backpropagation of the activation function.

Feedforward neural networks (FFNNs) are prominent models of Artificial Neural networks that can recognize and approximately compute models utilizing their advancement in a correlated layered design. They are comprised of neurons set, which performs as processing component, scattered over a list of entirely connected heap layers. MLP is a peculiar class of FFNN. In Multilayer perceptron, neurons have arranged in 1 direction. Data transition happens among three layers: input layer, hidden layer, and output layer. It explains the Multilayer perceptron network with 1 hidden layer. The inter-connection between those layers should be outlined by various weights [-1 to 1]. Every node in MLP will achieve 2 functions: one is activation, and another is a summation. The summation function is summed by the inputs, weights, and bias products.

$$S_j = \sum_{i=1}^{n} w_{ij} I_i + \beta_j \tag{22}$$

Where n is the no. of inputs, Ii represent input i, β_j is bias, and w_{ij} is weight connection.

Next, an activation function has been stimulated by using Eq. (13), various models of activation functions can be handled in Multilayer perceptron. The function has outlined in Eq. (14)

$$f_j (x) = \frac{1}{1 + e^{-S_j}} \tag{23}$$

Subsequently, the final result of neuron j can be acquired in Eq. (15)

Figure 5. Multilayer perceptron architecture

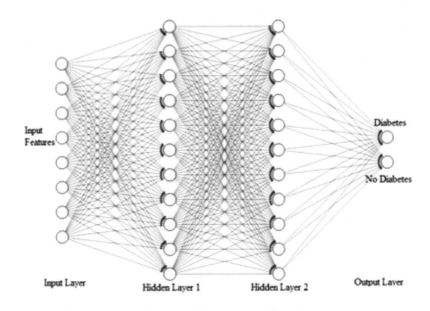

$$y_i = f_j \left(\sum_{i=1}^{n} \omega_{ij} I_i + \beta_j \right) \tag{24}$$

The framework of Artificial Neural Network is modeled, the learning step is observed and fine-tuned, then the network weights are modified. Those weights are rationalized to compute the result and decrease the error.

Advantage Verma et al. (2019)

- It is utilized as a metaphor for biological/medical neural networks.
- Compute competently, so that can parallelize simply.
- Computing the global value of machines.

Disadvantage Verma et al. (2019)

- Slow convergence.
- The training process can influence local minima.
- Difficult to scale.

EVALUATION METRICS

Accuracy

Accuracy is computed by the total sum of true positive and true negative over the sum of classification attributes of true and false values. It refers how much the classification model predicts correctly over all the predictions.

$$\text{Accuracy} = \frac{TP + TN}{TP + TN + FP + FN} \tag{25}$$

Sensitivity

Sensitivity is a metric which is used to assess how much is the model correctly predicting the patients with a disease out of the correct predictions it made.

$$\text{Sensitivity} = \frac{TP}{TP + TN} \tag{26}$$

Specificity

Specificity is a metric which is used to assess how much is the model correctly predicting the patients without disease out of the correct predictions it made.

$$\text{Specificity} = \frac{TN}{TP + TN} \tag{27}$$

RESULT AND DISCUSSION

The objective and motivation of the study are to build an efficient deep learning model that can predict the probability of having diabetes or not and increase the model efficiency with the help of activation function and introducing the dropout layer.

For the algorithm, the total number of data trained is 576 and the data tested are 192. For Proposed MLP, the correctly predicted data is 191 and wrongly predicted

Table 3. Accuracy of various algorithms

Algorithm	Accuracy (%)	Sensitivity (%)	Specificity (%)
SVM	85	85	84
Random Forest	89	88	88
Naive Bayes	92	90	91
Multilayer perceptron Neural Network	98	97	97

is 1, which is less maximum accuracy for the proposed model. Not only the accuracy sensitivity and the specificity which classifies the diseased and non-diseased correctly is also high compared to all. The investigation is carried out by selecting the parameters from the diabetes dataset. The performance analysis of machine learning and deep learning algorithms like support vector machines, naive Bayes, random forest, and multi-layer perceptron are compared along with the other work. From the result statistic represented, It is clear that Proposed MLP outperforms well among all the algorithms with high accuracy of 98%, and sensitivity and specificity of 97%. Proposed MLP uses the activation function and hidden layer feature for more accuracy and in less time. Figure 6 and Table 3 represent the accuracy of various algorithms performed in the diabetic dataset. This is observed that the accuracy of Multilayer perceptron of deep learning algorithm has higher accuracy of 98% than the accuracy of SVM of 85%, Random Forest of 89%, and Naive Bayes of 89%,

Figure 6. Accuracy comparison of various algorithms

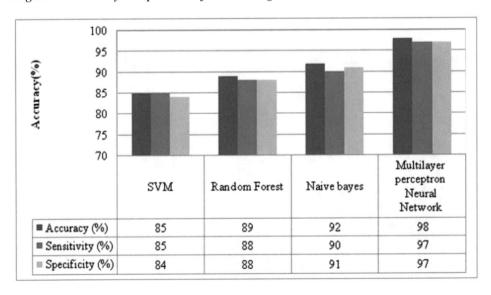

	SVM	Random Forest	Naive bayes	Multilayer perceptron Neural Network
■ Accuracy (%)	85	89	92	98
■ Sensitivity (%)	85	88	90	97
■ Specificity (%)	84	88	91	97

which is lower. Sensitivity and specificity also follow the same, high for Proposed MLP with 97% respectively

CONCLUSION

The experiment is done with various machine and deep learning algorithms on the PIMA India diabetes dataset collected from a UCI machine learning repository with 768 female records. The proposed multi-layer perceptron outperforms the benchmarking models with an accuracy of about 98% with the help of activation function with three layers input, hidden, and output layer. The Proposed MLP model exhibits its predominance in predicting the disease more accurately than other conventional approaches in the literature. The significance of predicting diabetes is the immediate demand of the health care sector in India, being the largest growing population of diabetes globally. Also, diabetes can be greatly controlled and treated better in humans at the early stage as it is difficult to treat diabetes at a critical stage.

As a future direction, the metaheuristic approach can be studied as an adaptive learning model built based on both machine and deep learning algorithms. Also, both the automated learning models shall be experimented on predicting the np-hard multi-class problem of finding the severity of the disease with a large dataset. Some of the bio-mimics optimization techniques can be deployed to increase the model's efficacy.

REFERENCES

Dey, S. K., Hossain, A., & Rahman, M. M. (2018). Implementation of a Web Application to Predict Diabetes Disease: An Approach Using Machine Learning Algorithm. *21st International Conference of Computer and Information Technology (ICCIT)*, 1-5. 10.1109/ICCITECHN.2018.8631968

Ayman, M., & Dhage, S. N. (2018). Diabetes Disease Prediction Using Machine Learning on Big Data of Healthcare. *2018 Fourth International Conference on Computing Communication Control and Automation (ICCUBEA)*, 1-6. 10.1109/ICCUBEA.2018.8697439

Sneha, J., & Borse, M. (2016). Detection and Prediction of Diabetes Mellitus Using Back-Propagation Neural Network. *2016 International Conference on Micro-Electronics and Telecommunication Engineering (ICMETE)*, 110-113. 10.1109/ICMETE.2016.11

Rahul, B., & Kulkarni, P. (2018). Analysis of Classifiers for Prediction of Type II Diabetes Mellitus. *2018 Fourth International Conference on Computing Communication Control and Automation (ICCUBEA)*, 1-6. 10.1109/ICCUBEA.2018.8697856

Saru, S., & Subashree, S. (2019). Analysis and Prediction of Diabetes Using Machine Learning. *International Journal of Emerging Technology and Innovative Engineering*, *5*(4).

Faruque, M., Asaduzzaman, & Sarker, I. (2019). Performance Analysis of Machine Learning Techniques to Predict Diabetes Mellitus. In *2019 International Conference on Electrical, Computer and Communication Engineering (ECCE)*. IEEE Xplore.

Yuvaraj, N., & SriPreethaa, K.R. (2019). Diabetes prediction in healthcare systems using machine learning algorithms on Hadoop cluster. *Cluster Computing, 22*, 1–9. doi:10.1007/s10586-017-1532-x

Verma, G., & Verma, H. (2020). A Multilayer Perceptron Neural Network Model For Predicting Diabetes. *International Journal of Grid and Distributed Computing*, *13*, 1018–1025.

Ashiquzzaman, A., Kawsar Tushar, A., Islam, R., Shon, D., Im, K., Park, J., Lim, D., & Kim, J. (2017). *Reduction of Overfitting in Diabetes Prediction Using Deep Learning Neural Network*. Computer Vision and Pattern Recognition.

Suresh, K., Obulesu, O., & Ramudu, B. V. (2020). Diabetes Prediction using Machine Learning Techniques. Helix-The Scientific Explorerǀ Peer Reviewed Bimonthly. *International Journal (Toronto, Ont.)*, *10*(02), 136–142.

Tigga, N. P., & Garg, S. (2020). Prediction of type 2 diabetes using machine learning classification methods. *Procedia Computer Science*, *167*, 706–716.

Sahoo, A. K., Pradhan, C., & Das, H. (2020). *Performance Evaluation of Different Machine Learning Methods and Deep-Learning Based Convolutional Neural Network for Health Decision Making* (Vol. 871). Nature Inspired Computing for Data Science - Studies in Computational Intelligence.

Parab, S., Rathod, P., Patil, D., & Chikkareddi, V. (2020). A Multilayer Hybrid Machine Learning Model for Diabetes Detection. In *ITM Web of Conferences* (Vol. 32). EDP Sciences.

Ladha, G. G., & Pippal, R. K. S. (2018, October). A computation analysis to predict diabetes based on data mining: a review. In *2018 3rd international conference on communication and electronics systems (ICCES)* (pp. 6-10). IEEE.

Aliberti, A., Pupillo, I., Terna, S., Macii, E., Di Cataldo, S., Patti, E., & Acquaviva, A. (2019). A multi-patient data-driven approach to blood glucose prediction. *IEEE Access: Practical Innovations, Open Solutions*, *7*, 69311–69325.

Xu, Z., & Wang, Z. (2019). A Risk Prediction Model for Type 2 Diabetes Based on Weighted Feature Selection of Random Forest and XGBoost Ensemble Classifier. *2019 Eleventh International Conference on Advanced Computational Intelligence (ICACI)*, 278-283. DOI: 10.1109/ICACI.2019.8778622

Tyler, N. S., Mosquera-Lopez, C. M., & Wilson, L. M. (2020). An artificial intelligence decision support system for the management of type 1 diabetes. Nat Metab, 2, 612–619.

Rahman, S. A., AlRashed, R. A., AlZunaytan, D. N., AlHarbi, N. J., AlThubaiti, S. A., & AlHejeelan, M. K. (2020). Chronic Diseases System Based on Machine Learning Techniques. *Int. J. Data.Science*, *1*(1), 18–36.

Daghistani, T., & Alshammari, R. (2020). Comparison of statistical logistic regression and randomforest machine learning techniques in predicting diabetes. *Journal of Advances in Information Technology, 11*(2).

Naz, H., & Ahuja, S. (2020). Deep learning approach for diabetes prediction using PIMA Indian dataset. *Journal of Diabetes and Metabolic Disorders*, *19*, 391–403.

Guttikonda, G., Katamaneni, M., & Pandala, M. (2019). Diabetes Data Prediction Using Spark and Analysis in Hue Over Big Data. *2019 3rd International Conference on Computing Methodologies and Communication (ICCMC)*, 1112-1117.

Preetha, S., Chandan, N., Darshan, N. K., & Gowrav, P. B. (2020). Diabetes Disease Prediction Using Machine Learning. *International Journal of Recent Trends in Engineering & Research*, *5*(6), 37–43.

Patil, R., Majumder, L., Jain, M., & Patil, V. (2020). Diabetes Disease Prediction Using Machine Learning. International Journal of Research in Engineering, Science and Management, 3(6), 292-295.

Soni, A. N. (2020). *Diabetes Mellitus Prediction Using Ensemble Machine Learning Techniques*. Available at SSRN 3642877..

Zhu, C., Idemudia, C. U., & Feng, W. (2019). Improved logistic regression model for diabetes prediction by integrating PCA and K-means techniques. *Informatics in Medicine Unlocked*, *17*, 100179.

Parte, R. S., Patil, A., Kad, A., & Kharat, S. (2019). Non-invasive method for diabetes detection using CNN and SVM classifier. *International Journal of Research in Engineering, Science and Management, 2*, 659-661.

Ameena, R. R., & Ashadevi, B. (2020). Predictive analysis of diabetic women patients using R. In *Systems Simulation and Modeling for Cloud Computing and Big Data Applications* (pp. 99–113). Academic Press.

Sarwar, M. A., Kamal, N., Hamid, W., & Shah, M. A. (2018, September). Prediction of diabetes using machine learning algorithms in healthcare. In *2018 24th international conference on automation and computing (ICAC)* (pp. 1-6). IEEE.

Chapter 2

Analysis of Cardiovascular Disease Prediction Using Model–Agnostic Explainable Artificial Intelligence Techniques

Selvani Deepthi Kavila

ⓘ https://orcid.org/0000-0001-5307-3113

Anil Neerukonda Institute of Technology and Sciences (Autonomous), India

Tanishk Venkat Mahesh Babu Gali

Anil Neerukonda Institute of Technology and Sciences (Autonomous), India

Jana Shafi

Prince Sattam Bin Abdul University, Saudi Arabia

Rajesh Bandaru

GITAM University (Deemed), India

ABSTRACT

The heart is mainly responsible for supplying oxygen and nutrients and pumping blood to the entire body. The diseases that affect the heart or capillaries are known as cardiovascular diseases. In predicting cardiovascular diseases, machine learning and neural network models play a vital role and help in reducing human effort. Though the complex algorithms in machine learning and neural networks help in giving accurate results, the interpretability behind the prediction has become difficult. To understand the reason behind the prediction, explainable artificial intelligence (XAI) is introduced. This chapter aims to perform different machine learning and neural network models for predicting cardiovascular diseases. For the interpretation behind the prediction, the authors used explainable artificial intelligence model-agnostic approaches. Based on experimentation results, the artificial neural network

DOI: 10.4018/978-1-6684-3791-9.ch002

(ANN) with multi-level model gives an accuracy of 87%, which is best compared to other models.

INTRODUCTION

Cardiovascular diseases (CVDs) also known as heart diseases are a leading cause of death worldwide, with an estimated 17.9 million people dying from CVDs. Cardiovascular diseases are a range of heart and vascular problems (Westerlund et al., 2021), (Virani et al., 2021). According to a World Health Organization (WHO) report, more than four out of five cardiovascular disease deaths are caused by myocardial infarction, and one-third of these deaths occur in people under the age of 70. Identifying high-risk individuals for cardiovascular disease and ensuring appropriate treatment can help prevent early deaths. The majority of CVDs can be prevented by avoiding risk factors such as excessive alcohol consumption, a poor diet, obesity, cigarette use, and physical inactivity (Ghosh et al., 2021).

Figure 1. Graph displaying relationship between age and heart disease frequency

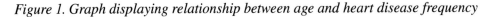
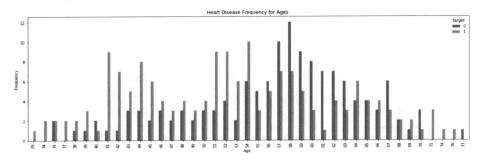

Figure 1 illustrates which age group are suffering more from heart diseases. The blue color of the graph indicates the people (in millions) not suffering from heart disease and orange indicates the people suffering from heart disease. It can be depicted that in the age group 29-54, people suffering from heart diseases are more compared to not suffering from the heart diseases. In contrast, for the people whose age is greater than 54, the people suffering from heart diseases are comparatively less.

Both the Figures 1 and 2 show general trends of occurrence of heart diseases with respect to age and gender.

Numerous machine-learning algorithms, such as the Support Vector Machine, the Decision Tree, and numerous more, have been suggested. While these algorithms provide great accuracy, they are not easily interpretable. In comparison, although techniques such as Naive-Bayes and Linear Regression can be studied, their accuracy

Figure 2. Graph displaying relationship between gender and cardiovascular disease percentage

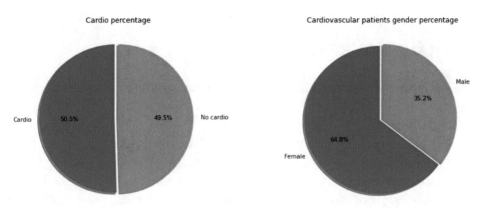

is limited (London, 2019), (Duval, 2019). While they are capable of analyzing sophisticated algorithms, they lack the ability to relate the data's properties (Kavila et al., 2021), (Pawar et al., 2020). Given that the majority of individuals are unable of comprehending sophisticated algorithms, it is critical to create a model that is understandable to the average person.

In healthcare, models must explain why they made a particular categorization and significantly reduce their accuracy numbers to do so. These are referred to as Explainable AI (XAI) approaches (Porto et al., 2021). We used the SHAP (Shapley Additive Explanations) and LIME (Local Interpretable Model-Agnostic Explanations) to implement these methods. The Model-Agnostic XAI technique's characteristics are intended to help visualize the qualities' contribution to classification. In this study we used methods such as Support Vector Machine with Normal Distribution Model (SVM-NDM), Logistic Regression (LR), K-Nearest Neighbors and Single-Layered Artificial Neural Networks (SL-ANN) and Multi-Layered Artificial Neural Networks (ML-ANN) to create an end-to-end interpretable Explainable Artificial Intelligence system for cardiovascular disease prediction. Our Major Contributions outlines:

1. Predicting the cardiovascular disease of the data points using machine learning and neural network models.
2. Displaying the interpretability behind the prediction with the help of SHAP and LIME technique plots.

The outline of the paper is as follows: Section 2 represent the overview of related research on Cardiovascular disease prediction. Subsequently, section 3 sketches out the proposed system and Section 4 describes the results and accuracies of the models and plotting model-agnostic explainable artificial intelligence techniques plot for a data point. Conclusion and Recommendations for future works are in section 5.

LITERATURE SURVEY

Various researchers have explained and experimented with different kinds of datasets to predict cardiovascular and other diseases and used various machine learning methods and tools.

An Dinh, Somya D. Mohanty, Amber Young, Stacey Miertschin (Dinh et al., 2019) have proposed a model exploring data-driven approaches that use supervised learning model to identify cardiovascular diseases and diabetes patients. With the help of feature sets and various time-frames for the data, various machine learning algorithms (gradient boosting, SVM, logistic regression, and random forest) are estimated for the classification performance and then combined the models to improve weighted group model and classification accuracy. To identify the key attributes within the patient data, information gained from tree-based models contributed to detecting at-risk patients in cardiovascular disease is used by the data-learned models. The proposed model has achieved an AU-ROC score of 83.1% on NHANES dataset.

Erico Tjoa et al (Tjoa & Guan, 2020) proposed a survey paper on XAI. As of late, computerized reasoning and AI overall have shown noteworthy exhibitions in numerous undertakings, from picture preparation to normal language handling, particularly with the approach of profound learning. Clarifications for machine choices and expectations are consequently expected to legitimize their dependability. This requires more noteworthy interpretability, which regularly implies the author need to comprehend the component hidden in the calculations. The Discovery of an illness at its beginning stage is regularly basic to the recuperation of patients or to keep the infection from progressing to more extreme stages. While AI techniques, fake neural organizations, mind machine interfaces and related subfields have as of late shown promising execution in performing clinical errands, they are not really awesome. Numerous papers have recommended various measures and systems to catch interpretability, and the subject reasonable man-made consciousness (XAI) has become an area of interest in ML research in the local area. The author applies the order into the clinical field. A few endeavors are made to validate interpretabilities numerically, some give visual clarifications, while others may zero in on the improvement in task execution subsequent to being given clarifications created by calculations.

Kumar G Dinesh, et al (Dinesh et al., 2018) used machine learning models to detect cardiovascular disease and it is a range of diseases that affect the arteries and heart. The proposed model helps to make choices about the changes to occur in risky patients, which reduce their threats. Among the proposed models i.e., Naïve Bayes, Random Forest, Gradient Boosting, the Logistic Regression model is performing well on the Cleveland heart dataset with an accuracy of 91.6%.

N. Yasnitsky, A. Dumler, A. N. Poleshuk et al. (Yasnitsky et al., 2015) has proposed a system to diagnose and predict the progression of the most widespread cardiovascular diseases. It captures the disease progression and recommends the correction in lifestyle for that patient after completing investigations on the recommendations obtained. The author observed that some of them are not only unhealthy but harmful for many. So, the presented system allows doctors to reveal those non-typical patients and to make individual recommendations for them.

Najmul Husan, Yukan Bao (Hasan & Bao, 2021) studied various feature selection methods for predicting cardiovascular disease, and they proposed a model to determine the features. The author used a two-step feature sub-set retrieving technique to obtain the features contributing to CVD in the model. The first step is considering three well-established feature selections (embedded, filter, wrapper) and in second step, Boolean process is used for extracting the feature sub-set by these three algorithms. The author's used algorithms like random forest, SVM, Naïve Bayes, and XGBoost models to find the accurate model. From the models, the XGBoost Classifier combined with the wrapper methods to get the accurate result.

N. G. Bhuvaneswari Amma (Amma, 2012) has presented work about the medical diagnostic system for cardiovascular disease risk prediction. The author took relative advantage of the genetic algorithm and neural network to build the system. For training the system on Cleveland heart dataset, a genetic-based neural network and Backpropagation are used. After training, the output were classified into five categories based on stage of the disease namely absent, low, medium, high and serious. The proposed neural network model has obtained an accuracy of 94.17%.

Qiang Huang et al. (Huang et al., 2020) proposed a non-linear local interpretable model for graphs using Hilbert-Schmidt Independence criterion lasso. A non-linear interpretable model is generated from its N-Hop Neighborhood and then computed the K most representative features to explain its prediction using HSIC Lasso. This model is known as GraphLIME. The author combined 10 noisy features with 2 real-world datasets and invented 2 classifiers by recursively training GraphSAGE or GAT classifers until both the training and testing accuracy was above 70%.

Radwa ElShawi et al. (ElShawi et al., 2021) have proposed a study on Interpretable machine learning techniques. Due to lack of intuition and explanation of their predictions in complex machine learning models. With the new general data protection regulation (GDPR), the plausibility and validity of predictions made by ML models have become vital. In this paper, the author presented the four primary quantitative measures for accessing the quality of interpretability techniques: similarity, Execution time, Trust, and Bias detection. The proposed models were Anchors, LORE, ILIME,

MAPLE etc. and found out that MAPLE was performing well on text data with 95% identity performance and ILIME is performing well on tabular data with 58% trust.

Siddhika Arunachalem (Arunachalam, 2020) represent in the paper that, Machine Learning plays a vital role in identifying cardiovascular disease and, if specified in advance, can provide significant insights to doctors who can then adapt their treatment and diagnosis for each patient. In the proposed methods (Gradient Boost classifier, Random Forest Classifier, Extra Trees Classifier, MLP Classifier) applied on Cleveland Dataset, initially, the features are selected from the records. Data pre-processing takes place, which utilizes methods like removing missing data and noisy data, fill the default values, attribute classification for prediction, and decision-making at different levels. Classification, sensitivity, accuracy, and specificity analysis is used to get the accurate model. Among all the proposed models the MLP classifier is more accurate with an accuracy of 91.7%.

PROPOSED SYSTEM

The Neural Network architecture (figures 6 and 7) and feature selection of the proposed models is different from the existing systems that makes the proposed

Figure 3. System architecture control flow(Direction) from CVD Prediction Model to Output

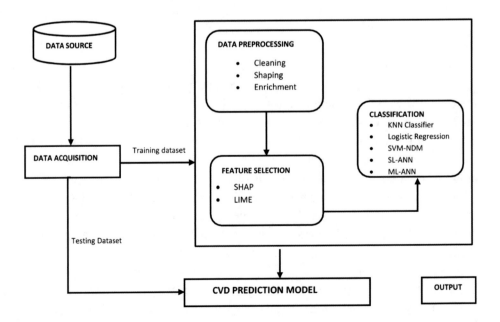

system more accurate compared to existing methods. Various Machine Learning, Neural Network and XAI Models were used for training the cardiovascular disease dataset. The training of the proposed models is as shown in the Figure 3 that involves five significant steps. They are:

1. Data Acquisition
2. Data Pre-processing
3. Feature Selection
4. Training Classification Methods
5. Testing Data

Data Acquisition

Data Acquisition is used to identify and gather data-related problems. Here, we identified the different data origins and acquires the data from various sources. The quantity and quality of acquired data will play a vital role in determining the accuracy of output. The more data points, the more cases the algorithms tend to learn. The dataset for cardiovascular disease is collected from the Kaggle website, which has approximately 70000 data points. There are 14 attributes in the dataset. They are: id, age, gender, height, weight, ap_hi, ap_low, cholesterol, glucose, smoke, alcohol, active, pulse and cardio. ap_hi and ap_lo refers to the Systolic blood pressure and Diastolic blood pressure respectively. The unit for age attribute in the dataset is

Figure 4. Sample datapoints of cardiovascular disease patients acquired from Kaggle website

	id	age	gender	height	weight	ap_hi	ap_lo	cholesterol	gluc	smoke	alco	active	cardio
2	0	18393	2	168	62	110	80	1	1	0	0	1	0
3	1	20228	1	156	85	140	90	3	1	0	0	1	1
4	2	18857	1	165	64	130	70	3	1	0	0	0	1
5	3	17623	2	169	82	150	100	1	1	0	0	1	1
6	4	17474	1	156	56	100	60	1	1	0	0	0	0
7	8	21914	1	151	67	120	80	2	2	0	0	0	0
8	9	22113	1	157	93	130	80	3	1	0	0	1	0
9	12	22584	2	178	95	130	90	3	3	0	0	1	1
10	13	17668	1	158	71	110	70	1	1	0	0	1	0
11	14	19834	1	164	68	110	60	1	1	0	0	0	0
12	15	22530	1	169	80	120	80	1	1	0	0	1	0
13	16	18815	2	173	60	120	80	1	1	0	0	1	0
14	18	14791	2	165	60	120	80	1	1	0	0	0	0
15	21	19809	1	158	78	110	70	1	1	0	0	1	0
16	23	14532	2	181	95	130	90	1	1	1	1	1	0
17	24	16782	2	172	112	120	80	1	1	0	0	0	1
18	25	21296	1	170	75	130	70	1	1	0	0	0	0
19	27	16747	1	158	52	110	70	1	3	0	0	1	0
20	28	17482	1	154	68	100	70	1	1	0	0	0	0
21	29	21755	2	162	56	120	70	1	1	1	0	1	0

number of days and can be converted to years by dividing with 365. An attribute named "pulse" is added to dataset by subtracting ap_lo from ap_hi.

Data Pre-Processing

Data Pre-Processing is mainly used to know the characteristics of the data and to understand the format and quality of data. The data cleaning must be done and converted into a usable data type (mostly data frames). In this process, the data wrangling procedure selects the features to use in the model. Removing unnecessary data points (like points having null values etc.) is required to deal with quality issues. If the attribute encounters null values, then it is replaced by the mean of the feature.

Feature Selection

Feature Scaling using Standard Scaler class

Feature Selection is used to find the features that contribute more to the given model. To acquire these features, we have to find the outliers present in the data and adjust them to the interquartile range. Outliers mean the bounds of the given points. Generally, outliers don't contribute to the model much, so they should be either removed or minimized. We suggest that outliers should not remove from the data type. So, one of the best ways to reduce is using the interquartile range. The interquartile range is the difference between the 25th and 75th percentile of the data of a given feature.

Feature Selection using Explainable Artificial Intelligence (XAI) tools

Explainable Artificial Intelligence (XAI) tools are used for finding the individual feature contribution in the given dataset. In this paper, the given dataset consists of 14 features. Six features (age, ap_lo, ap_hi, weight, cholesterol, pulse) were selected using EDA (Exploratory Data Analysis) and heatmap plot as shown in figure 5 and their contributions were plotted using XAI tools in the section Local Interpretable Model-Agnostic Explanations (LIME) Plots and Shapley Additive Explanations (SHAP) Plots and the working of XAI techniques is described in the section Feature Contribution Visualization using SHAP and Feature Contribution Visualization using LIME.

Figure 5. Heatmap of cardiovascular disease dataset

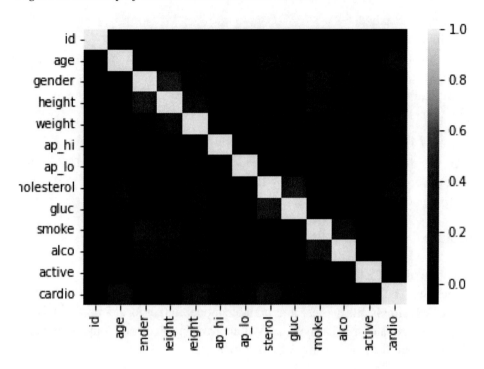

Feature Contribution Visualization using SHAP

We used the SHAP tool, which is an Explainable AI tool introduced by Lundberg and Lee. SHAP stands for Shapley Additive Explanations. The idea behind SHAP is a cooperative game theory (Rathi, 2019). It means SHAP values are found out for each feature, indicating the contribution towards the model. The main intuition behind Shapley values is that we want to compare how the correlation would perform with v/s without a specific feature. In this way, we can find out how this feature contributed to the model. The Shapley values are calculated for a feature correlation in each subset. Then averaging all of these contributions gives us marginal contribution of a feature to model, also known as marginal value.

Formula for calculating Shapley values,

$$\$_i\left(f, x\right) = \sum_{z' \subseteq x'} \frac{\left|z'\right|!\left(M - \left|z'\right| - 1\right)!}{M!}\left[f_x\left(z'\right) - f_x\left(z' / i\right)\right] \quad (1)$$

In the Above formula,

$\mathcal{S}_i$: Shapley value for feature i.

f: Blackbox model.

x: Input Datapoint.

z' : Subset.

x' : set of all subsets.

M: total number of features.

$f_x\left(z'\right)$: Blackbox model output with feature.

$f_x\left(z' \mathbin{/} i\right)$: Blackbox model output without feature.

In this dataset Kernel SHAP technique is used for calculating SHAP Values. The time complexity for calculating the SHAP value for all features is 2^n, where 'n' is number of features.

Feature Contribution Visualization using LIME

The basic idea of LIME is that we just focus into the local area of the individual predictions. Thus, we can create a simple explanation that makes sense in that local area. LIME simply fits a linear interpretable model in that local area which is also called as surrogate. It is basically a local approximation of our complex model in this local area. It works on any Blackbox model.

Formula for calculating LIME values,

$$\xi\left(x\right) = \arg\min{}_{g \int G} L\left(f, g, \pi_x\right) + \Omega\left(g\right) \tag{2}$$

In the above formula,

x : Input Variables.

g : Simple Interpretable model (Sparse Linear model).

G : Family of Interpretable models.

f : Complexity model.

π_x : Proximity

$\Omega\left(g\right)$: The Omega is a complexity measure and this optimization problem is a minimization problem we want to minimize the complexity.

$L\left(f, g, \pi_x\right)$: Loss Function

$$L\left(f, g, \pi_x\right) = \sum{}_{z, z' \epsilon\, Z} \pi_x\left(z\right)\left(f\left(z\right) - g\left(z'\right)\right)^2 \tag{3}$$

The loss function for optimizing a linear model is basically the sum of squared distances between the label which comes from complex model and the prediction of simple model g. Additionally, proximity is added to weight the loss. A sparse linear model g is used, the advantage of using it is sparse linear models aim to produce as many zero weights as possible.

Training Classification Methods

K-Nearest Neighbors model

K-Nearest Neighbors model is a supervised and lazy algorithm. A lazy algorithm means the training of data doesn't take place and what it generally does during training time is store the inputs and outputs of the points in the given dataset. KNN classifier classifies its nearest neighbors based on the criteria of Euclidean distance between two points.

Euclidean Distance Formula,

$$D(X, Y) = \sqrt{\sum_{i=1}^{n} \left(Y_i - X_i\right)^2} \tag{4}$$

In the above formula,

X, Y are any two points in the given dataset.

D (X, Y): Distance between the points X and Y.

n: Number of features.

Y_i, X_i feature values of the points Y, X respectively (where i=1 to n).

The basic idea of the KNN Algorithm is as follows:

1. Select a point from the dataset
2. Consider a value of K where KϵN where N is set of Natural Numbers (Using the K value, the output is predicted. Generally, the K-value is taken odd number so that there will be no tie-breaks in classification).
3. In the test data, for each point do the following steps:
    a. Compute the distance between the testing data point and each point of training data by using equation (1).
    b. Sort the data points in ascending order as per the distance.
    c. Select the first K rows from the sorted array.
    d. Based on the highest count of K-Nearest points, a class is assigned.

Logistic Regression (LR)

Logistic Regression is a classification and supervised algorithm. Logistic Regression classifies the data by calculating the probability using the sigmoid function, and the output score in Logistic Regression is between 0 and 1.

Sigmoid Function,

$$f(x) = \frac{1}{1+e^{-z}} \tag{5}$$

In the above formula,

Z: function with combination of weights and input values.

Log - Loss Function,

$$L(x) = \frac{-1}{N}\left(\sum_{i=1}^{N}\left[Y_i \log P_i + \left(1-Y_i\right)\log\left(1-P_i\right)\right]\right) \tag{6}$$

In the above formula,

N: number of input samples.

Y_i: Actual output of the ith sample.

P_i: Probability predicted for the ith sample.

The basic idea of Logistic Regression Algorithm is as follows:

- Step 1: Select a point from the dataset.
- Step 2: Initially set the random weight values.
- Step 3: Calculate the probability value using equation (3).
- Step 4: Update the weight values.
- Step 5: calculate the loss value using equation (4) and repeat above steps for every data point until the loss is minimized.

Support Vector Machine with Normal Distribution Model (SVM-NDM)

SVM-NDM is a supervised machine learning algorithm used for classification problems. In N-dimensional space (where N is the number of features)., we plot each data item as a data point in which each feature's value is a particular coordinate. Then, we perform classification by finding the hyper-plane that differentiates the two classes (Naga Srinivasu et al., 2020) (Guleria et al., 2022). The hyperplane (Kernel) used in this dataset is RBF (Gaussian) Kernel.

$$K\left(X_1, X_2\right) = e^{-\left(\frac{\|X_1 - X_2\|^2}{2\tilde{A}^2}\right)} \tag{7}$$

In the above formula,

K (X_1, X_2): Similarity between points X_1, X_2.

'σ': Variance.

$\|X_1 - X_2\|$: Euclidean Distance between two points X_1 and X_2.

The basic idea of SVM Algorithm is as follows:

- Step 1: Plot the Dataset Points on the cartesian plane.
- Step 2: Choose the kernel as Gaussian (RBF).
- Step 3: Calculate the similarity between the points by using equation (5).
- Step 4: The points are similar if there is less distance between them.
- Step 5: Repeat the above steps for all the points.

Artificial Neural Network Model (ANN)

An Artificial Neural Network (ANN), likewise alluded to as a "neural network" (NN). It performs calculations and mathematical models by memic of neurons. Its capacities as a solitary neuron of the human cerebrum. It has different levels and each level has different perceptrons. The result relies upon the weight appended to each perceptron. It likewise has different information layers that perform calculations and reassigning of weights and an output layer that produces the result.

Relu Function,

$$y = \max\left(0, x\right) \tag{8}$$

In the above formula,

x is the input variable.

max $(0, x)$ function returns the maximum value among and x.

Adam Optimizer,

$$w_{t+1} = w_t - \alpha m_t \tag{9}$$

In the above formula,

w_t : Weights at time t (present weights)

α : learning rate

m_t : sum of gradients at time t

$$m_t = \beta\,m_{t-1} + \left(1 - \beta\right)\left[\frac{\partial \mathrm{L}}{\partial w_t}\right] \tag{10}$$

In the above formula,

β: Moving average parameter (0.9 constant value)

$\partial \mathrm{L}$: Loss Function derivative

∂w_t : Weights derivative at time t

Single-layered Artificial Neural Network (SL-ANN)

The basic idea of ANN Model is as follows:

Figure 6. Architecture of single layered artificial neural network

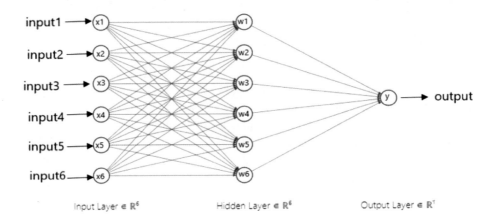

1. Dividing dataset to various training and testing proportions.
2. Creating the model:
   a. The input layer consists of six features.
   b. One hidden layer with six nodes and Relu as activation function.
   c. One node in output layer with sigmoid as activation function.
   d. The loss function used is binary_crossentropy and is calculated using equation (4), optimizer function is adam using equation (7) and learning rate is 0.001.
3. The training in each epoch is done by multiplying weights with input values and passing the result to equation (6).
4. Train the data for 50 epochs with batch size as 1.

Multi-layered Artificial Neural Network (ML-ANN)

The basic idea of ML-ANN Model is as follows:

Figure 7. Architecture of multi-layered artificial neural network

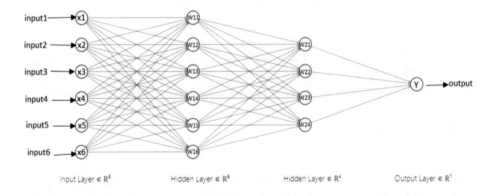

1. Dividing dataset to various training and testing proportions.
2. Creating the model:
   a. The input layer consists of six features.
   b. Two hidden layers with six nodes in hidden layer-1, four nodes in hidden layer-2 and Relu as activation function.
   c. One node in output layer with sigmoid as activation function.
   d. The loss function used is binary_crossentropy and is calculated using equation (4), optimizer function is adam using equation (7) and learning rate is 0.001.

3. The training in each epoch is done by multiplying weights with input values and passing the result to equation (6).
4. Train the data for 100 epochs with batch size as 10.

PERFORMANCE ANALYSIS AND RESULTS

For evaluating the model, we used standard measures like precision and recall. Accuracy is the ratio of correct predictions to that the number of predictions. The precision is the number of patients correctly found having cardiovascular disease out of total patients having it. The recall measures how many patients correctly found having a cardiovascular disease out of the entire cardiovascular disease patients (Pasha et al., 2020). The F-measure is a weighted mean of precision and recall. It is also known as a balanced F-score.

$$Precision\ (P) = \frac{No\ of\ patients\ identified\ correctly\ having\ cardiovascular\ disease}{No.\ of\ patients\ having\ cardiovascular\ disease} \quad (11)$$

$$Recall\ (R) = \frac{No.\ of\ patients\ identified\ correctly\ having\ cardiovascular\ disease}{No.of\ patients\ identified\ with\ cardiovascular\ disease} \quad (12)$$

$$F - measure = \frac{2PR}{P + R} \quad (13)$$

We categorized the dataset into four sets, namely yes or no and suffering from cardiovascular disease or not suffering from cardiovascular disease as shown in

Table 1. Displaying the categorized datasets

Predicted /Actual	Suffering from Cardiovascular disease	Not Suffering from Cardiovascular disease
Suffering from Cardiovascular disease	T_p	F_p
Not Suffering from Cardiovascular disease	F_n	T_n

Table 1. We compared the training model using accuracy, precision, recall, and f-measure metrics.

Where, T_p, F_n, F_p and T_n are true positives, false negatives, false positives and true negatives respectively.

Table 2. Displaying the categorized datasets for trained models

MODEL	T_p	F_p	F_n	T_n	TOTAL
KNN	3772	1729	2709	4578	12788
LR	4388	1466	2093	4841	12788
SVM-NDM	4516	1554	1965	4753	12788
SL-ANN	4943	1127	1463	5255	12788
ML-ANN	5564	506	1087	5631	12788

Accuracies of the Model's

Calculate the accuracy by using K–fold cross-validation method, and it is used to identify the Over fitting / Under fitting of the data. In this method, we divided the data into k-sets, then fits the model using k-1 folds and validates it with the Kth fold. The minimum, maximum and average accuracy of the combination of folds are given as output.

Table 3. Accuracy table for KNN algorithm

K- Value	Train – Test Split		Accuracy		
	Training Percentage	Testing Percentage	Min Accuracy	Max Accuracy	Avg Accuracy
11	60%	40%	70.46%	72.03%	71.23%
11	70%	30%	70.37%	72.56%	71.27%
11	80%	20%	70.19%	72.39%	71.14%

Table 4. Accuracy table for logistic regression algorithm

Train – Test Split		Accuracy		
Training Percentage	Testing Percentage	Min Accuracy	Max Accuracy	Avg Accuracy
60%	40%	71.22%	74.19%	72.30%
70%	30%	71.60%	73.23%	72.44%
80%	20%	72.19%	74.39%	73.29%

Table 5. Accuracy table for SVM-NDM

Kernel Type	Train – Test Split		Accuracy		
	Training Percentage	Testing Percentage	Min Accuracy	Max Accuracy	Avg Accuracy
Gaussian	60%	40%	71.48%	74.40%	72.94%
Gaussian	70%	30%	72.25%	75.00%	74.38%
Gaussian	80%	20%	72.85%	74.29%	72.85%

Table 6. Accuracy table for SL-ANN

Layer Architecture	Train – Test Split		Accuracy		
	Training Percentage	Testing Percentage	Min Accuracy	Max Accuracy	Avg Accuracy
Single layer	60%	40%	76.48%	79.40%	77.94%
Single layer	70%	30%	78.95%	80.00%	79.46%
Single layer	80%	20%	78.41%	79.29%	78.85%

Table 7. Accuracy table for ML-ANN

Layer Architecture	Train – Test Split		Accuracy		
	Training Percentage	Testing Percentage	Min Accuracy	Max Accuracy	Avg Accuracy
Two hidden layers	60%	40%	83.02%	85.40%	84.21%
Two hidden layers	70%	30%	86.45%	87.00%	86.72%
Two hidden layers	80%	20%	84.14%	86.12%	85.13%

Table 8. Comparing model's accuracies

Name of the model	Accuracy Score
ML-ANN	87
SL-ANN	80
SVM-NDM	75
LR	74.39
KNN	72.56

Comparing Accuracies of the Experimented Models

Based on the results of the experimented models, Multi-Layered Artificial Neural Networks (ML-ANN) is the best model which gives an accuracy of 87%, Single-Layered Artificial Neural Networks (SL-ANN) gives an accuracy of 80%, Support Vector Machine with Normal Distribution Model (SVM-NDM) and Logistic Regression (LR) gives similar accuracy of 75% and 74.39% respectively whereas K-Nearest Neighbors (KNN) is giving least performance among othe models with 72.56% accuracy.

Figure 8. Graph displaying comparison of accuracies among experimented models

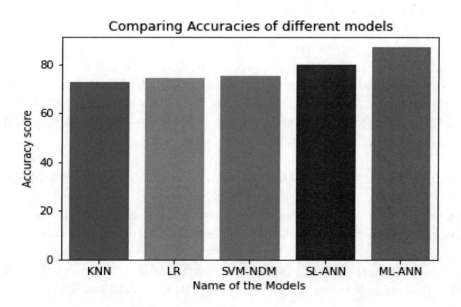

Model-Agnostic Explainable Artificial Intelligence technique plots

We considered the 1st Test point for the visualization of Model-Agnostic Explainable Artificial Intelligence technique plots. The Actual Output of the 1st point is **"1"**. The characteristics of the 1st Test point are as shown in the Table 9.

Table 9. 1st test point characteristics

Characteristics	Value
Age	57
Weight	70
Ap_hi (Systolic Blood Pressure)	140
Ap_low (Diastolic Blood Pressure)	80
Cholesterol	1
Pulse	60
Actual Output	1

While Plotting the Model-Agnostic Explainable Artificial Intelligence technique plots, the data with 70% / 30% Train – Test Split is considered, as it is more accurate compared to splitting data in other percentages.

Local Interpretable Model-Agnostic Explanations (LIME) Plots

The LIME PLOT gives the probability values, which indicates the probability of patient suffering from cardiovascular disease and probability of patient not suffering from cardiovascular disease. The Orange Color in the PLOT shows that the features have a high impact, suggesting that cardiovascular disease affects the person. The Blue Color in the PLOT indicates that the features have a low impact, implying that person is not suffering from cardiovascular disease.

LIME PLOT for 1st point KNN Algorithm (70% /30% Train-Test Split)

Figure 9 clearly states that the person has a probability of 73% to be suffered from the cardiovascular disease which almost predicts the actual output, in contradiction the model also predicts a probability of 27% to be not suffered from cardiovascular disease. The features ap_lo, ap_hi and cholesterol contribute to the classification class "1", whereas the age and pulse are contributing to the classification class "0".

Figure 9. LIME Plot for KNN Model

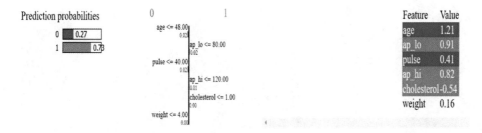

LIME PLOT for 1st point LR Algorithm (70% /30% Train-Test Split)

Figure 10. LIME Plot for LR Model

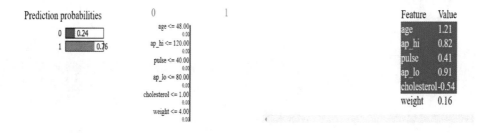

Figure 10 clearly states that the person has a probability of 76% to be suffered from the cardiovascular disease which almost predicts the actual output, in contradiction the model also predicts a probability of 24% to be not suffered from cardiovascular disease. The features age, ap_lo, ap_hi, pulse and cholesterol contribute to the classification class "1".

LIME PLOT for 1st point SVC-NDM Algorithm (70% /30% Train-Test Split)

Figure 11 clearly states that the person has a probability of 81% to be suffered from the cardiovascular disease which almost predicts the actual output, in contradiction the model also predicts a probability of 19% to be not suffered from cardiovascular disease. The features age, ap_lo, pulse, ap_hi and cholesterol contribute to the classification class "1".

Figure 11. LIME Plot for SVC-NDM Model

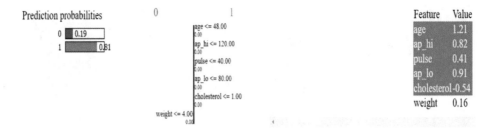

LIME PLOT for 1st point SL-ANN Algorithm (70% /30% Train-Test Split)

Figure 12. LIME Plot for SL-ANN Model

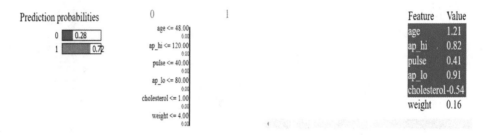

Figure 12 clearly states that the person has a probability of 72% to be suffered from the cardiovascular disease which almost predicts the actual output, in contradiction the model also predicts a probability of 28% to be not suffered from cardiovascular disease. The features age, ap_lo, ap_hi, pulse and cholesterol contribute to the classification class "1",

LIME PLOT for 1st point ML-ANN Algorithm (70% /30% Train-Test Split)

Figure 13 clearly states that the person has a probability of 100% to be suffered from the cardiovascular disease which predicts the actual output.

The ML-ANN, SVM-NDM LIME Plot is more accurate than other model LIME plots as the models predict 100% and 81% probability for the correct output, whereas the models KNN, LR, SL-ANN predict 73%, 76% and 72% probability respectively.

Figure 13. LIME Plot for ML-ANN Model

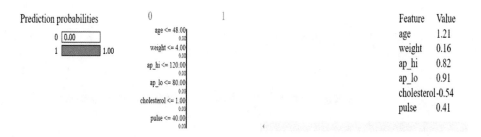

Shapley Additive Explanations (SHAP) Plots

The Base Value in the SHAP PLOT is the minimum value, which indicates that the patient is suffering from cardiovascular disease. The Red Color in the PLOT shows that the features have a high impact, suggesting that cardiovascular disease affects the person. The Blue Color in the PLOT indicates that the features have a low impact, implying that person is not suffering from cardiovascular disease.

SHAP PLOT for 1st point KNN Algorithm (70% /30% Train-Test Split)

Figure 14. SHAP Plot for KNN Model

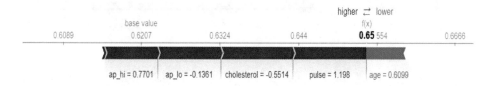

Figure 14 clearly states that the features ap_hi, ap_lo, cholesterol, and pulse contribute to the classification class "1", whereas the age attribute contradicts the classification class "1". The SHAP value $(f(x) = 0.65)$ is greater than the base value (0.6207), so the model predicts output as class 1, which is the same as actual output, and the feature pulse is contributing more for the prediction in this model. where $f(x)$ is the SHAP Value for the data point.

SHAP PLOT for 1ˢᵗ point LR Algorithm (70% / 30% Train-Test Split)

Figure 15. SHAP Plot for LR Model

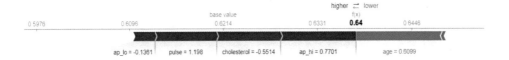

Figure 15 clearly states that the features ap_hi, ap_lo, cholesterol, and pulse contribute to "1", whereas the age attribute contradicts the classification class "1". The output value (f(x) = 0.64) is greater than the base value (0.6214), so the model predicts output as class 1, which is the same as actual output, and the feature ap_hi is contributing more for the prediction in this model.

SHAP PLOT for 1ˢᵗ point SVM-NDM Algorithm (70% / 30% Train-Test Split)

Figure 16. SHAP Plot for SVC-NDM Model

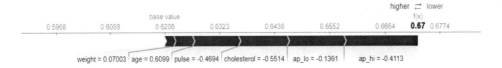

Figure 16 clearly states that the features ap_hi, ap_lo, cholesterol, weight, age, and pulse contribute to the classification class "1". The output value (f(x) = 0.67) is greater than the base value (0.6206), so the model predicts output as class 1, which is the same as actual output, and the feature ap_hi is contributing more for the prediction in this model.

SHAP PLOT for 1ˢᵗ point SL-ANN Algorithm (70% / 30% Train-Test Split)

Figure 17 clearly states that the features ap_hi, ap_lo, cholesterol, weight and pulse contribute to "1", whereas the age attribute contradicts the classification class "1". The output value (f(x) = 0.70) is greater than the base value (0.6237), so the model

Figure 17. SHAP Plot for SL-ANN Model

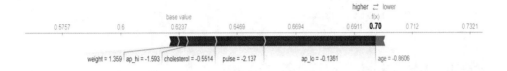

predicts output as class 1, which is the same as actual output, and the feature ap_lo is contributing more for the prediction in this model.

SHAP PLOT for 1st point ML-ANN Algorithm (70% / 30% Train-Test Split)

Figure 18. SHAP Plot for ML-ANN Model

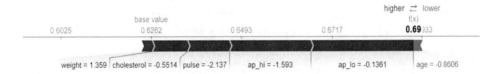

Figure 18 clearly states that the features ap_hi, ap_lo, cholesterol, weight and pulse contribute to "1", whereas the age attribute contradicts the classification class "1". The output value (f(x) = 0.69) is greater than the base value (0.6262), so the model predicts output as class 1, which is the same as actual output, and the feature ap_lo is contributing more for the prediction in this model.

The ML-ANN, SL-ANN, SVM-NDM SHAP Plot is more accurate than other model SHAP plots, and all the features contribute in ML-ANN, SL-ANN, SVM-NDM Plot, whereas the feature "weight" does not contribute in the remaining model SHAP plots.

Comparison of Shapley Additive Explanations (SHAP) and Local Interpretable Model-Agnostic Explanations (LIME)

Each Model has its own drawbacks. While the visualizations in the Local Interpretable Model-Agnostic Explanations (LIME) are easily understandable compared to the Shapley Additive Explanations (SHAP) and the time taken to visualize LIME Plot is also less than time taken to visualize SHAP Plot, the SHAP Plots are more accurate as individual feature contribution is clearly shown for every model whereas in few model's LIME Plots the feature contribution is not shown and LIME technique cannot interpret some of the models like XGBoost Classifier, SHAP Plots can be used to interpret most of the models.

CONCLUSION AND FUTURE SCOPE

In this research, we used K-Nearest Neighbors, Logistic Regression, Support Vector Machine with Normal Distribution, Single-Layered Artificial Neural Networks and Multi-Layered Artificial Neural Networks to forecast the health care records of cardiovascular disease patients. Based on those methods, a prediction model is generated and in order to acquire better justifications for the predictions Model-Agnostic Explainable Artificial Intelligence (XAI) techniques i.e., SHAP and LIME are used. To evaluate the model's performance, we used performance metrics like f-1 score, precision, recall and accuracy, and found out that the ML-ANN (Multi-Layered Artificial Neural Networks) is performing well which gives an accuracy of 87%. In the future, we will compare those methods with other methods like advanced deep-learning techniques using performance metrics, and Explainability can also be extended by using other Explainable AI techniques.

REFERENCES

Adadi, A., & Berrada, M. (2020). Explainable AI for healthcare: from black box to interpretable models. In *Embedded Systems and Artificial Intelligence* (pp. 327–337). Springer. doi:10.1007/978-981-15-0947-6_31

Amma, N. B. (2012, February). Cardiovascular disease prediction system using genetic algorithm and neural network. In *2012 International Conference on Computing, Communication and Applications* (pp. 1-5). IEEE. 10.1109/ICCCA.2012.6179185

Arunachalam, S. (2020). Cardiovascular disease prediction model using machine learning algorithms. *International Journal for Research in Applied Science and Engineering Technology*, 8(6), 1006–1019. doi:10.22214/ijraset.2020.6164

Dinesh, K. G., Arumugaraj, K., Santhosh, K. D., & Mareeswari, V. (2018, March). Prediction of cardiovascular disease using machine learning algorithms. In *2018 International Conference on Current Trends towards Converging Technologies (ICCTCT)* (pp. 1-7). IEEE. 10.1109/ICCTCT.2018.8550857

Dinh, A., Miertschin, S., Young, A., & Mohanty, S. D. (2019). A data-driven approach to predicting diabetes and cardiovascular disease with machine learning. *BMC Medical Informatics and Decision Making*, *19*(1), 1–15. doi:10.118612911-019-0918-5 PMID:31694707

Duval, A. (2019). Explainable artificial intelligence (XAI). MA4K9 Scholarly Report, Mathematics Institute, The University of Warwick.

ElShawi, R., Sherif, Y., Al-Mallah, M., & Sakr, S. (2021). Interpretability in healthcare: A comparative study of local machine learning interpretability techniques. *Computational Intelligence*, *37*(4), 1633–1650. doi:10.1111/coin.12410

Ghosh, P., Azam, S., Jonkman, M., Karim, A., Shamrat, F. J. M., Ignatious, E., Shultana, S., Beeravolu, A. R., & De Boer, F. (2021). Efficient prediction of cardiovascular disease using machine learning algorithms with relief and LASSO feature selection techniques. *IEEE Access: Practical Innovations, Open Solutions*, *9*, 19304–19326. doi:10.1109/ACCESS.2021.3053759

Guleria, P., Ahmed, S., Alhumam, A., & Srinivasu, P. N. (2022, January). Empirical Study on Classifiers for Earlier Prediction of COVID-19 Infection Cure and Death Rate in the Indian States. In Healthcare (Vol. 10, No. 1, p. 85). Multidisciplinary Digital Publishing Institute.

Hasan, N., & Bao, Y. (2021). Comparing different feature selection algorithms for cardiovascular disease prediction. *Health and Technology*, *11*(1), 49–62. doi:10.100712553-020-00499-2

Huang, Q., Yamada, M., Tian, Y., Singh, D., Yin, D., & Chang, Y. (2020). *Graphlime: Local interpretable model explanations for graph neural networks.* arXiv preprint arXiv:2001.06216.

Kavila, S. D., Muddana, M. K., Bharath, N., Sai Teja, N. K. S., Kumar, N. T., & Swaroop, L. J. (2021). *Explainable Artificial Intelligence to Predict Cardiovascular Diseases. International Journal of Emerging Technologies and Innovative Research*, 8.

London, A. J. (2019). Artificial intelligence and black-box medical decisions: Accuracy versus explainability. *The Hastings Center Report*, *49*(1), 15–21. doi:10.1002/hast.973 PMID:30790315

Naga Srinivasu, P., Srinivasa Rao, T., Dicu, A. M., Mnerie, C. A., & Olariu, I. (2020). A comparative review of optimisation techniques in segmentation of brain MR images. *Journal of Intelligent & Fuzzy Systems*, *38*(5), 6031–6043. doi:10.3233/JIFS-179688

Pasha, S. N., Ramesh, D., Mohmmad, S., Harshavardhan, A., & Shabana. (2020, December). Cardiovascular disease prediction using deep learning techniques. *IOP Conference Series. Materials Science and Engineering, 981*(2), 022006. doi:10.1088/1757-899X/981/2/022006

Pawar, U., O'Shea, D., Rea, S., & O'Reilly, R. (2020). Explainable AI in Healthcare. *2020 International Conference on Cyber Situational Awareness, Data Analytics and Assessment (CyberSA)*, 1-2. 10.1109/CyberSA49311.2020.9139655

Porto, R., Molina, J. M., Berlanga, A., & Patricio, M. A. (2021). Minimum Relevant Features to Obtain Explainable Systems for Predicting Cardiovascular Disease Using the Statlog Data Set. *Applied Sciences (Basel, Switzerland), 11*(3), 1285. doi:10.3390/app11031285

Rathi, S. (2019). *Generating counterfactual and contrastive explanations using SHAP*. arXiv preprint arXiv:1906.09293.

Tjoa, E., & Guan, C. (2020). A survey on explainable artificial intelligence (xai): Toward medical xai. *IEEE Transactions on Neural Networks and Learning Systems, 32*(11), 4793–4813. doi:10.1109/TNNLS.2020.3027314 PMID:33079674

Virani, S. S., Alonso, A., Aparicio, H. J., Benjamin, E. J., Bittencourt, M. S., Callaway, C. W., Carson, A. P., Chamberlain, A. M., Cheng, S., Delling, F. N., Elkind, M. S. V., Evenson, K. R., Ferguson, J. F., Gupta, D. K., Khan, S. S., Kissela, B. M., Knutson, K. L., Lee, C. D., Lewis, T. T., ... Tsao, C. W. (2021). Heart disease and stroke statistics—2021 update: A report from the American Heart Association. *Circulation, 143*(8), e254–e743. doi:10.1161/CIR.0000000000000950 PMID:33501848

Westerlund, A. M., Hawe, J. S., Heinig, M., & Schunkert, H. (2021). Risk Prediction of Cardiovascular Events by Exploration of Molecular Data with Explainable Artificial Intelligence. *International Journal of Molecular Sciences, 22*(19), 10291. doi:10.3390/ijms221910291 PMID:34638627

Yasnitsky, L. N., Dumler, A. A., Poleshchuk, A. N., Bogdanov, C. V., & Cherepanov, F. M. (2015). Artificial neural networks for obtaining new medical knowledge: Diagnostics and prediction of cardiovascular disease progression. *Biology and Medicine (Aligarh), 7*(2), 95.

Chapter 3
Role of Deep Learning in Medical Image Super-Resolution

Wazir Muhammad
Balochistan University of Engineering and Technology, Khuzdar, Pakistan

Manoj Gupta
JECRC University, Jaipur, India

Zuhaibuddin Bhutto
Balochistan University of Engineering and Technology, Khuzdar, Pakistan

ABSTRACT

Recently, deep learning-based convolutional neural networks method for image super-resolution has achieved remarkable performance in various fields including security surveillance, satellite imaging, and medical image enhancement. Although these approaches obtained improved performance in medical images, existing works only used a pre-processing step and hand-designed filter methods to improve the quality of medical images. Pre-processing step and hand-designed-based reconstructed medical image results are very blurry and introduce new noises in the images. Due to this, sometimes medical practitioners make wrong decisions, which are very dangerous for human beings. In this chapter, the authors explain that the hand-designed as well as deep learning-based approaches, including some image quality assessment metrics to open the gate to verify the images with different approaches, depend on the single image approach. Furthermore, they discuss some important types of medical images and their properties.

DOI: 10.4018/978-1-6684-3791-9.ch003

INTRODUCTION

Reconstructing the visually pleasing high-resolution (HR) images from the low-quality or low-resolution ones is a challenging classical problem in image enhancement. This restoration process is called an image super-resolution (SR), which depends on pre-or post-processing steps to boost the perceptual quality of the recovered output image. In the field of medical images, upscaling the LR image into the desired HR image is no easy task due to some physical limitations of imaging systems and noise factor, jagged ringing artifact, and blurring output. Hand-designed filter approaches have already resolved these issues, but performances are not satisfactory. Recently, Artificial Intelligence (AI) has been involved in medical imaging and reconstructs the visually pleasing quality of the MRI image compared to earlier approaches. However, AI is a very new idea, which was begun in the 1940s. The name of artificial intelligence was invented in 1956 by John McCarthy. In other words, AI is used for computer algorithms that can mimic the human cognitive level. The most recent success of AI has been enabled by massive increases in both computer power and data availability. AI implementation in medical imaging improves the quality of clinical practice and supports the clinical decision (Hosny, Parmar, Quackenbush, Schwartz, & Aerts, 2018; Vickers, 2017; C. Wang, Zhu, Hong, & Zheng, 2019). Currently, machine learning technologies have matured to the point where they can meet clinical criteria. The development in information and data has been linked to improved illness knowledge and comprehension, thanks in part to advances in technologies that induce quantitative and qualitative measures of physiological labels. Indeed, the promise of machine learning as a platform for combining data from various references into an intertwined system may greatly benefit highly competent worker's decision-making processes. When machine learning was still in its infancy, it was hypothesized that the capability to gather and store massive quantities of information in a knowledge base would determine the success of an intelligent system that could learn and improve (Clancey & Shortliffe, 1984). Deep learning (DL) is an area of AI that has exploded more popular in recent decades. Because of its adaptability, high performance, strong generalization capability, and diverse applications. A significant volume of medical data and the development of increasingly powerful computers have sparked interest in medical imaging enhancement.

A Deep Convolutional Neural Network (DCNN) is a type of CNN neural network type approach that could enlarge the input image to awesome gadgets withinside the image and distinguish one from the different. In evaluating different types of methods, CNN calls for considerably fewer pre-processing steps. The structure of a CNN is stimulated via way of means of the organization of the Visual Cortex, which is connected to the sample of neurons in withinside the brain. Different neurons respond to stimuli best in the Receptive Field, a tiny area of the field of view. Several comparable fields may be stacked on the pinnacle of every different from spanning the entire field of vision. Recently, with the advancement of image enhancement technology, especially in a medical image, SR has performed valuable clinical applications. MRI image gives a rich, detailed information of high resolution in medical images and their applications (Greenspan, 2009; Van Ouwerk & Computing, 2006). The main function of MRI is to obtain the sagittal plane, transverse plane, different inclined plane, and coronal plane (Huang, Shao, & Frangi, 2019) information. The medical images enhancement in terms of (resolution) is limited by different enlargement parameters, like scanning type hardware up-gradation, signal-to-noise ratio (SNR), moving objects, limited scanning time of hardware, technical and economic factors (J. Zhu, Yang, & Lio, 2019;), and image motility of organs. These factors decrease the perceptual quality of the medical images and generate very blurred images, having jagged ringing artifacts and diminishing the visibility of important pathological details. The primary goal of image SR is to reconstruct the highly pleasing quality of output MRI images from the degraded version of quality input MRI images, which is the typically ill-posed problem (X. Wang et al., 2018).

Researchers have discussed a variety of image SR approaches. Such approaches can be classified into three main groupings: interpolation, reconstruction, and learning type methods (Dou et al., 2018). The interpolation-based methods are included as a bicubic interpolation (Li & Orchard, 2001), bilinear interpolation (Keys & processing, 1981), nearest-neighbor interpolation, and some other derivates of these approaches (Shao & Zhao, 2007; L. Zhang & Wu, 2006). Design architecture of interpolation is easy and simple to implement. The main issue is that it does not reconstruct the high-frequency details. In the reconstruction method (Keys & processing, 1981), the proposed maximum a posteriori probability (MAP) type approach constrains the solutions space with the implementation of prior knowledge. Recently, DCNN-based approaches have achieved remarkable progress in the medical imaging and computer vision tasks to solve the SR problem (Dong, Loy, He, & Tang, 2014). The most important thing of deep learning-based models is that they can extract more contextual information from the original input LR medical image to recover the details of the HR medical output image. Furthermore, deep CNN-based models can efficiently achieve and automatically learn the rich features information hierarchically (Kim, Lee, & Lee, 2016; Lai, Huang, Ahuja, & Yang, 2017). This book chapter focuses on medical image enhancement using deep learning-based approaches to reconstruct the HR images. The major contribution of the proposed book chapter is summarized as under:

- The authors are present different types of medical images and their simulation operation in MATLAB.

- We discuss different software packages and medical image filtering techniques to remove the noise.
- Finally, we discuss the relationship between deep learning and medical imaging modalities with CNN architectures.

The remaining section of our book chapter is arranged into different sections. Section 2 discusses the various types of medical images. Section number 3rd presents the different properties of medical images. Medical image denoising and Filtering techniques are discussed in section 4. Sections 5 and 6 discuss the Medical image formats and Software used for medical image analyses. Section 7 and 8 discuss the deep learning platform and medical imaging modalities. Quality metrics are discussed in section 10, and Brain MRI image super-resolution techniques are present in section11. Section 12 discussed the requirement for deep Learning in Medical Imaging. Finally, the Deep-learning framework for brain MRI image and SR are discussed in section13. The quantitative comparison of MRI Medical Images is explained in 14 sections. The conclusion part with future directions is discussed in the 15th section.

TYPES OF MEDICAL IMAGES

Binary Medical Images

Pixels make up a binary image, which can only have one of two colors: black or white. 1-Bit refers to a pixel that is made up of two colors. Binary image or also known as bi-level or two-level image in Figure 1. Each pixel value is represented by a single unit bit, either a 0 or a 1. Additionally, Monochrome, Black-and-white, or monochromatic are the common terms used for Binary images (Srinivasu PN et al., 2020).

Gray Scale Medical Images

A monochromatic range of colors covering black and white is known as grayscale. As a result, a grayscale image contains no color and only grayscale hues. Grayscale information can be stored as a black and white image, as seen in Figure 2. This is due to each value of pixels being assigned a brightness, irrespective of color channels. Almost all file formats of images include at least 8-bit grayscale, which provides each pixel a brightness range of 28 or 256 levels. Several formats offer 16-bit grayscale, which has 216 or 65,536 levels of brightness.

Figure 1. Convert gray scale brain MRI image into binary image

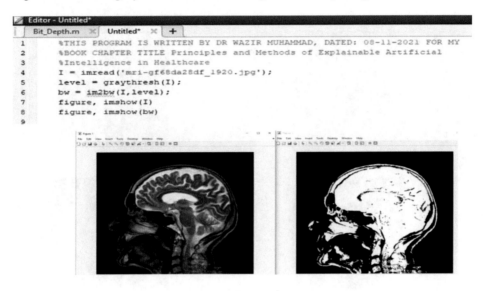

Figure 2. Convert false color medical X-ray image into grayscale image

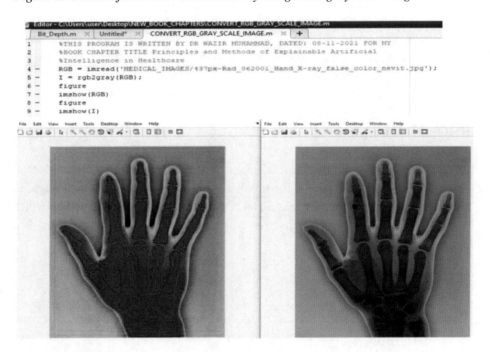

Figure 3. Extract the three colors from the original false color medical X-ray image

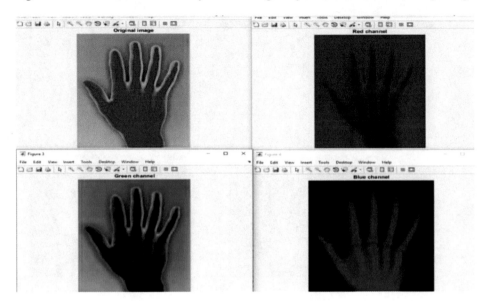

Color Medical Images

A digital or color image is one in which the color information is stored in each pixel. For visually pleasing results, each pixel must have three color channels. All channels read as a coordinate with some space of colors, as shown in Figure 3. However, the RGB color space is generally applied in the CPU monitor display.

PROPERTIES OF MEDICAL IMAGES

Image is the combination of several pixels and is represented in spatial domain and time domain. Additionally, the number of pixels is available in the image is a real number because it is easy to store and compress. Therefore, the medical image has various properties, but we discussed the main common properties of medical images are as under:

Bit Depth

The color information available in the medical image is called Bit depth. Bit depth is higher, which means more color information is available in the image. Sometimes,

Table 1. A detailed explanation of bit depth calculation

S.NO	Value of n	$Bit\,Depth = 2^n$	Output
1.	1	$Bit\,Depth = 2^1 = 2$	The medical image would produce 2 shades of grayscale.
2.	2	$Bit\,Depth = 2^2 = 4$	The medical image would produce 4 shades of grayscale.
3.	3	$Bit\,Depth = 2^3 = 8$	The medical image would produce 8 shades of grayscale.
4.	10	$Bit\,Depth = 2^{10} = 1024$	The medical image would produce 1,024 shades of grayscale.
5.	12	$Bit\,Depth = 2^{12} = 4096$	The medical image would produce 4,096 shades of grayscale.

some shades are available in medical images is called Bit Depth. Mathematically, Bit depth can be calculated as:

$$Bit\,Depth = 2^n, \tag{1}$$

where the integer number 2 indicates the image in black and white and n is the power of gray shades.

The medical DR, CT, MRI are generated with the bit depth of the range of the order of 10 or 12. The different ranges of bit depths are calculated in Table 1.

Voxel

In computer 3D graphics, a Voxel is a value of three-dimensional regular grid space. Now a day's, voxel is mostly used to analyze scientific and medical data. The main difference between pixel (2D) and voxel is the (3D) dimension. Pixels have an absolute position, but voxel has a relative position. Finally, the voxel has a volume, but the pixel does not have any volume. The voxel of an image is shown in Figure 4.

Pixel

A pixel or picture element (Foley & Van Dam, 1982) is the basic building block of a medical image and is represented as a square or dot on the computer screen. The pixel color combination depends on the type of graphics card and the type of display monitor. The display monitor screen has more pixels per inch, gives a better result.

Figure 4. Voxel result of original false color image

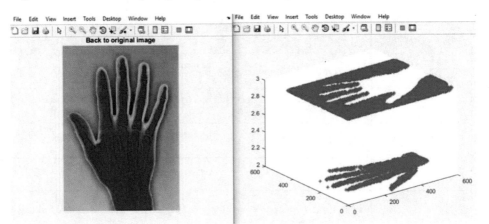

Histogram

In the field of image processing, histogram technique normally shows the pixel's intensity values. To put it another way, a histogram is a type of graph where all pixels are available with various intensities. An 8-bit grayscale image has a unique value of intensities of 256, and a histogram shows these grayscale values. In the case of color images, the intensities values are individually shown as red, green, and blue color channels.

Cross-Correlation

Correlation is a most powerful technique for detecting the position of an object in extremely noisy images. The cross correlation between two matrices of images describes the possible displacements between similar input images. Mathematically, cross-correlation is defined as:

$$C = F^{-1}\left[F\left(I\right).F\left(p\right)^{*}\right], \tag{2}$$

The input image is denoted as I and the target pattern image as a p and Fourier Transform of these images denoted as F and the Correlation and Conjugate complex denoted as C, and *.

Natural Scene Statistics (NSS)

According to the information theory, natural scene statistics can utilize to define the natural task with the behavior of the ideal observer. The most important application of the NSS model is the prediction of the perceived quality of the image. For example, the Visual Information Fidelity (VIF) technique is widely used in the image and video processing industries to measure perceptual quality, particularly after compression, which can degrade the appearance of a visual signal. The idea is that distortion modifies scene statistics and that changes in scene statistics affect the visual system. In the streaming television market, the VIF format is frequently used. BRISQUE and NIQE, are two more common image quality models based on natural scene statistics, and both are no-reference quality matrices.

MEDICAL IMAGE DENOISING AND FILTERS

The field of medical image processing and its filtering techniques play a vital role in daily life, but the main problem is acquiring the images from different sources. The acquired images are usually affected by unwanted signals/noises such as salt and pepper type noise, Gaussian noise, periodic noise, and speckle noise. The acquired noiseless image is an impossible task (Bhateja, Tiwari, & Srivastava, 2015). This section discusses different statistical approaches to enhance the quality of medical images using filtering approaches.

Types of Noises in Images

There are many types of noises available in digital signal and image processing. Here we discuss some main types of noises are as under:

Gaussian Noise

This type of noise appears during the acquisition process, and it also has sensor noise due to its temperature and low level of illumination, as shown in Figure 5.

Salt-and-Pepper Noise

Salt-and-pepper type noise is also called impulsive noise or Fat-tail-distributed type noise (Naga Srinivasu P, et al. 2020). An Image has a darker pixel accessible in the vibrant areas and greater vivid pixels accessible in the darkish areas as shown in Figure 6. Such type of noise appears during conversions, such as analog to digital

Figure 5. Original images with Gaussian type noise

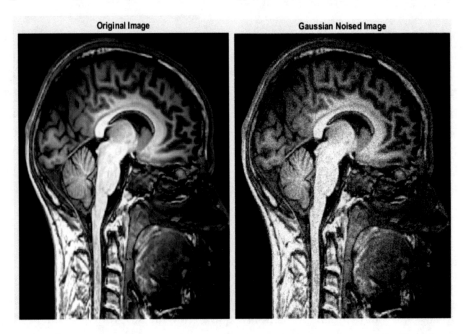

conversion and bit error in the transmission. The filtering techniques like, mean, median, and interpolation are used to reduce the noise level.

Mean Filter

A mean filter, also known as an average filter, is a windowed linear class filter that smooths out signals (image). The filter functions as a low-pass filter. The primary principle behind a filter is to take an average of any signal (image) constituent in its immediate vicinity. The MATLAB code and the filter's resultant output are shown in Figure 7.

Median Filter

The median filter is a category of non-linear filtering, and its main task is to reduce the noise from the image and data. To reduce the noise is a pre-processing procedure in medical image enhancement. It is extensively used in medical image processing, and it also has applications in signal processing, as shown in Figure 8.

Figure 6. Original image with salt-and-pepper noise

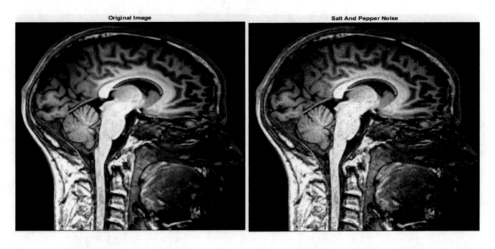

Figure 7. Mean filter used to remove the noise

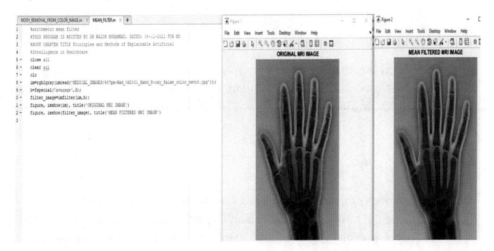

MEDICAL IMAGE FORMATS

There are many formats available for medical images, but we discuss some of them due to limited space, and a detailed explanation of these formats is presented in Table 2.

Figure 8. Median filter used to remove the noise

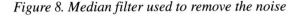

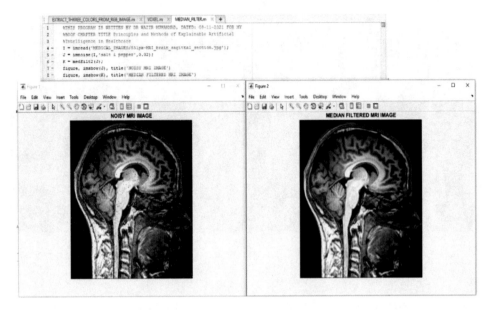

Analyze

Analyze is a fixed-length medical image format. It stored 348-byte binary information. The data type is used in this format is an unsigned integer of 8-bit, signed integer range is 16 to 32-bit, float type of data is 32-64 bit, and complex type data is used 64 bits only.

NIfTI

The Neuroimaging Informatics Technology Initiative (NIFTI) envisioned the NIfTI format replacing the ANALYZE 7.5 Format. Its origins are in neuroimaging science, but it can also be used in other domains. The format includes two affine coordinate definitions that link each voxel index (i,j,k) to a specific spatial location (x,y,z), and nibabel is a python library for reading nifti files. The "oro.nifti" is an R package for reading nifti data. The same formatting is used by DICOM, and the primary difference between DICOM and NIfTI is that in NIfTI the raw image data is saved as a 3d image, whereas in DICOM, the raw image data is saved as 2d image slices. Because NIFTI is modeled as a three-dimensional image, it is better than DICOM for several machine learning applications. It's easier to manage a single NIFTI file than hundreds of DICOM files. Nifti only keeps two files per 3D image, but DICOM maintains hundreds.

Table 2. Summary of medical image file formats

Image File Format	Data Stored	Image Extension	Types of Data
Analyze	484 byte	.imgand .hdr	8, 16, 32, and 64-bit
Nifti	352 byte	.nii	8, 16, 32, 64, and 128-bit
Minc	Extended binary format	.mnc	8, 16, 32, and 64-bit
Dicom	VLBF	.dcm	8, 16, and 32-bit

Minc

Any 2D or 3D image data, such as MRI, PET, CT, or histology, is often represented using Minc file format. The ability of Minc to express an irregularly spaced time axis is one advantage for PET data. Diffusion tensors and deformation fields are derived data that can be represented with Minc.

DICOM

DICOM is a trendy structure of clinical pictures used for the alternate and administration of scientific imaging statistics and its associated information. DICOM is the most extensively used popular for storing and transferring scientific images, allowing numerous manufacturers' scanners, servers, workstations, printers, community hardware, and image archiving and verbal exchange structures to work together. It has been extensively typical by way of hospitals, and it is beginning to make inroads into smaller functions like dentist and doctor's workplaces.

OpenCV

OpenCV is another application to analyze the natural and medical image enhancement with different basic operations. Initially, OpenCV was developed by the Intel Corporation. OpenCV is a free library under the license of Apache 2. In 1999 Intel research team was officially launched the OpenCV project with real CPU-supported applications. Additionally, the new alpha version of OpenCV was presented at the 2000 IEEE conference on Computer Vision and Pattern Recognition. The further five beta versions were released between 2001 to 2005. The most important and dominant second version was launched in 2009. In 2011, OpenCV launched real-time operations with GPU support. The major applications of OpenCV including as Egomotion estimation, motion understanding, motion tracking, Facial recognition, image segmentation and recognition, gesture recognition, mobile robotics. The main machine learning libraries are supported as a k-nearest neighbor algorithm, random forest, artificial neural networks, decision tree learning, support vector machine, and deep neural networks.

MEDICAL IMAGING SOFTWARE

Everyone is talking about electronic medicine or the e-health system these days, but only a few have come up with a comprehensive definition of this relatively new term. This term, which was rarely in use before 1999, has become a broad "buzzword," used to encompass practically everything about technology and medicine? The word is considered to have been coined by industry leaders and marketers rather than academics.

Pros and Cons of Medical Imaging Software

- Ease of access and use.
- No need to wait in the queue as well as for appointments.
- Reduce the demand for physical consultations.
- Improve the overall patients' outcomes.
- fewer chances of mistakes when results are evaluated by software.
- Medical practitioners save more time with the help of software because every patient registration can consume more time.
- It is easy to communicate patient's electronic health record (HER) to referring doctors because all information of patients are available in the system
- Uses of software patients have received a high quality of care.
- Medical imaging software is more expensive results as compared to single-doctor practices because the software has a more initial cost.
- Personal information of patients is not secure and may be used by hackers.
- Learning process takes more time to train the whole medical staff to properly use the software.

ITK-SNAP

ITK-SNAP is a medical software used for 3D MRI images for segmentation. The design of the software is the ten-year collaboration between the University of Pennsylvania and the University of Utah's, whose main purpose was to develop a dedicated tool as a single function for segmentation purposes as illustrated in Figure 9, it is free and open-source software.

Figure 9. Segmentation of a skull in ITK-SNAP software

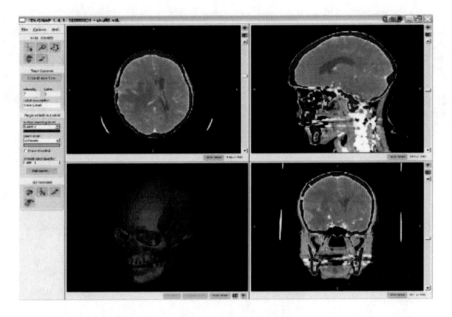

ImageJ

ImageJ is a Java-based medical image software licensed by the national institute of health. All ImageJ packages are under the BSD-2 license. The main screenshot of ImageJ is shown in Figure 10.

SimpleITK

SimpleITK is a simplified version of Insight Segmentation and Registration Toolkit (ITK) as shown in Figure 11. It is used the language of C++, C#, Java, Python, R, Ruby, Lua, and Tcl. SimpleITK supports all three major operating systems like Microsoft Windows, Linux, and macOS.

MITK

MITK is open-source software for medical imaging interaction as a toolkit and is freely available for researchers as shown in Figure 12.

Figure 10. Screenshot of ImageJ software

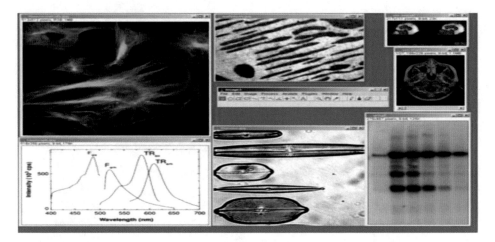

FreeSurfer

Anders Dale, Doug Greve, Martin Sereno, and Bruce Fischl created FreeSurfer, a brain imaging software suite. FreeSurfer is a collection of applications with the

Figure 11. Screenshot of SimpleITK software

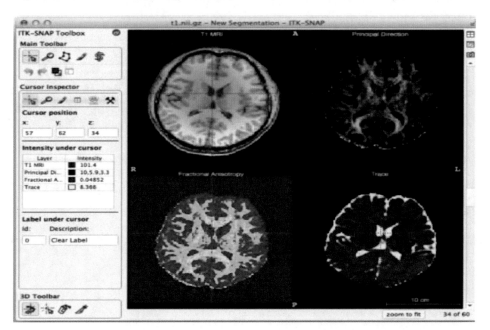

Figure 12. Screenshot of MITK software

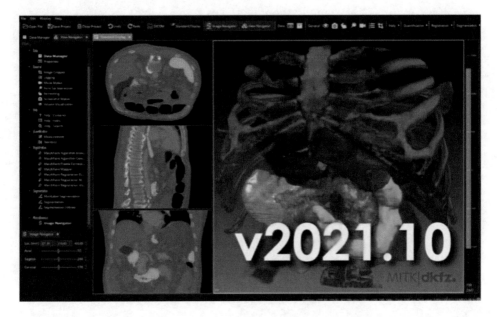

same goal: to analyze MRI scans of brain tissue. It is a useful tool for FBM because it includes volume and surface analysis options, as shown in Figure 13.

3D SLICER

3D SLICER is an open-source free software package of imaging analysis and visualization. Slicer is used in many medical applications, including breast cancer, lung cancer, prostate cancer, neurosurgery, and cardiovascular disease, as shown in Figure 14.

DEEP LEARNING PLATFORM FOR MEDICAL IMAGE

Recently, brain MRI deep learning-based medical image is partially accessed by publicly available programming framework. Many software developers maintain the framework to fulfill the end-user requirements. The most used deep learning-based frameworks are as under.

- TensorFlow (Abadi et al., 2016) is a deep learning free-access library. The Googles Brain team initially creates it for production and research purposes.

TensorFlow was released under the license of Apache in 2015 (Metz, 2015). It is supported C++ and Python interfaces.

Figure 13. Screenshot of FreeSurfer software

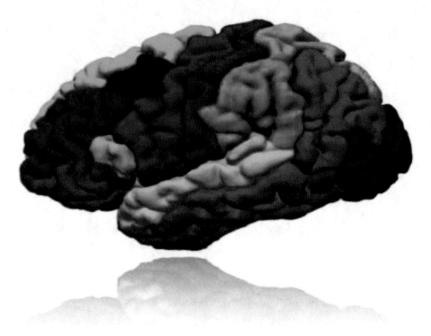

Figure 14. Screenshot of 3D SLICER software

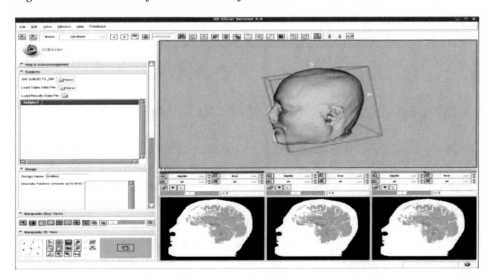

Table 3. Comparative assessment of existing computer vision-based research works on benchmark datasets for healthcare and rehabilitation treatment (Ahad, Antar, & Shahid, 2019)

Dataset	Method/Model	Accuracy (%)
MSRAction3D (Tran & Sorokin, 2008)	Convolutional Neural Networks (ConvNets)	100
	reviews + Portable Format for Analytics (PFA)	98.2
	Decision-Level Fusion (SUM)	98.2
MSR Daily Activity3D (Rodriguez, Ahmed, & Shah, 2008)	τ-test	95.63
	DL-GSGC + Total Productive Maintenance (TPM)	95
	3D joint + CS-MLtp	92.5
	Depth Volumetric Spatial Feature Representation (VSFR)	89.7
UCF-Kinect (Ellis, Masood, Tappen, LaViola, & Sukthankar, 2013)	Hierarchical model	98.7
Multiview 3D Event (Wei, Zhao, Zheng, & Zhu, 2013)	4D human-object interaction (4DHOI)	87
UT-Kinect (Xia, Chen, & Aggarwal, 2012)	Grassman manifold	95.25
UTD-MHAD (C. Chen, Jafari, & Kehtarnavaz, 2015)	Convolutional Neural Networks (CNN)	99.54
AHA-3D (Aung et al., 2015)	Kolmogorov-Smirnov test	88.29

- Keras (Chollet, 2015) is an open-source framework developed by a Google engineer and was initially released in 2015 written in Python platform.
- It is supported by multiple backends, including Theano, Cognitive Toolkit, TensorFlow, and PlaidML.
- PyTorch (Paszke et al., 2017) was once exceptionally developed using Facebook's AI lookup lab (FAIR). It is an open-source ML Torch-based library used for picture and laptop imaginative and prescient tasks. PyTorch has supported Python as properly as C++ interface environments.

The remaining platform information was summarized in Table 5.

MEDICAL IMAGING MODALITIES

The term modalities are mostly used in radiology to refer to one type of imaging, such as CT scan imaging. The medical imaging modalities are broadly classified into two

Table 4. Artificial intelligence-based healthcare datasets

	NLM's MedPix
General health and scientific research	The Cancer Imaging Archive (TCIA)
	Re3Data
	V7 COVID-19 X-Ray dataset
COVID-19 datasets	COVID-19 image dataset
	COVID-19 CT scans
	CT Medical Images
	Deep Lesion
CT datasets	Public Lung Database
	VIA Group Public Databases
	OASIS Brains Datasets
MRI datasets	MRNet: Knee MRI's
	IVDM3Seg
	NIH Database of 100,000 Chest X-Rays
	ChestX-Det-Dataset
X-Ray datasets	CheXpert
	SCR database: Segmentation in Chest Radiographs
	MURA: MSK Xrays
	OpenNEURO
Dataset aggregators	Kaggle
	UCI Machine Learning Repository

categories (1) Structural Medical Imaging Modalities and (2) Functional Medical Imaging Modalities. The subcategories of structural and functional modalities are discussed as under:

Magnetic Resonance Imaging (MRI):

MRI is the radiological type imaging technique, which provides the physiological process and anatomy of images of the body. To develop the images of body organs, doctors use high magnetic fields-based scanners to reconstruct the MRI images. MRI scanners use high magnetic fields, magnetic field gradients, and radio waves to create images of the body's organs. MRI scans are different from CT and PET scans since they do not use ionized radiation or X-rays. MRI of the human head with forehead and nose appears at the head's back as shown in Figure 15.

Table 5. Presents the different deep learning-based CNN platforms for brain MRI image SR

Name of Library	Operating System	Written In	Cuda supported	Parallel processing execution	Pretrained Model	CNN	RNN
TensorFlow	Windows, Linux, MacOs, Rasbian, Webapp, Mobile	C++, Python, Cuda	✓	✓	✓	✓	✓
Keras	Windows, Linux, MacOs	Python	✓	✓	✓	✓	✓
PyTorch	Windows, Linux, MacOs	C++, Python, Cuda	✓	✓	✓	✓	✓
MXNet	Window, Linux, Mac, Mobile, Webapp	C++, Python, Julia, R, Scala, Perl, Go	✓	✓	✓	✓	✓
Deeplearning4j	Window, Linux, Mac, Mobile	C++, Python, Perl, Cuda, java, Scala, Closure	✓	✓	✓	✓	✓
Microsoft CNTK	Window, Linux	C++	✓	✓	✓	✓	✓

T1 MRI/T1/T1 Image//T1W1/T1 Sequence

T1W is an abbreviation of T1-Weighted image. It is one of the fundamental sequences of pulses in MRI and determines variations in the T1 rest instances of specific tissues. Clinically, T1 Images are typically higher for overall performance than everyday anatomy images. T1 sequences of images are provided the best contrast of HR images, as shown in Figure 16.

T2-Weighted Image

T2 or T2*-Weighted MRI imaging sequence to measure the effectiveness of hemorrhages and hemosiderin deposits (Chavhan, Babyn, Thomas, Shroff, & Haacke, 2009). These images are built from the MRI images and characterized by the spin-spin relaxation time as shown in Figure 17.

Figure 15. MRI of human head with forehead

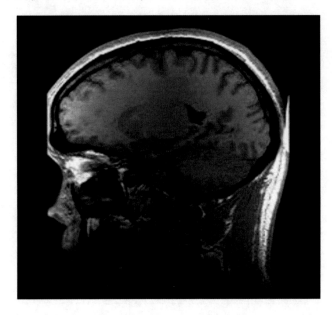

Figure 16. Sagittal T1-weighted brain MRI with gadolinium contrast

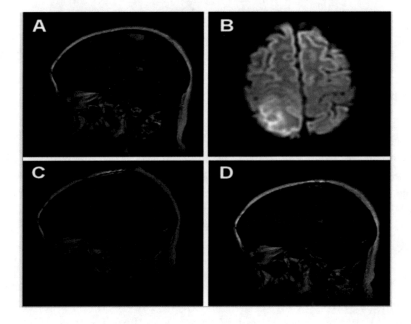

Figure 17. T2-weighted imaging of the brain

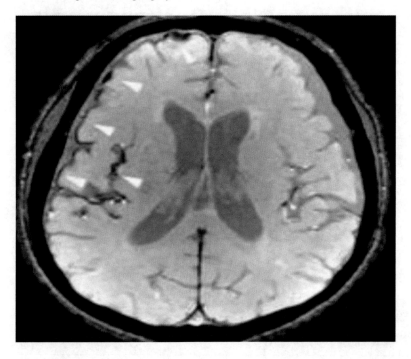

Proton Density Image

Proton density images are related to the number of nuclei in the area being imaged. The tissues of images with higher density or concentration of several protons reconstruct the strong signals and appear brighter than the original image. It also minimizes the impact of T1 and T2 sequences as shown in Figure 18.

MEDICAL IMAGING DATASETS

Many training datasets for medical image enhancements are available in the literature, but here we discuss some important datasets to train the model. Recent work used T1-weighted MRI images obtained from Kirby 21 (Landman et al., 2011). Shi et al. proposed to generate the LR image using the Gaussian blur technique with standard deviation is unity before a downscaling factor 2× (Shi, Cheng, Wang, Yap, & Shen, 2015). A particular listing of benchmark clinical picture datasets are proposed with the aid of Raza et al. (Raza & Singh, 2021) as shown in Table 3,4, and 6.

Figure 18. T1 and T2 sequences of proton density image

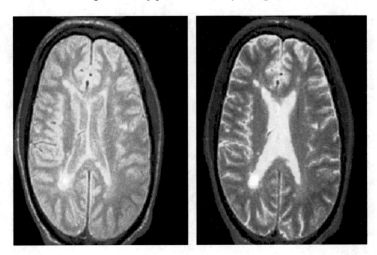

Table 6. List of BMID

S.No.	Dataset	Modalities	Open Access	Paid	Limited Access
1.	ABIDE	MRI	√		
2.	ADNI	MRI		√	
3.	BCDR	Mammography	√		
4.	CIVM	3D-MRM			√
5.	DDSM	Mammography	√		
6.	NBIA	CT, PET, MRI, etc.	√		√
7.	TCIA	Collection of MRI, CT, etc.	√		√
8.	IDA		√		
9.	MedPix	Variety of imaging data	√		
10.	DRIVE	2D color images of the retina	√		
11.	TCGA	Histopathology slide images	√		
12.	OASIS	MRI and PET	√		
13.	DICOM	MRI, CT, etc.	√		
14.	DermNet	Photo dermatology			√
15.	ISDIS	Dermoscopy, telemedicine, spectroscopy, etc		√	

QUALITY METRICS IN MEDICAL IMAGES

Measurements based on the subjective perception of the human visual system are known as qualitative metrics. It is also utilized to find unnoticed faults in compression methods' performance. When using quality metrics to evaluate the quality of a compression method, the original image is utilized as a reference image to evaluate the quality of the reconstructed image. The following are some of the most widely used qualitative metrics:

Mean Square Error

Mean Square Errors the cumulative squared error between the reconstructed and original image is represented by MSE. The smaller the MSE number, the smaller the error.

$$MSE = \frac{1}{MN} \sum_{y=1}^{M} \sum_{x=1}^{N} \left[I\left(x, y\right) - I\left(x, y\right)' \right]^{2}, \qquad (3)$$

where the number of pixels in the x and y axis of the image is denoted as M and N. Original image denoted by I and recovered image is denoted by I'. If the value of $I\left(x, y\right) = I\left(x, y\right)'$, then MSE should be zero.

Signal to Noise Ratio (SNR)

It is the ratio of signal to noise power. SNR identifies how the original image was corrupted by noise. Mathematically, it can be calculated as:

$$SNR = 10 \log_{10} \frac{VAR\left(I\right)}{MSE\left(I, I'\right)} \qquad (4)$$

where the variance and mean square error of an original image are denoted by VAR and MSE.

Figure 19. The pictorial representation of 3 x 3 matrices interpolated by 6 x 6 matrices

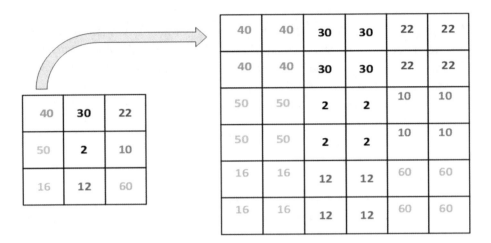

Peak Signal to Noise Ratio (PSNR)

We used the peak signal-to-noise ratio to compare two images in decibels. The quality of the original and compressed image is compared using this ratio. The greater the PSNR number, the better the reconstructed image quality.

$$PSNR = 10 \ \log_{10} \frac{\left(2^n - 1\right)}{\sqrt{MSE}}, \qquad \left(5\right)$$

where n is a maximum pixel value.

BRAIN MRI IMAGE SUPER-RESOLUTION ALGORITHMS

Recently brain MRI image super-resolution achieved remarkable performance and speedup the processing time. Many algorithms are available in the literature, but here we discuss the most important algorithms for brain MRI image SR.

Nearest Neighbor Interpolation Brain MRI Image SR Method

The nearest neighbor interpolation approach is very simple, and the interpolated pixel is replaced by the nearest pixel. This approach has less computational cost, and

Figure 20. Upscale the LR image using the nearest neighbor interpolation method

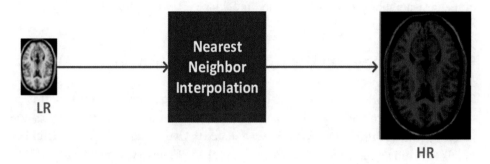

implementations are very easy, but some information is lost at the edges. The main operation of the nearest neighbor interpolation-based approach is shown in Figure 19.

Mathematically,

The original size of the image, Io: H x W

Scaled Image size, S: H' x W'

Input to output row scale factor:

$$J_r = \begin{cases} \dfrac{H}{H'}, & ifH > H' \\ \dfrac{H-1}{H'}, & ifH < H' \end{cases} \tag{6}$$

Input to output column scale factor:

$$J_c = \begin{cases} \dfrac{W}{W'}, & ifW > W' \\ \dfrac{W-1}{W'}, & ifW < W' \end{cases} \tag{7}$$

For each value of (r', c') inS, the corresponding fractional pixel location in Io is:

$$(r_f, c_f) = \left(J_r . r' . J_c . c' \right) \tag{8}$$

Figure 20 applies the conventional nearest-neighbor interpolation method to upscale the low-resolution brain MRI image. The reconstructed HR image result is still not satisfactory from a human perception point of view. The main drawbacks of nearest-neighbor interpolation are the blocky or imaging denoising in the reconstructed image.

Bilinear Interpolation Brain MRI Image SR Method

Bilinear interpolation is used to interpolate the two functions of variables. It is an extended version of linear type interpolation and performs the interpolation operation in one direction. Bilinear interpolation calculated the weighted average of 4 neighbor pixels to estimate the final value (Press, Teukolsky, Flannery, & Vetterling, 1992). For example, to calculate the function value of f at the point (G, H). It is supposed that the value of f at the four-quadrant point $Y_{11} = (G_1, H_1)$, $Y_{12} = (G_1, H_2)$, $Y_{21} = (G_2, H_1)$ and $Y_{22} = (G_2, H_2)$.

First, we perform the interpolation in a horizontal direction

$$f\left(G, H_1\right) \approx \frac{G_2 - G}{G_2 - G_1} f\left(Y_{11}\right) + \frac{G - G_1}{G_2 - G_1} f\left(Y_{21}\right),$$

$$f\left(G, H_2\right) \approx \frac{G_2 - G}{G_2 - G_1} f\left(Y_{12}\right) + \frac{G - G_1}{G_2 - G_1} f\left(Y_{22}\right).$$

Next, we proceed with interpolation on the vertical direction to obtain the desired estimate:

$$f\left(G, H\right) \approx \frac{H_2 - H}{H_2 - H_1} f\left(G, H_1\right) + \frac{H - H_1}{H_2 - H_1} f\left(G, H_2\right)$$

$$= \frac{H_2 - H}{H_2 - H_1}\left[\frac{G_2 - G}{G_2 - G_1} f\left(Y_{11}\right) + \frac{G - G_1}{G_2 - G_1} f\left(Y_{21}\right)\right] + \frac{H - H_1}{H_2 - H_1}\left[\frac{G_2 - G}{G_2 - G_1} f\left(Y_{12}\right) + \frac{G - G_1}{G_2 - G_1} f\left(Y_{22}\right)\right]$$

$$= \frac{1}{\left(G_2 - G_1\right)\left(G_2 - G_1\right)}\left(f\left(Y_{11}\right)\left(G_2 - G\right)\left(H_2 - H\right) + f\left(Y_{21}\right)\left(G - G_1\right)\left(H_2 - H\right) + f\left(Y_{12}\right)\left(G_2 - G\right)\left(H - H_1\right) + f\left(Y_{22}\right)\left(G - G_1\right)\left(H - H_1\right)\right)$$

$$= \frac{1}{\left(G_2 - G_1\right)\left(H_2 - H_1\right)} \begin{bmatrix} G_2 - G_1 & G - G_1 \end{bmatrix} \begin{bmatrix} f\left(Y_{11}\right) & f\left(Y_{12}\right) \\ f\left(Y_{21}\right) & f\left(Y_{22}\right) \end{bmatrix} \begin{bmatrix} G_2 - G_1 & G - G_1 \end{bmatrix} \quad (9)$$

The above discussion is related to the Bilinear Interpolation method to reconstruct the HR image. The resultant HR image is better than the Nearest neighbor interpolation but has not achieved the best result. The main severe drawbacks of Bilinear Interpolation are the blurring problems, particularly in the edge regions.

Bicubic Interpolation Technique for Brain MRI Image SR

Bicubic interpolation is also a pre-processing step technique to upscale the LR image into HR. It takes an average (weighted) of 16 neighbors of pixels to estimate the reconstructed value (Press et al., 1992). It provides better and sharp results as compared to previous interpolation methods. It has more computational cost as well as processing time. This approach provides the best results among other interpolation techniques if computational cost is no problem.

$$g\left(x, z\right) = \frac{1}{16} \sum_{i=-1}^{2} \sum_{m=-1}^{2} f\left(x + l, z + m\right) u\left(dx\right) u\left(dz\right), \quad (10)$$

where $f\left(p + l, q + m\right)$ is the value of the gray pixel, $u\left(dp\right)$ is known as changes in the $x - axis$ direction and $u\left(dq\right)$ is the changes in the $y - direction$.

$$f\left(x - 1, z - 1\right) f\left(x - 1, z\right) f\left(x - 1, z + 1\right) f\left(x - 1, z + 2\right)$$

$$f\left(x, z - 1\right) f\left(x, z\right) f\left(x, z + 1\right) f\left(x, z + 2\right)$$

$$f\left(x + 1, z - 1\right) f\left(x + 1, z\right) f\left(x + 1, z + 1\right) f\left(x + 1, z + 2\right)$$

$$f\left(x + 2, z - 1\right) f\left(x + 2, z\right) f\left(x + 2, z + 1\right) f\left(x + 2, z + 2\right)$$

Figure 21. All interpolation techniques apply to a brain tumor MRI Image

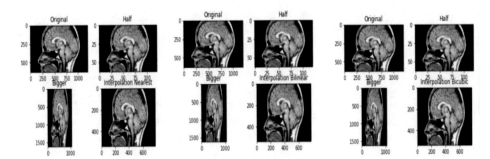

In Figure 21, we apply the Bicubic Interpolation method to reconstruct the HR image. The resultant HR image is better than previous interpolation techniques, but computational cost is the main hindrance.

REQUIREMENT FOR DEEP LEARNING IN MEDICAL IMAGING

Limited dataset availability for algorithm training and validation due to the lack of standardized digital scientific records, as nicely as an extreme felony and moral constraint to shield affected person privacy, which is presently obstructing the massive use of deep getting to know methods in the discipline of scientific imaging. Harmonized facts transmission protocols such as Digital Imaging and Communication in Medicine (DICOM) and digital information storage are trendy in scientific imaging, partly addressing the first issue, however, private restrictions are as strict. The deployment of technological know-how options that simultaneously fulfill the needs for information protection and use is required to forestall patient secrecy breaches while boosting scientific find out about on huge datasets to enhance affected person care. With an emphasis on scientific imaging applications, we provide an overview of current and next-generation methodologies for combined, secure, and privacy-preserving synthetic intelligence, as properly as attainable assault and future potentialities in clinical imaging and beyond.

DEEP LEARNING FRAMEWORK FOR BRAIN MRI IMAGE SUPER-RESOLUTION

In an earlier section, we discussed the hand-designed approaches to upscale the LR image. These approaches are very simple, but they can not provide the best result and reconstructed images having jagged ringing type artifacts present in the image. New deep learning-based approaches provide fast processing time with the best human visually pleasing image quality. In this part, we have covered the recent deep learning approaches that enhance the quality of medical image SR.

Chen et al., (Y. Chen et al., 2018) suggested the dense-based architecture concept known as DCSRN to generate the high-quality features from medical (MRI) images. The authors used the set of convolutional, batch normalization with exponential linear units (ELU) action functions. A single convolution layer is used as the first and last layer to reconstruct the HR brain image Zhao et al., (Zhao, Zhang, Zhang, & Zou, 2019) proposed the deep CNN model used a channel splitting network (CSN) approach to reduce the problem of reconstructing the HR image. The proposed CSN model is classified into two parts, i.e., residual/Resnet part, and dense/DenseNet part. The function of the residual part is used to support the features, though the DenseNet part is used to explore the latest features. Du et al., (Du et al., 2020) proposed a dilation-based CNN architecture known as DCED based brain MRI image SR network architecture to enhance the low resolution of MRI ones. To extract the high-frequency features, the authors are used a three-dimensional dilated convolution operation as an Encoder. To interpret the features information, they used inverse convolution operation (deconvolution) to alleviate the gridding effect and reconstruct the fine details. Furthermore, symmetrically connection-based blocks are used to integrate the encoders and decoders. The resultant output of every block is finally gone through the CNN layer to obtain the detailed hierarchical output features. To enhance the low quality of MRI images and speed up their performance Alom et al., present the fast medical image super-resolution (FMISR) (S. Zhang, Liang, Pan, & Zheng, 2018). In this approach, three CNN layers extract the feature information. This approach also supports a better environment for retinal-type image segmentations. The main deep CNN methods support the medical image brain MRI image super-resolution and COVID-19 image as shown in Figure 22.

QUANTITATIVE COMPARISON OF MRI MEDICAL IMAGES

This sub-section discusses the justification that MRI SR methods have improved performance than earlier approaches. Figure 23, clearly shows that the Residual dense network for medical magnetic resonance images super-resolution (MRDN) (D. Zhu & Qiu, 2021) obtained better performance in terms of PSNR and faster CPU speed than other methods. Furthermore, the computational cost of different medical image SR evaluates k parameters. In Figure 24, data is obtained from the recent paper (L. Wang, Zhu, He, Jia, & Du, 2022).

Figure 22. Shows a different medical image framework for COVID-19 and image SR architecture using the deep learning framework in (a) Progressive BPN for COVID-CT SR (PBPN)(Song, Zhao, Hui, & Jiang, 2021), (b) Multi-window based method proposed by (Qiu, Cheng, Wang, & Zhang, 2021), and (c)MIRN method proposed by (Qiu, Zheng, Zhu, & Huang, 2021)

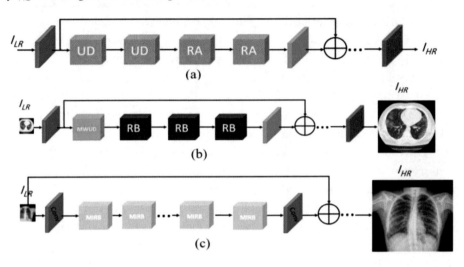

Figure 23. Quantitative comparison performance in terms of PSNR versus CPU running time of the Set5 test dataset with enlargement factor 2x

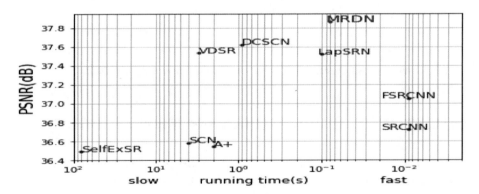

Figure 24. Quantitative comparison of PSNR versus network k parameters of MRI SR algorithms on enlargement scale-factor 2x on Kirby21 dataset

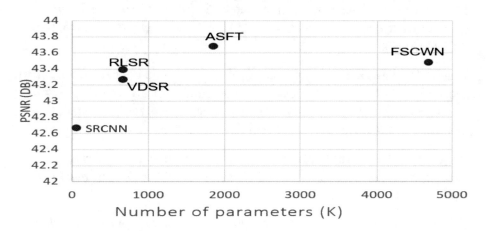

CONCLUSION

In this book, chapter authors present the concept of deep learning with medical enhancement using different hand-designed filter techniques and deep CNN-based image super-resolution. The authors have also discussed more detailed information about the latest software involved in medical image enhancement. Furthermore, we provide information about different medical image datasets for using deep CNN during the training and testing purposes with different medical image formats available for research purposes. Finally, we present the quantitative comparison of PSNR, CPU processing time, and Network parameters. These results clearly show that the deep CNN-based method for medical image enhancement also achieves superior performance than previous methods. For future directions, we select the different areas of the medical image using generative adversarial network (GAN) techniques to increase the perceptual quality of the medical image.

REFERENCES

Abadi, M., Barham, P., Chen, J., Chen, Z., Davis, A., Dean, J., & Isard, M. (2016). *Tensorflow: A system for large-scale machine learning.* Paper presented at the 12th USENIX symposium on operating systems design and implementation (OSDI 16).

Ahad, M. A. R., Antar, A. D., & Shahid, O. (2019). *Vision-based Action Understanding for Assistive Healthcare: A Short Review.* Paper presented at the CVPR Workshops.

Aung, M. S., Kaltwang, S., Romera-Paredes, B., Martinez, B., Singh, A., Cella, M., & Shafizadeh, M. (2015). The automatic detection of chronic pain-related expression: Requirements, challenges, and the multimodal EmoPain dataset. *IEEE Transactions on Affective Computing*, *7*(4), 435–451. doi:10.1109/TAFFC.2015.2462830 PMID:30906508

Bhateja, V., Tiwari, H., & Srivastava, A. (2015). A non-local means filtering algorithm for restoration of Rician distributed MRI. *Emerging ICT for Bridging the Future-Proceedings of the 49th Annual Convention of the Computer Society of India CSI.* 10.1007/978-3-319-13731-5_1

Chavhan, G. B., Babyn, P. S., Thomas, B., Shroff, M. M., & Haacke, E. (2009). *Principles, techniques, and applications of T2*-based MR imaging and its special applications.* Academic Press.

Chen, C., Jafari, R., & Kehtarnavaz, N. (2015). *UTD-MHAD: A multimodal dataset for human action recognition utilizing a depth camera and a wearable inertial sensor.* Paper presented at the 2015 IEEE International conference on image processing (ICIP). 10.1109/ICIP.2015.7350781

Chen, Y., Xie, Y., Zhou, Z., Shi, F., Christodoulou, A. G., & Li, D. (2018). *Brain MRI super resolution using 3D deep densely connected neural networks.* Paper presented at the 2018 IEEE 15th International Symposium on Biomedical Imaging (ISBI 2018). 10.1109/ISBI.2018.8363679

Chollet, F. (2015). *Keras.* https://keras.io

Clancey, W. J., & Shortliffe, E. H. (1984). Readings in medical artificial intelligence: The first decade. Addison-Wesley Longman Publishing Co., Inc.

Dong, C., Loy, C. C., He, K., & Tang, X. (2014). *Learning a deep convolutional network for image super-resolution.* Paper presented at the European conference on computer vision. 10.1007/978-3-319-10593-2_13

Dou, Q., Wei, S., Yang, X., Wu, W., Liu, K. (2018). *Medical image super-resolution via minimum error regression model selection using random forest.* Academic Press.

Du, J., Wang, L., Liu, Y., Zhou, Z., He, Z., & Jia, Y. (2020). *Brain MRI Super-Resolution Using 3D Dilated Convolutional Encoder–Decoder Network.* Academic Press.

Ellis, C., Masood, S. Z., Tappen, M. F., LaViola, J. J. Jr, & Sukthankar, R. (2013). Exploring the trade-off between accuracy and observational latency in action recognition. *International Journal of Computer Vision, 101*(3), 420–436. doi:10.100711263-012-0550-7

Foley, J. D., & Van Dam, A. (1982). Fundamentals of interactive computer graphics. Addison-Wesley Longman Publishing Co., Inc.

Greenspan, H. (2009). *Super-resolution in medical imaging.* Academic Press.

Hosny, A., Parmar, C., Quackenbush, J., Schwartz, L. H., & Aerts, H. J. (2018). Artificial intelligence in radiology. *Nature Reviews. Cancer, 18*(8), 500–510. doi:10.103841568-018-0016-5 PMID:29777175

Huang, Y., Shao, L., & Frangi, A. F. (2019). *Simultaneous super-resolution and cross-modality synthesis in magnetic resonance imaging Deep Learning and Convolutional Neural Networks for Medical Imaging and Clinical Informatics.* Springer.

Keys, R. (1981). *Cubic convolution interpolation for digital image processing.* Academic Press.

Kim, J., Lee, J. K., & Lee, K. M. (2016). Accurate image super-resolution using very deep convolutional networks. *Proceedings of the IEEE conference on computer vision and pattern recognition.* 10.1109/CVPR.2016.182

Lai, W.-S., Huang, J.-B., Ahuja, N., & Yang, M.-H. (2017). Deep laplacian pyramid networks for fast and accurate super-resolution. *Proceedings of the IEEE conference on computer vision and pattern recognition.* 10.1109/CVPR.2017.618

Landman, B. A., Huang, A. J., Gifford, A., Vikram, D. S., Lim, I. A. L., Farrell, J. A., . . . Jarso, S. (2011). *Multi-parametric neuroimaging reproducibility: a 3-T resource study.* Academic Press.

Li, X., & Orchard, M. (2001). *New edge-directed interpolation.* Academic Press.

Metz, C. (2015). *Google just open sourced tensorflow, its artificial intelligence engine.* Academic Press.

Naga Srinivasu, P., Srinivasa Rao, T., Srinivas, G., & Prasad Reddy, P. V. G. D. (2020). A computationally efficient skull scraping approach for brain MR image. *Recent Adv Comput Sci Commun, 13*(5), 833–844. doi:10.2174/22132759126661 90809111928

Ofli, F., Chaudhry, R., Kurillo, G., Vidal, R., & Bajcsy, R. (2013). *Berkeley mhad: A comprehensive multimodal human action database.* Paper presented at the 2013 IEEE Workshop on Applications of Computer Vision (WACV). 10.1109/WACV.2013.6474999

Paszke, A., Gross, S., Chintala, S., Chanan, G., Yang, E., DeVito, Z., Lerer, A. (2017). *Automatic differentiation in pytorch.* Academic Press.

Press, W. H., Teukolsky, S. A., Flannery, B. P., & Vetterling, W. T. (1992). Numerical recipes in Fortran 77: volume 1, volume 1 of Fortran numerical recipes: The art of scientific computing. Cambridge University Press.

Qiu, D., Cheng, Y., Wang, X., & Zhang, X. (2021). Multi-window back-projection residual networks for reconstructing COVID-19 CT super-resolution images. *Computer Methods and Programs in Biomedicine, 200,* 105934. doi:10.1016/j.cmpb.2021.105934 PMID:33454574

Qiu, D., Zheng, L., Zhu, J., & Huang, D. (2021). Multiple improved residual networks for medical image super-resolution. *Future Generation Computer Systems, 116,* 200–208. doi:10.1016/j.future.2020.11.001

Raza, K., & Singh, N. K. (2021). A tour of unsupervised deep learning for medical image analysis. *Current Medical Imaging, 17*(9), 1059–1077. doi:10.2174/157340 5617666210127154257 PMID:33504314

Rodriguez, M. D., Ahmed, J., & Shah, M. (2008). *Action mach a spatio-temporal maximum average correlation height filter for action recognition.* Paper presented at the 2008 IEEE conference on computer vision and pattern recognition. 10.1109/CVPR.2008.4587727

Shao, L., & Zhao, M. (2007). *Order statistic filters for image interpolation.* Paper presented at the 2007 IEEE International Conference on Multimedia and Expo. 10.1109/ICME.2007.4284684

Shi, F., Cheng, J., Wang, L., Yap, P.-T., & Shen, D. (2015). *LRTV: MR image super-resolution with low-rank and total variation regularizations.* Academic Press.

Song, Z., Zhao, X., Hui, Y., & Jiang, H. (2021). Progressive back-projection network for COVID-CT super-resolution. *Computer Methods and Programs in Biomedicine, 208,* 106193. doi:10.1016/j.cmpb.2021.106193 PMID:34107373

Srinivasu, P. N., Rao, T. S., & Balas, V. E. (2020). Volumetric estimation of the damaged area in the human brain from 2D MR image. *International Journal of Information System Modeling and Design, 11*(1), 74–92. doi:10.4018/IJISMD.2020010105

Tran, D., & Sorokin, A. (2008). *Human activity recognition with metric learning.* Paper presented at the European conference on computer vision.

Van Ouwerkerk, J. (2006). *Image super-resolution survey.* Academic Press.

Vickers, N. J. (2017). Animal communication: When i'm calling you, will you answer too? *Current Biology*, *27*(14), R713–R715. doi:10.1016/j.cub.2017.05.064 PMID:28743020

Wang, C., Zhu, X., Hong, J. C., & Zheng, D. (2019). Artificial intelligence in radiotherapy treatment planning: Present and future. *Technology in Cancer Research & Treatment*, *18*, 1533033819873922. doi:10.1177/1533033819873922 PMID:31495281

Wang, L., Zhu, H., He, Z., Jia, Y., & Du, J. (2022). Adjacent slices feature transformer network for single anisotropic 3D brain MRI image super-resolution. *Biomedical Signal Processing and Control*, *72*, 103339. doi:10.1016/j.bspc.2021.103339

Wang, X., Zhou, D., Zeng, N., Yu, X., Hu, S. (2018). *Super-resolution image reconstruction using surface fitting with hierarchical structure.* Academic Press.

Wei, P., Zhao, Y., Zheng, N., & Zhu, S.-C. (2013). Modeling 4d human-object interactions for event and object recognition. *Proceedings of the IEEE International Conference on Computer Vision.* 10.1109/ICCV.2013.406

Xia, L., Chen, C.-C., & Aggarwal, J. K. (2012). *View invariant human action recognition using histograms of 3d joints.* Paper presented at the 2012 IEEE computer society conference on computer vision and pattern recognition workshops. 10.1109/CVPRW.2012.6239233

Zhang, L., & Wu, X. (2006). *An edge-guided image interpolation algorithm via directional filtering and data fusion.* Academic Press.

Zhang, S., Liang, G., Pan, S., & Zheng, L. (2018). *A fast medical image super resolution method based on deep learning network.* Academic Press.

Zhao, X., Zhang, Y., Zhang, T., & Zou, X. (2019). *Channel splitting network for single MR image super-resolution.* Academic Press.

Zhu, D., & Qiu, D. (2021). Residual dense network for medical magnetic resonance images super-resolution. *Computer Methods and Programs in Biomedicine*, *209*, 106330. doi:10.1016/j.cmpb.2021.106330 PMID:34388684

Zhu, J., Yang, G., & Lio, P. (2019). *How can we make gan perform better in single medical image super-resolution? A lesion focused multi-scale approach.* Paper presented at the 2019 IEEE 16th International Symposium on Biomedical Imaging (ISBI 2019). 10.1109/ISBI.2019.8759517

APPENDIX: LIST OF ABBREVIATIONS

AI = Artificial Intelligence
CNN = Convolutional Neural Network
MRI = Magnetic Resonance Imaging
MAP = Maximum a posteriori probability
HR = High-Resolution
LR = Low-Resolution
RGB = Red Green Blue
YCbCr = Luma Blue Chroma Red Chroma
HSV = Hue Saturation and Value
CT = Computed Tomography
NIfTI = Neuroimaging Informatics Technology Initiative
PET = Positron emission tomography
CT = Computed Tomography
DICOM = Digital Imaging and Communications in Medicine
MSE = Mean Square Error
PSNR = Peak Signal to Noise Ratio
SNR = Signal to Noise Ratio
FMISR = Fast Medical Image Super-Resolution
CNTK = Microsoft Cognitive Toolkit
MITK = Medical Imaging Interaction Toolkit
PICSL = Penn Image Computing and Science Laboratory

Chapter 4
Analyzing and Forecasting of COVID-19 Situation Using FbProphet Model Algorithms

S. Geetha
BNM Institute of Technology, India

Ayush Sengar
CMR Institute of Technology, India

M. Farida Begam
CMR Institute of Technology, India

Joshua Samuel Raj
CMR Institute of Technology, India

Ayush Dubey
CMR Institute of Technology, India

ABSTRACT

SARS-CoV-2 (n-coronavirus) is a global pandemic that has killed millions of people all over the world. In severe situations, it can induce pneumonia and severe acute respiratory syndrome (SARS), which can lead to death. It's an asymptomatic sickness that makes life and work more difficult for us. This research focused on the current state of the coronavirus pandemic and forecasted the global situation, as well as its impacts and future status. The authors used the FbProphet model to forecast new covid cases and deaths for the month of August utilizing various information representation and machine learning algorithms. They hope the findings will aid scientists, researchers, and laypeople in predicting and analyzing the effects of the epidemic. Finally, they conclude that the virus's second wave was around four times stronger than the first. They also looked at the trajectory of COVID-19 instances (monthly and weekly) and discovered that the number of cases rises more during the weekdays, which could be due to the weekend lockout.

DOI: 10.4018/978-1-6684-3791-9.ch004

INTRODUCTION

The World Health Organization declared the Coronavirus Pandemic to be a worldwide health disaster of concern in 2020 in the month of March. This epidemic, which first originated in Wuhan City of China in December 2019, has wreaked havoc across the globe. On the 30th of January 2020, the first case in a long time was accounted for, with the total number of cases exceeding 4 million (Darapaneni et al., 2020). Over 80,000 people have died as a result of the pandemic, with 3 million people recovering. Proactive measures adopted by experts include a long-term lockdown of the country, rapid separation of cases, and application-based tracking of contaminated people. Intended for a improved consideration of COVID-19's development in the world, a focus scheduled the development then development of occurrences in India might not be unnoticed (Tiwari et al., 2020).

In March of 2020, the World Health Organization (WHO) proclaimed the Coronavirus Disease to be a universal health calamity of anxiety. This disease, which began in Wuhan City in November 2019, has struck havoc around the world. The first scenario in a long time was accounted for on January 30, 2020, with a total number of scenarios topping 4 million (Darapaneni et al., 2020). The disease has claimed the lives of nearly 80,000 people, with 3 million people recovering. Experts recommend a long-term a state of isolation of the country, fast scenario isolation, and application-based surveillance of contaminated persons as proactive measures. A focus scheduled the development of disease in the globe in order to improve the consideration of disease's development in the world. (Tiwari et al., 2020).

Working with time series data can be tedious, and the many ways for creating copies can be finicky. It's especially true when working with data that has a lot of seasonal variations (Kumar et al., 2020). SARIMAX and other traditional time series models have a variety of data restrictions. As a result, the average data analyst has a significant learning curve when it comes to time series analysis. So, in 2017, a group of Facebook researchers published "Forecasting at Scale," an open-source initiative that provides data analysts and data scientists with quick, powerful, and accessible time-series modelling (Inbaraj et al., 2017).

To comprehend something like, a compartmentalised ideal, Susceptible -Infected -Quarantine-Recover (SIQR) is cast-off. The retrieval and replication rates of absolute disclosed confident scenarios in the Nationboth topped 75% and 25 days, respectively (Alok Tiwari et al., 2020). SIQR can be used to increase the model's robustness by employing a weighted border method, and it can be designed to maintain the model stable. AI calculations can be applied to a load model based on data from different nations, allowing for precise inspection (Geetha et al., 2021).

The Covid disease which started in Asian countries, swiftly spread to other nations, with thousands of scenarios documented throughout the world. As of May 8, 2020,

56,342 positive scenarios had been identified in India. India will have challenges in preventing the spread of Covid 2, a deadly respiratory ailment (Geetha et al., 2019). The Indian Office of Wellbeing and Domestic Wellbeing has voiced concern about the present eruption and has made significant paces to prevent disease from spreading further (Beulah et al., 2020). Both the federal and state governments are involved. In addition, the Indian government instituted a 55-day a state of isolation across the Nation on March 25, 2020, to prevent the sickness from spreading. This has a direct impact on the economy of the Nation since it is closed contemporary areas, as persons are nowadays uncertain to do commercial in the stuck zones (Rahimi et al., 2017).

At the time of writing, disease had spread to over 200 countries throughout the world, with over 36 million confirmed scenarios. Several studies have been published on the topic of global disease forecast (Wan et al., 2009). The most important subject areas in this work were highlighted using keyword analysis. In addition, a number of traits were uncovered that may be useful in future research. In addition, the most useful models utilised by researchers to predict the disease were recognised in this study. A thorough scient metric analysis was performed as a useful tool for bibliometric analyses and reviews. This includes keywords and subject categories, as well as the classification of forecasting models (Immorlica et al., 2020). Introduction section is followed with literature review, proposed methodology, results and finally concluded with conclusion.

LITERATURE REVIEW

We assessed disease progress in the most afflicted Indian states, Tamil Nadu, Andhra Pradesh, and Maharashtra, as of 29-Aug-20, and built a forecast model to forecast disease feast behaviour in the following calendar months (Choudhary et al., 2018). With festivals approaching, there is little to do until immunisation is available. In states where the number of scenarios has already peaked, there is a considerable likelihood of a resurgence. If social remoteness and other switch events are not properly trailed in the upcoming calendar month, there is a significant risk of a repeat in the number of scenarios (Satrio et al., 2021).

The Covid sickness 2019 (disease) commenced in Hubei Province, Wuhan, Asian countries, in November 2019. This flare-up has created a through out the world disease, with about 28 million illnesses and 0.95 million deaths. On January 30, 2020, India saw its first confirmed scenario. Over a huge number of people have been positively identified thus far, with 77,588 deaths and close to 3 .1 million retrievals (Roosa et al., 2020). The Indian government implemented a tough rough a state of isolation in IV stages, starting on March 26th and lasted nearly three calendar months till May 31st. Republic of India ranks first in terms of the number of confident instances. With almost 90,000 incidents recorded every day, India is just second to the United States. Despite the fact that a high confident scenarios are reported every day, the amount of people who die is extremely low (57 for per million people) (Maleki et al., 2017). The disease scenarios in nations are evaluated using a arithmetical performance in this study, which includes scenarios up through August 22, 2020. (Van et al., 2014).

Fig 1 Illustrate the different rediction model for finding the corona virus. Numerical conditions are frequently used in the general public to depict the landscape and impact of throughout the world diseases (Anastassopoulou et al., 2020). Its version SIQR is widely recognised as the best displaying strategy for disease, in which irresistible confinement plays a significant part (Ji et al., 2020). One a few jammed countries, such as Italy, Brazil employ this proven technique of dealing with the infection's implications (Chaudhry et al., 2020 and Melika et al., 2017).

Trainings on the application of switch regulations and the influence of a state of isolation on the broadcast of disease, notably in India, have been taken into account (Shipra et al., 2012). Despite this, no study has examined how distant the illness has advanced in relations of epidemiologic limits. The current study investigated an emergence of disease in India using the SIQR paradigm. Boundaries and indicators are set to measure global development and disease development (Saeed et al., 2011). Seasonal cycles and emergencies influence the expansion of large-scale volume fracturing in shale oil horizontal wells, as well as production, making production forecasting challenging (Saeed et al., 2012). According to the findings, the Prophet algorithm has a higher forecast accuracy and is more reliable. The results show that the Prophet algorithm has a higher forecast accuracy and is more accurate for complex shale oil production (Pablo et al., 2014).

In a basic online choice issue, a decision-maker aiming to maximize her value inspects a sequence of arriving items to learn their values (derived from known distributions) and selects when to finish the process by taking the current item (Yossi et al., 2018). The purpose is to demonstrate a "prophet inequality," which states that if she has foreknowledge of all values, she can do roughly as well as a prophet. Threshold-based algorithms, which are commonly used to solve prophet inequalities, no longer guarantee adequate performance when dealing with linear correlations, which is a significant challenge. This stumbling block is tied to another "augmentations" issue that may be of interest in and of itself (Moshe et al., 2014). We'd like to be notified when a forecast model fails to perform as predicted. When a forecast model doesn't work as planned, we'd like to be able to fine-tune the method's parameters to fit the situation. In order to fine-tune these tactics, you'll need a thorough understanding of how time series models work in general (Bateni et al., 2015). The first input variables to automate ARIMA are, for example, the

Figure 1. Illustration of corona virus prediction with different models

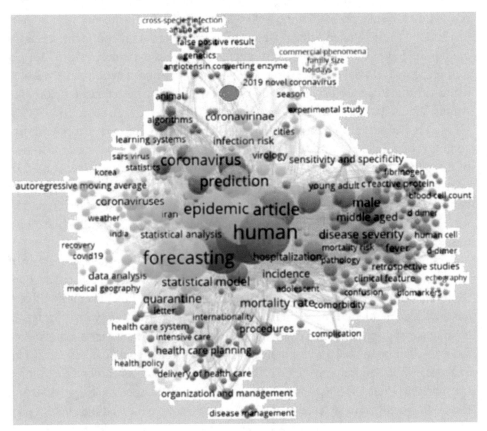

maximum values of the differencing, auto-regressive components, and moving average components. A typical analyst will have no idea how to alter these instructions to prevent the behavior, and this is the type of expertise that is difficult to acquire and scale. The Prophet package has easy-to-adjust settings (Domagoj et al., 2020). Even if you aren't familiar with forecast models, you can use this to make accurate forecasts (Moses et al., 2017).

PROPOSED METHODOLOGY

A necessity and unique contributions of this study is completely related and can be used as a set of Principles and Methods for Healthcare sectors with the help of Explainable Artificial Intelligence. Any organisation must be able to recognise time-based patterns. Questions such as how much goods to keep on hand, how

Table 1. Overall summary of literature survey

Reference Number	Contributions from the research work
12.	A comparison analysis of the forecast results from the SIR and FbProphet models and in this research that, if a total of 5.2% of India's populace gets infected by Covid, the disease's nationwide spread will peak by the end of November 2020.
13.	There is a considerable chance of a recurrence in the number of scenarios if social distance and other control measures are not carefully followed in the coming calendar months.
14.	The Government of India imposed a harsh cross-Nation a state of isolation in four stages, commencing on March 25th and lasting for almost two calendar months, ending on May 31st.
15.	Furthermore, the Nation had began a regular process, which included the opening of all activities and institutions.
16.	Despite this, no study has examined how distant the illness has advanced in terms of epidemiologic limits.
17.	This model is a popular computational tool for assessing and forecasting illness development.
18.	Its form SIQR is widely recognized as the best displaying strategy for disease, in which desirable internment plays a significant part.
19.	By means of the previous design, this technique is sed to find limits for measuring the growth and expansion of possessions in an area
20.	Only a few impacted countries, such as Brazil, employ this proven technique of dealing with the infection's implications.
21.	Revisions on the implementation of switch regulations and the influence of a state of isolation on the communication of illness, notably in India, have been taken into account.
22.	Our nation is a second one to the nation of United States in terms of the amount of confident scenarios reported each day, with over 90,000 scenarios recorded every day.
23.	The current study investigated the emergence of disease in India using the SIQR paradigm. Boundaries and indicators are set to track global development and disease progression.
24.	The Indian Health Welfare had taken actions to stop the disease from dispersal more.
25.	To regulate the increase as well as the quick advancement, a number of methods would be necessary, counting computational showcasing, truthful devices, and entitative inquiries.
26.	In order to achieve this goal, the US governments are captivating a list of actions and accepting a insufficient war standards.
27.	There are a few assumptions in this model, as with any numerical model. To improve the model's resilience, a mechanism including a weighted boundary can be designed to prevent the illness.
28.	AI calculations can be used on traditional information from numerous nations, permitting for extra exact and precise review and prediction.
29.	The disease which started in Asian countries, swiftly spread to other nations, with thousands of scenarios documented throughout the world. As of May 8, 2020, 56,32 confident scenarios had been recognized. India might face challenges in evading sanctions.

much foot traffic to expect in your store, and how many passengers will fly are all crucial period sequence complications to address. This is wherefore period sequence

Figure 2. Block illustration for the planned method

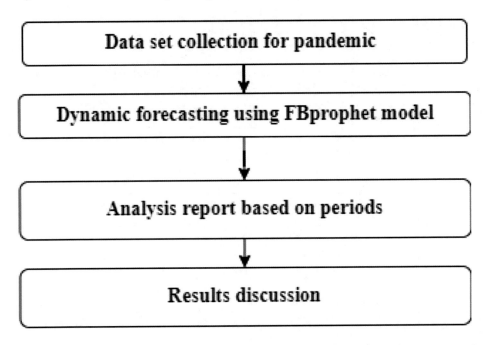

forecast is a technique that every data scientist should be familiar with (Shuchi et al., 2010). [30]. The situation is combined hooked on the data discipline ecology, from weather forecast to product sales, making the situation a necessary addition to a data expert's skill set. Data sequence is a great method to get started on real-world tasks. Time sequence are easy to understand and can assist you in entering the bigger field of machine learning. The dataset has day-by-day near data on the amount of impacted scenarios by disease, the period begins the 2020 and closes in August 2021. It should be noticed that this period was described by everyday information concerning scenarios in India on some random day which is an aggregate number (Shuchi et al., 2015). [31]. Fig 2 presents the block illustration of planned method.

FbProphet

This research work analyses a pattern system as seen by FBprophet of diseases, which can give significant knowledge for the public skilled specialists (Jose et al., 2017). In the future examination, we intend to combine this exploration with Deep Learning models like the Deep Sequential Prediction Model (DSPM) and contrast it with the FBprophet results with refining the forecast models to additionally work on the expectation of the spread of this infection (Jose et al., 2019).

Prophet may detect change points either automatically or manually. You may also vary the strength of the change points to change the growth function and the amount of data taken into account in automatic changepoint identification (Jose et al., 2019).

There are three primary alternatives for the growth function:

Linear Growth: This is Prophet's default option. It employs a series linear equation with slope value that vary across points. When direct growth is used, the growth time will look like the middle school formula

$$y = mx1 + b \tag{1}$$

with the exception that the slopes(m) and offsets(b) are mutable and will alteration value at respectively point. The term "logistic growth" is used when the term "growth" is used (Ilias et al., 2018).

Definition

In 2017, Facebook made FbProphet, a time-series forecasting tool, open-source (Ilias et al., 2016). It operates on the additive model principle. The non-linearities of the FbProphet are based on several seasons and other parameters. So,

$$I1 + R1 + S1 = S0 + I0 + R0 \tag{2}$$

The S1 (Susceptible) I1 (infected) R1 (Respiratory) aims to receive key values about the disease. The following are the set of questions that improves the innovation model of finding the present public of the disease and forecasting new covid scenarios and deaths by utilizing various information representation and machine learning algorithms (Ilias et al., 2018).

Q1: Is the illness transmissible?

The quantity of ill people at the start is I0. Susceptible people are represented by the letter Ss. However, we're curious as to whether or not this figure will continue to climb. We expect "Ss" to decrease with time because dS/dt 1 is now less than 0. So,

$$Ss \leq sS0 \ di/dt_1 < I1 \ (\beta 1S0 - \gamma 1) \tag{3}$$

if, Sickness spreads, then *di/dtv >0 i. e if sS0> γ/β1=1/qq* $\tag{4}$

The percentage of infected people who come into touch with the general public during their infectious period is known as the contact ratio. As we did earlier in this study, we define the parameter R = S0/ here. As a result, if R is more than one, the disease will spread (Paul et al., 2017).

Q2: On any given day, what is the maximum amount of infectious mediators, often known as the peak?

Not only can Facebook Prophet forecast future trends, but it also assists in the identification and filling in of missing factors. Equation for the FbProphet model:

$$Y1(t)=g1(t)+s1(t)+h1(t)+\varepsilon t \tag{5}$$

g_I (t) is used to study non-periodic trends in time series (Paul et al., 2019). [39]. s_I denotes the regularity of a weekly or annual change (t). The effect of an uneven day or days, such as a break, is referred to as h_I (t). The error word t is used to refer to unobserved factors. In this analysis, only non-periodic time-series modifications were taken into account.

RESULTS AND DISCUSSIONS

This segment presents the test consequences of the disease pattern anticipating four scenarios dependent on authentic disease information (Soheil et al., 2018). Week by week disease patterns and model execution is additionally investigated to comprehend model adequacy. We plotted day by day pestilence trademark bends for every nation to comprehend the illness practices (Hossein et al., 2017). These bends present just counterfeit information designs yet didn't affirm the genuine diseases each day (Hossein et al., 2018). This might happen because of the changes in information qualities of accessible information and real data. At times there is a plausible of few out of every odd tainted individual that couldn't be tried or affirmed (Michal et al., 2015). Changing age and sex seroprevalence was 8.5 percent (95 percent CI 7 percent -10.7 percent). Individually, participants with hypertension and diabetes had uncorrected seroprevalences of 16.2 percent (95 percent CI: 9.3–25.9) and 10.8 percent (95 percent CI: 5.5-18.3), respectively (Moran et al., 2016). When we changed the test execution, the seroprevalence was 6.2 percent (95 percent CI 4.2–8.18). A history of self-revealed signs and instruction was largely related with positive status (p 0.05). (Ezra et al., 2020).

Weekly Covid Scenarios

Fig 3 chart says us that the amount of covid scenarios rises during the weekdays, which can be related with the efficacy of vacation a state of isolations.

Figure 3. Illustration of Weekly precious covid scenario

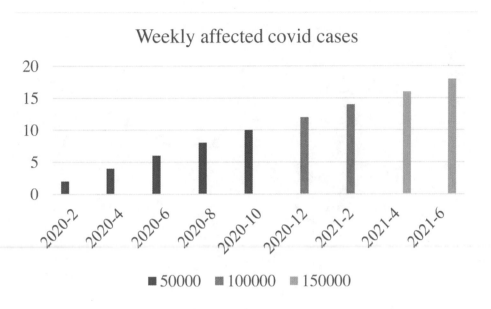

Monthly Covid Scenarios

- Real Scenarios in Blue line
- Red Line: Predicted Scenarios Mean Value
- The range of projected scenarios is shown in background,

The new covid instances are depicted in Fig 4 graph. As can be seen from the graph, the first wave peaked in 2020-09, and the second wave peaked in 2021-05, with the second wave being nearly four times stronger than the first. The number of infected people is depicted in Figure 4. The blue related gives the top and inferior limit of the predictable instances, the graph resonates with the actual scenarios and seems to break only when the scenarios reach their maximum, but it offers us an indication that fresh examples will emerge in the next calendar month, i.e. 2021-08.

Monthly Covid Deaths

- Real Deaths in Blueline
- Red Line: Predicted Deaths Mean Value
- The Range of Predicted Deaths is depicted in chart

Figure 4. Illustration of Monthly affected covid scenarios

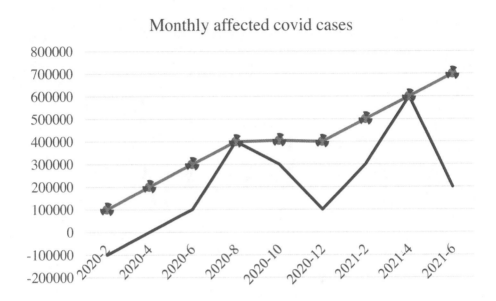

The new covid deaths are depicted in Fig 4 graph. As can be seen from the graph, the first wave peaked in 2020-09, while the second wave peaked in 2021-05, with the second wave being nearly four periods tougher than the primary. We too forecast original demises for the coming calendar month, i.e. 2021-28. The background indicates the limits of predictable demises. Graphs show scenarios climbed by four epochs, demises increased in the same proportion that the worst-hit dated lasted around one calendar month.

The calendar monthly trend original scenarios and deaths grew in the same ratio for both the first and second waves, as shown in Fig 5, and the worst-hit period lasted around one calendar month.

Fig 6 time series displays the Monthly New affected covid cases death in integer with Prophet model.

Fig 7 period sequence has a proportion of distortion, as can observe. We may re-sample it day by day and add the results to create a new sequence with less noise and thus make it easier to model. To address the problem of poor real effect or heavy workload of shale oil production forecast by conventional reservoir engineering, reservoir numerical simulation, and other methods, a new shale oil production forecast methodology based on the Prophet algorithm is provided. It's easier to find the inherent law from a small amount of data. The authors compare the results with long-term and short-term memory neural networks (LSTM) and the ARPS production decline model in this study, which uses data from production wells in

Figure 5. Diagram of scheduled new precious covid bags in number

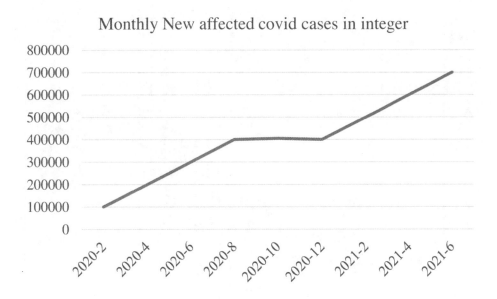

the Huanjiang, A reservoir in 2015. We updated the model day by day in fig 8 and combined the results to build a new series with less noise. The striking proliferation

Figure 6. Diagram of monthly original pretentious covid bags decease in number with prophet model

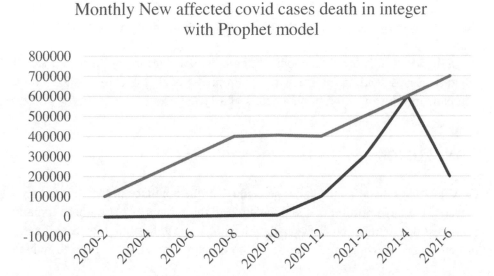

Figure 7. Illustration of monthly covid scenarios in number with prophet model with variations

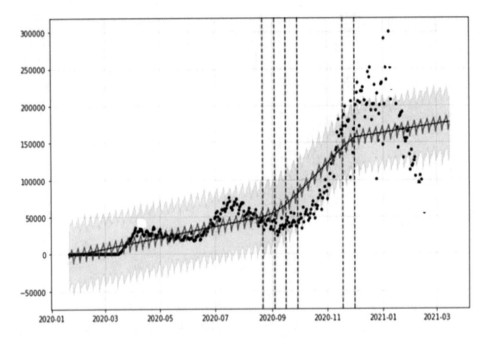

figure of 1.2 is gradually increasing after peaking in the first 15 days of March. It is estimated that for every well-known scenario in India, there could be 10–50 unknown instances using this method. There are a few assumptions in this model, as with any numerical model.

In fig 9, We displayed the model with a Monthly New affected covid scenarios death in integer with FB Prophet model by adjusting Fitness calendar monthly seasonality.

In fig 10, We displayed the model different models for forecast of New affected covid scenarios death in integer with FB Prophet model. Table 2 provided with a comparison value of different parameters of affected people.

CONCLUSION

COVID-19 has made a substantial percentage of the populace in India's provinces powerless. a large portion of the population in the provinces of southern India is powerless due to infection. To keep their health, we need to strengthen basic health principles and provide quick access to the immune reaction. we need to reduce

Figure 8. Drawing of monthly original affected covid bags death in number with FB prophet model

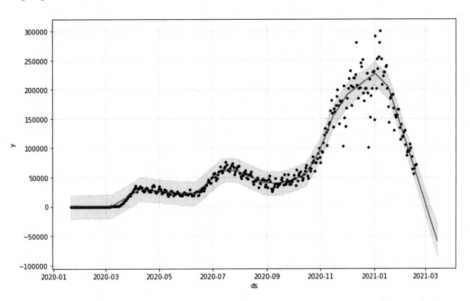

Figure 9. Drawing of monthly original affected covid bags death in number with FB prophet model by adjusting fitness calendar monthly seasonality

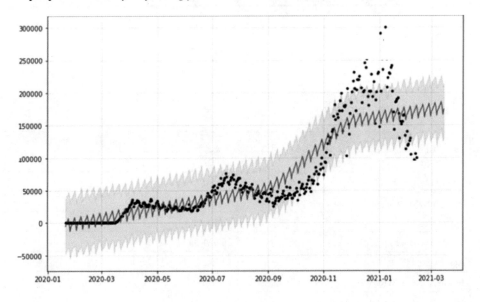

population density and provide proper housing. according to the study, public health officials, corporations and local communities should work together to improve ventilation and to limit urbanization to prevent future viral infections. air quality and lifestyle, working with appropriate govt, enterprise, and community health authorities, are key factors in preventing future viral infections.

Figure 10. Illustration of different models for forecast of original affected covid scenarios death in integer with FB prophet model

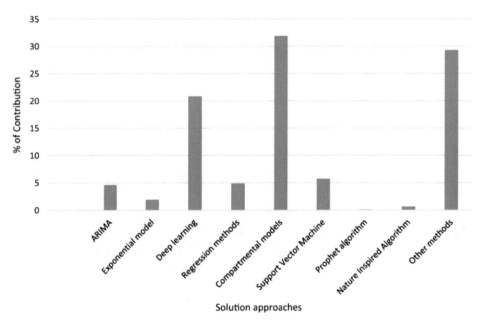

Table 2. Results summary

Parameters	Data values
Median Age	28.209
The whole quantity of people fully vaccinated	74854875
Persons vaccinated per hundred:	22.202
Population:	1.38001409
Total vaccinations per hundred:	26.624
Results from INDIA	12 June
People Vaccinated (dose)	306612781
Hospital beds available per thousand:	0.54

ACKNOWLEDGMENT

Neither a public, private, or non-profit funding source provided specific funding for this research.

REFERENCES

Darapaneni, N., Jain, P., Khattar, R., Chawla, M., Vaish, R., & Paduri, A. R. (2020, December). Analysis and Prediction of COVID-19 Pandemic in India. In *2020 2nd International Conference on Advances in Computing, Communication Control and Networking (ICACCCN)* (pp. 291-296). IEEE.

Tiwari, A. (2020). Modeling and analysis of COVID-19 epidemic in India. *Journal of Safety Science and Resilience*, *1*(2), 135–140. doi:10.1016/j.jnlssr.2020.11.005

Kumar, S. U., Kumar, D. T., Christopher, B. P., & Doss, C. (2020). The rise and impact of COVID-19 in India. *Frontiers in Medicine*, *7*, 250.

Inbaraj, L. R., George, C. E., & Chandrasingh, S. (2021). Seroprevalence of COVID-19 infection in a rural district of South India: A population-based seroepidemiological study. *PLoS One*, *16*(3), e0249247.

Tiwari, A. (2020). Modelling and analysis of COVID-19 epidemic in India. *Journal of Safety Science and Resilience*, *1*(2), 135–140. doi:10.1016/j.jnlssr.2020.11.005

Geetha, S., Nanda, P., Joshua Samuel Raj, R., & Prince, T. (2021). Early Recognition of Herb Sickness Using SVM. In *Intelligence in Big Data Technologies—Beyond the Hype* (pp. 543–550). Springer. doi:10.1007/978-981-15-5285-4_54

Geetha, S., Deepalakshmi, P., & Pande, S. (2019, December). Managing Crop for Indian Farming Using IOT. In *2019 IEEE International Conference on Clean Energy and Energy Efficient Electronics Circuit for Sustainable Development (INCCES)* (pp. 1-5). IEEE. 10.1109/INCCES47820.2019.9167699

Beulah, J. R., Cyril, C. P. D., Geetha, S., Irene, D. S., & Nadu, T. (2021). Towards Improved Detection of Intrusions with Constraint-Based Clustering (CBC). *International Journal of Computer Networks and Applications*, *8*(1), 28–43. doi:10.22247/ijcna/2021/207980

Rahimi, I., Chen, F., & Gandomi, A. H. (2021). A review on COVID-19 forecasting models. *Neural Computing & Applications*, 1–11. PMID:33564213

Wan, X., Zou, Y., Wang, J., & Wang, W. (2021, August). Prediction of shale oil production based on Prophet algorithm. *Journal of Physics: Conference Series, 2009*(1), 012056. doi:10.1088/1742-6596/2009/1/012056

Immorlica, N., Singla, S., & Waggoner, B. (2020, July). Prophet inequalities with linear correlations and augmentations. In *Proceedings of the 21st ACM Conference on Economics and Computation* (pp. 159-185). 10.1145/3391403.3399452

Choudhary, A. (2018). *Generate quick and accurate time series forecasts using Facebook's Prophet (with Python & R codes)*. Analytics Vidya.

Satrio, C. B. A., Darmawan, W., Nadia, B. U., & Hanafiah, N. (2021). Time series analysis and forecasting of coronavirus disease in Indonesia using ARIMA model and PROPHET. *Procedia Computer Science, 179*, 524–532.

Roosa, K., Lee, Y., Luo, R., Kirpich, A., Rothenberg, R., Hyman, J. M., ... Chowell, G. (2020). Real-time forecasts of the COVID-19 epidemic in China from February 5th to February 24th, 2020. *Infectious Disease Modelling, 5*, 256–263.

Maleki, M., & Arellano-Valle, R. B. (2017). Maximum a-posteriori estimation of autoregressive processes based on finite mixtures of scale-mixtures of skew-normal distributions. *Journal of Statistical Computation and Simulation, 87*(6), 1061–1083.

Eck, N. J. V., & Waltman, L. (2014). Visualizing bibliometric networks. In *Measuring scholarly impact* (pp. 285–320). Springer.

Anastassopoulou, C., Russo, L., Tsakris, A., & Siettos, C. (2020). Data-based analysis, modelling and forecasting of the COVID-19 outbreak. *PLoS One, 15*(3), e0230405.

Ji, D., Zhang, D., Xu, J., Chen, Z., Yang, T., Zhao, P., ... Qin, E. (2020). Prediction for progression risk in patients with COVID-19 pneumonia: The CALL score. *Clinical Infectious Diseases, 71*(6), 1393–1399.

Chaudhry, R. (2020). Coronavirus disease (2019) (COVID-19): Forecast of an emerging urgency in Pakistan. *Cureus, 12*(5).

Abolhassani, M., Ehsani, S., Esfandiari, H., Hajiaghayi, M., Kleinberg, R., & Lucier, B. (2017, June). Beating 1-1/e for ordered prophets. In *Proceedings of the 49th Annual ACM SIGACT Symposium on Theory of Computing* (pp. 61-71). ACM.

Agrawal, S., Ding, Y., Saberi, A., & Ye, Y. (2012). Price of correlations in stochastic optimization. *Operations Research, 60*(1), 150–162.

Alaei, S. (2014). Bayesian combinatorial auctions: Expanding single buyer mechanisms to many buyers. *SIAM Journal on Computing, 43*(2), 930–972.

Alaei, S., Hajiaghayi, M., & Liaghat, V. (2012, June). Online prophet-inequality matching with applications to ad allocation. In *Proceedings of the 13th ACM Conference on Electronic Commerce* (pp. 18-35). ACM.

Rubinstein, A., Wang, J. Z., & Weinberg, S. M. (2019). *Optimal single-choice prophet inequalities from samples.* arXiv preprint arXiv:1911.07945.

Azar, Y., Chiplunkar, A., & Kaplan, H. (2018, June). Prophet secretary: Surpassing the 1-1/e barrier. In *Proceedings of the 2018 ACM Conference on Economics and Computation* (pp. 303-318). ACM.

Babaioff, M., Immorlica, N., Lucier, B., & Weinberg, S. M. (2020). A simple and approximately optimal mechanism for an additive buyer. *Journal of the Association for Computing Machinery, 67*(4), 1–40.

Bateni, M., Dehghani, S., Hajiaghayi, M., & Seddighin, S. (2015). Revenue maximization for selling multiple correlated items. In *Algorithms-ESA 2015* (pp. 95–105). Springer.

Bradac, D., Gupta, A., Singla, S., & Zuzic, G. (2019). *Robust algorithms for the secretary problem.* arXiv preprint arXiv:1911.07352.

Charikar, M., Steinhardt, J., & Valiant, G. (2017, June). Learning from untrusted data. In *Proceedings of the 49th Annual ACM SIGACT Symposium on Theory of Computing* (pp. 47-60). ACM.

Chawla, S., Hartline, J. D., Malec, D. L., & Sivan, B. (2010, June). Multi-parameter mechanism design and sequential posted pricing. In *Proceedings of the forty-second ACM symposium on Theory of computing* (pp. 311-320). ACM.

Chawla, S., Malec, D., & Sivan, B. (2015). The power of randomness in bayesian optimal mechanism design. *Games and Economic Behavior, 91*, 297–317.

Correa, J., Foncea, P., Hoeksma, R., Oosterwijk, T., & Vredeveld, T. (2017, June). Posted price mechanisms for a random stream of customers. In *Proceedings of the 2017 ACM Conference on Economics and Computation* (pp. 169-186). ACM.

Ezra, T., Feldman, M., Gravin, N., & Tang, Z. G. (2020, July). Online stochastic max-weight matching: Prophet inequality for vertex and edge arrival models. In *Proceedings of the 21st ACM Conference on Economics and Computation* (pp. 769-787). ACM.

Correa, J., Saona, R., & Ziliotto, B. (2021). Prophet secretary through blind strategies. *Mathematical Programming, 190*(1), 483–521.

Diakonikolas, I. (2018). *Algorithmic high-dimensional robust statistics*. http://www. iliasdiakonikolas. org/simons-tutorial-robust. html

Diakonikolas, I., Kamath, G., Kane, D., Li, J., Moitra, A., & Stewart, A. (2019). Robust estimators in high-dimensions without the computational intractability. *SIAM Journal on Computing*, *48*(2), 742–864.

Diakonikolas, I., Kamath, G., Kane, D. M., Li, J., Moitra, A., & Stewart, A. (2018). Robustly learning a gaussian: Getting optimal error, efficiently. In *Proceedings of the Twenty-Ninth Annual ACM-SIAM Symposium on Discrete Algorithms* (pp. 2683-2702). Society for Industrial and Applied Mathematics.

Dutting, P., Feldman, M., Kesselheim, T., & Lucier, B. (2020). Prophet inequalities made easy: Stochastic optimization by pricing nonstochastic inputs. *SIAM Journal on Computing*, *49*(3), 540–582.

Dütting, P., & Kesselheim, T. (2019, June). Posted pricing and prophet inequalities with inaccurate priors. In *Proceedings of the 2019 ACM Conference on Economics and Computation* (pp. 111-129). ACM.

Ehsani, S., Hajiaghayi, M., Kesselheim, T., & Singla, S. (2018). Prophet secretary for combinatorial auctions and matroids. In *Proceedings of the twenty-ninth annual acm-siam symposium on discrete algorithms* (pp. 700-714). Society for Industrial and Applied Mathematics.

Ezra, T., Feldman, M., & Nehama, I. (2018). *Prophets and secretaries with overbooking*. arXiv preprint arXiv:1805.05094.

Esfandiari, H., Korula, N., & Mirrokni, V. (2018). Allocation with traffic spikes: Mixing adversarial and stochastic models. *ACM Transactions on Economics and Computation*, *6*(3-4), 1–23.

Feldman, M., Gravin, N., & Lucier, B. (2014, December). Combinatorial auctions via posted prices. In *Proceedings of the twenty-sixth annual ACM-SIAM symposium on Discrete algorithms* (pp. 123-135). Society for Industrial and Applied Mathematics.

Feldman, M., Svensson, O., & Zenklusen, R. (2016). Online contention resolution schemes. In *Proceedings of the twenty-seventh annual ACM-SIAM symposium on Discrete algorithms* (pp. 1014-1033). Society for Industrial and Applied Mathematics.

Ezra, T., Feldman, M., Gravin, N., & Tang, Z. G. (2020, July). Online stochastic max-weight matching: Prophet inequality for vertex and edge arrival models. In *Proceedings of the 21st ACM Conference on Economics and Computation* (pp. 769-787). ACM.

Chapter 5

Role of Explainable Artificial Intelligence (XAI) in Prediction of Non-Communicable Diseases (NCDs)

Jana Shafi

ⓘ https://orcid.org/0000-0001-6859-670X

Prince Sattam bin Abdul Aziz University, Saudi Arabia

Selvani Deepthi Kavila

ⓘ https://orcid.org/0000-0001-5307-3113

Anil Neerukonda Institute of Technology and Sciences, India

Shamayita Basu

University of Kalyani, India

ABSTRACT

Explainable artificial intelligence (XAI) concentrated on methods and models that simplify the comprehending and analysis of the ML models operation. Using XAI, systems deliver the essential facts to defend outcomes, mostly when unpredicted conclusions are made. It also certifies that there is an auditable and demonstrable way to guard algorithmic judgments including the factors of unbiased and being principled, which lead to building trust. Swift upsurge of non-communicable diseases (NCDs) turns out to be one of the severe health matters and one of the leading origins of death globally. In this chapter, the authors discussed XAI in healthcare, its benefits, and the deep Shapley additive explanations (DeepSHAP)-based deep neural network (DeepNN) framework provided with a feature selection method for prediction and explanation of non-communicable diseases followed by case study discussion about detection and progression of Alzheimer's disease (AD) with the help of XAI-based predictive models.

DOI: 10.4018/978-1-6684-3791-9.ch005

Figure 1. XAI vs. AI

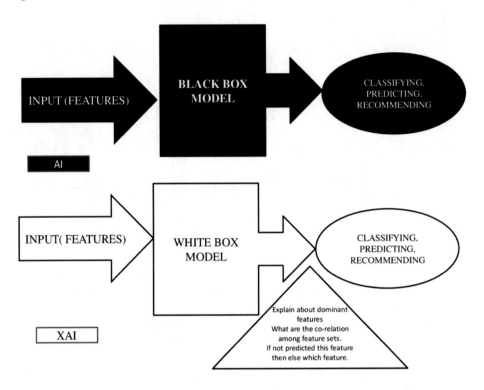

INTRODUCTION

Today Explainable Artificial Intelligence (XAI) is an evolving topic in Artificial Intelligence (AI). It encompasses a group of procedures and methods that permit humans to understand and believe in the output get by algorithms machine learning (ML). XAI can be used to define a model of AI, its estimated influence, and potential prejudices. It supports precision of characterizing model, equality, transparency, and results in AI-based decision making (Gunning & Aha, 2019). With advanced Artificial Intelligence, users are faced with knowing and tracking how the algorithm gets output, which leaves behind engineers and data scientists who are the owners of the algorithm can only comprehend or describe what exactly is processing in AI algorithm that reached exact output. As explanation is vital for precarious applications, for example, security, wellbeing, commandment, mandate, etc., it is essential to trust and have a clear viewpoint (Gohel.P.et.al, 2017).

This added function of "able to explain" modernizes AI research and is acknowledged as Explainable AI (XAI). Figure 1 illustrates how XAI can add to AI by replying to the "wh" queries absent in the old model of AI. Therefore, XAI has been a subject of great interest from grave applications such as healthcare, security, law and order, and many others where the answers were explained (i.e., responses to "wh" queries), which is equally important to get answers. This XAI research has become a top priority (Gohel.P.et.al, 2017).

Significance: Explainable AI

XAI is helpful to comprehend and describe machine learning algorithms (ML), deep learning also neural networks. ML models are assumed as black-boxes that are difficult to understand. Neural networks (NN) in deep learning models face comprehension difficulties for a human. In addition, the Artificial Intelligence model performance can drift or worsen due to the difference between production data and training data (Adadi & Berrada, 2018), thus making it critical for a corporate/ commercial business to always observe and take care of its models to encourage AI explainability meanwhile computing the commerce effect of applying similar algorithms. XAI supports encouraging client expectation, it's model associability as well productive AI use. It also diminishes agreement, authorization, safety, and reputational threats of AI production. It is essential for executing responsible AI. A process for the comprehensive execution in AI means in existent establishments with impartiality, model explainability, and taking responsibility. AI to get help being responsible requires establishments to set in ethical values into requests and methods by constructing AI systems founded on faith and transparency.

XAI Benefits

- **Dropping Rate of Errors:** Decision-based, highly sensitive areas, for example, Healthcare, Business, Authorised, etc., are the ones who got extremely affected by the result of incorrect forecasts. Oversight over the outcomes decreases the effect of incorrect results as well as recognizing the origin cause leading to refining the fundamental model.
- **Diminishing Model Influence being partial:** Models of AI have exposed major signs of unfairness. Instances include gender Partiality for Apple Cards, Racial Prejudice by Autonomous Vehicles, Gender, and by Amazon Rekognition. Understandable coordination can cut the impact of such partial guesses rooting by clarifying decision-making conditions.
- **Control and Liability:** Models of AI constantly have any amount of error with their estimates, and permitting an individual to be in control and liable for those mistakes can make the overall system more well-organized
- **Program of Self-confidence:** Each implication, with its description, inclines to escalate the system's confidence. More or less user serious system

structures, for example, Autonomous automobiles, Medicinal Analysis, the Investment sector, etc., weights great Program of Self-confidence from the user for ideal operation.

- **Code Agreement:** Growing burden from the governing organizations means that corporations have to become accustomed and use XAI to fulfill with the ruling classes hastily (Birlasoft. (n.d.)).

EXPLAINABLE AI IN HEALTHCARE

Smart Health lifted the entire healthcare industry together with the shared wearable devices and Internet of Things (IoT) (Awotunde et al., 2021). Various studies have shown the prediction of diseases can help in acting as first aid, such as Cervical cancer detection (Ijaz, Attique and Son, 2020), Hypertension, Diabetes (Ijaz, Alfian, Syafrudin and Rhee, 2018), and segmentation of liver (Naga Srinivasu et al., 2021). The Health of human beings is of vital importance in the world. AI techniques have been implemented to predict medical-related outcomes and enhance data tools of healthcare due to the flooded amount of data-driven from electronic health records of patients (Davagdorj et al., 2021). Machine learning (ML) is a subgroup of AI that studies data without describing precedence. Old-fashioned machine learning very much hangs on difficult feature engineering work.

Conversely, these methods cannot identify composite forms of Electronic Health data Records with great aspects, thereby producing less performance. Deep learning (DL) approaches let machines automatically learn the complex connections of the features and drive relevant information from data records. In addition, lately, innovative Deep learning models, for instance, transformers also auto-encoders, have proved potential for expressing complex clinical data records of several methods. These models have pointedly upgraded downstream jobs, for instance, looking for related patients, expecting onset disease, and profound appearance. As DL algorithms integrate high-level relations among input patterns with various neurons via a multi-layer nonlinear structure, they are characteristically considered as black-box models. To explain, justify, and believe the DL model prediction for highly risked medicinal uses, health experts have to comprehend the way model comes up with a prediction output. These explanations are essential to make sure equality and responsibility in the process of making the medical decision as a solo mistaken estimate output from the model may lead to severe medical blunders. In recent times, The European Union's General Data Protection Regulation (GDPR) endorsed involve establishments use clinical patient data records for categorizations also references to deliver explanations on-call.

Adequate AI models explanations permit medicinal specialists to recognize and faith these AI-based medical decision support systems. Therefore, the study on XAI in healthcare is growing. The utmost current AI architecture is set by Deep Learning (DL), which includes a neural network (NN) which are hundreds of "neuron" layers or fundamental processing units, is used. The DL architectures complication marks as "black boxes", so it is almost difficult to find the precise method for which the system gives exact responses. Artificial intelligence applications in the medical field are quickly rising. But the contribution of deep learning constructions turns the attention on the processes of responsibility. Known for the extensive DL solutions usage, this issue will become gradually sensed in outlook. It must be highlighted that in healthcare, the liability, or in charge, of the expert is of main significance: any medicinal verdict must be essential to be defensible a posteriori, perhaps via objective proof.

The similar must be correct when the output of AI processing type adds to the medical decision, for which the "black box" architectures are barely companionable with the healthcare area. Moreover meanwhile, all software-based applications are required to be qualified. The criticality of this technique is assumed in the aspect of an unexplained algorithm. Clinicians are glad to practice neural networks in the utmost difficult or stimulating diagnoses, but they require understanding in what way they come to their assumptions to confirm the description. XAI systems can clarify the decision's logic, describe the strengths and faults of decision making, and be responsible for understandings their upcoming actions ("The big causes of death from non-communicable disease," 2016).

XAI IN NON-COMMUNICABLE DISEASES

A non-communicable disease (NCD) exists as a sickness nontransmissible from one to another being. These contain autoimmune illnesses, Parkinson's, strokes, mostly all heart illnesses, cancers, diabetes, chronic kidney disease, osteoarthritis, osteoporosis, Alzheimer's disease, cataracts, and many more (Administrator, 2017). NCD is a worldwide concern facing the human race. As per the NCDs international grade article by the agency World Health Organization (WHO), the primary origin of demises responsible around forty million people each year, which equals seventy percent of the fifty-seven million demises worldwide ("Noncommunicable diseases country profiles 2018," n.d.). In actuality, NCDs are the prominent root of fifteen million early demises that happened among adults of thirty and seventy ages per annum.

The NCDs' highest ranges belong to cardiovascular ailments, kind of diabetes mellitus, all types of cancers, and chronic breathing ailments. Unusually, heart-related cardiovascular disease (CVD) is presumed foremost with a maximum sum around eighteen million, tailed by cancers diseases of nine million, breathing diseases of around four million, and followed by diabetes holds around one and half million people for expiries owing to NCDs yearly Lancet (London, England). NCDs are determined by services of regulating and non- regulating risk features. It is well known that regulating risk features consist of dreadful tobacco, alcohol usage, various eco-friendly f, harmful intakes, and physical idleness, all leading to stoutness, hypertension, and elevated lipid. Opposite to this, non- regulating risks involve age, gender, and heredities ("Noncommunicable diseases progress monitor 2017," 2017) (Kathirvel & Thakur Rapporteurs, 2018). By chance, around eighty percent of heart-related diseases, diabetes, stroke, and about forty percent of type cancers can be stopped if the chief threat causes were removed (Chen et al., 2018), ("Action plan for the prevention and control of NCDs in the WHO European region 2016–2025," 2017).

Maximum NCDs are every so often detected at a late phase. If NCDs can be anticipated formerly when it takes place, Particular medical engagements can be in use by persons and thus decreasing harm of suffering patients. Henceforward, it requires a decision support system to be established, aiding the NCDs progress for identifying high in danger patients and reducing the bereavement ratio. In recent times, the practice of AI in healthcare has been swiftly growing.

Although, reactions in decision-making bear from several hitches. On the way to coping with these difficulties, progressive focused dataset and ML methods are recurrently established in the latest studies (Davagdorj et al., 2019)- (Davagdorj et al., 2020). Moreover, several systems cannot switch high aspect datasets and choose major patterns to calculate a broad load due to the absence of a smart model (Davagdorj et al., 2021)– ("Noncommunicable diseases country profiles 2018," n.d.). In a research ("Noncommunicable diseases country profiles 2018," n.d.), a smart medical-care controlling system used for heart ailment forecast collective deep learning with feature fusion was suggested.

Next, inappropriate, repeated attributes removed are based on its features data achievement method. The provisional approach of probability computing an exact feature weight for each class promotes the outcomes of the system. Lastly, the deep joint learning (DL) model was skilled for the forecast of a heart ailment; it also gained higher correctness than other related approaches. Consequently, the greatest of the current works are well-thought-of the correctness plus false-positive rate for measuring the outcomes of classification procedures. The lack of other outcomes actions, such as time of model building, precision, and rate of misclassification, must be considered key constraints in classifier performance assessment (Panigrahi et al., 2021).

Furthermore, time-series information investigation is vital for health trade supervision of prolonged diseases to health specialists who could examine the heart patient's records while creating advanced analysis. In a research (El-Sappagh et al., 2021), writers used a group of economic types of time-series comprising its patient's past treatment records, as well demographics to forecast Alzheimer's disease(AD) progress using ML models of support vector machine (SVM), k-nearest neighbor (KNN), RF, logistic regression (LR), and decision tree methods. In their consequences, the initial union of concurrent diseases and medicine features, along with others, exposed substantial analytical control with all ML models. The ML-based RF model had gotten the finest analytical outcome.

Similarly, difficult AI models, for instance, DL and co-operative methods, add higher presentation for improving the analysis and cure of many chronic syndromes (Davagdorj et al., 2020), (Davagdorj et al., 2020). In broad, correct estimation presentation and explaining are dual main standards of the greatest verdict support structure (Carvalho et al., 2019). Correct prediction and its presentation in the course of testing can fix up trust marks in the DL model. Regardless of their accurate estimate, a mutual problem of this recent research is connected to their black-box prototype. Therefore, the users have no clue about methods used in predictions, as well it is difficult to imply them in practical applications of healthcare.

Usually, healthcare physicians/experts don't support black box-based models outcomes (Carvalho et al., 2019) – (Elshawi et al., 2019). Meanwhile, choosing an appropriate feature set is critical to eliminate repeated feature set that adds various aids. In uses of healthcare, a group of major model feature selections is a crucial process. Numerical research anticipated feature selection procedures, such as data information gain, correlation coefficients, and gain ratio. Still, there are no interactions between the features in these methods, leading to not being fit for using them straight to healthcare applications (Davagdorj et al., 2020).

PREDICTION: NON-COMMUNICABLE DISEASES (NCDs)

In the machine learning and data science field, the difficult step is to select features for data pre-processing. So tri-stage filter-based is one of the frameworks for disease detection (Mandal et al., 2021). For classification, direct input of raw data at times, learning algorithms do not execute well (Mandal et al., 2021). The deep neural network (DNN) technique is AI motivated by the function of the human brain structure. NN, a neural network, is a set of interrelated neurons that train collectively to accomplish a certain task. DeepSHAP based on a DNN is introduced, which provided a dataset feature selection method to form an exact decision provision system that can be explainable to solve the earlier discussed issues.

In this research, the used dataset belongs to the National Health and Nutrition Examination Survey (NHANES) to form NCDs' analytical and understandable decision care model. For building the correct and understandable NCDs structure, this model is driven through Deep Shapley Additive Explanations (DeepSHAP) (Chen et al., 2020, for varied types of models, which have a structure for layer-wise circulation of SHAP (Lundberg et al., 2017) standards that form based on DL significant features (DeepLIFT) (Shrikumar et al.,2019). SHAP is a combined structure built on the value of Shapley. It describes example x assessing the role of every set feature in the model prediction.

The planned structure includes three modules. In the initial module, descriptive features are prepared for cleaning dataset and elastic net (EN), an inserted feature selection method. The next module is trained when the DNN classifier is tuned using the hyper-parameters with the selected feature subclass. In the final module, dual types of model descriptions are delivered by the approach DeepSHAP: First, it explains the related risk in the view based on population that affects the model's prediction. Second, it aims to explain from a human point of a particular instance (Davagdorj et al., 2021). In this approach, the complete procedure of demonstrating, selecting features, training, hyperparameter tuning, model assessment, along explanations took into account.

Three diverse groups of major features are produced from the derive dataset for building NCDs decision support models. The produced features set is designated by support vector regression-based recursive feature removal (SVR-RFE), consecutive backward feature selection set with random forest (SBFS-RF), and suggested EN-based feature set selection methods. To discover the combination of the ideal features in every subgroup, features are reserved when they make the most of the ML model outcome. Later, these subsets feature the training of all types of ML classifiers. This also advises that ML algorithms used in this model can be interchangeable based on the required domain.

In the meantime, ML classifiers are adjusted with their reliable hyper-parameters to advance the model performance prediction avoiding the over-fitting problem at the same time. A contrast of investigational consequences is performed among the DNN and modern standard models in authentication and test datasets. Various measures such as accuracy, specificity, recall, precision, f-scores, and area under the curve (AUC) are used (Davagdorj et al., 2021).

The DeepSHAP structure provided an EN feature set selection method to create a precise and understandable decision-based support AI structure illustrated in FIGURE 2. This structure integrates three modules: dataset pre-processing using feature set collection, estimated model construction, and comparison.

Figure 2. Prediction model for NCDs

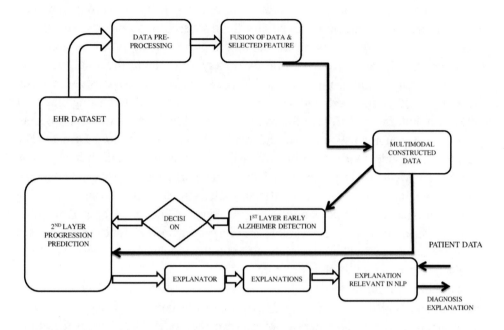

Case Study: XAI Based Framework for Alzheimer's Disease

Mental-based Alzheimer's disease (AD) comes under the category of NCD. This irremediable syndrome is regarded as an unusual build-up of amyloid plaques and neurofibrillary knots in the function of the human brain, causing its progressive memory deterioration, intellectual and linguistic abilities, with behavioral alterations. Its analysis and development of uncovering disease have been rigorously researched. However, investigated studies regularly have a slight outcome on scientific exercise mostly due to the subsequent explanations:

1. maximum work subject to generally on a single mode, particularly in neuroimaging;
2. detection of analysis and its progression mostly studied distinctly as individual complications;
3. prevailing work focus mostly on improving the detection ML performance of its multifaceted algorithms and models, despite the fact ignoring their need of explainability.

Medical doctors tussle to understand these models since it is tough to believe them. According to new research, (El-Sappagh et al., 2021) build a precise and expressible

Alzheimer's disease analysis and progression model for detection. This approach provides medical practitioners with exact true verdicts, including a group of related justifications for each judgment. Explicitly, this discussed model incorporates eleven modalities of around a thousand for hundred topics from the AD, Neuroimaging Initiative (ADNI) dataset from real-life: two ninety-four analytically usual, two fifty-four steady mild cognitive impairment (MCI), two thirty-two progressive MCI, and two sixty-eight Alzheimer's Disease. It is a model of a two-layer using classifier of ML random forest (RF) (*see* figure 3). The initial level in the model brings out a multiclass grouping used in the initial identification of Alzheimer's Disease. The next uses the model to identify binary classing to perceive probable mild cognitive impairment MCI-to-AD evolution in 3 years since the analysis started. The model performance is improved with significant indicators carefully chosen from a big group from areas of biological and clinical procedures. Concerning the explainability component, this model makes available, for every layer, universal and example-based justifications of the Random Forest classifier via the Shapley Additive ex Plantations (SHAP) feature set attribution structure.

Furthermore, the model is implemented with twenty-two interpreters centered on models of decision trees also fuzzy rule systems to offer complimentary explanations for each Random Forest judgment in every layer of the model. Also, these justifications are signified in AI-based natural language procedures to aid medical doctors in comprehending the estimates. They discussed AI model attains cross-validation correctness of around 93.9% with an F1score of 93.9% in the model's initial layer. In contrast, the situation attains cross-validation correctness with 87.0% and around 87.09% F1-Score in the second layer of the model. The subsequent structure is correct, honest, responsible, and pathologically appropriate, appreciations to the delivered reasons and justifications that are most reliable and Alzheimer's Disease (AD) medical research. The discussed system (El-Sappagh et al., 2021) can improve the medical insights of Alzheimer's Disease(AD) analysis and progression courses by offering thorough understandings of different modalities on the syndrome threat.

Figure 3 displays a complete explanation of the XAI structure. The first phase is pre-processing to arrange and advance the quality of the used dataset. This includes the resulting next four sub-procedures.

- *Multimodal fusion:* The Alzheimer's Disease (AD) setting is multimodal in reality, in which numerous feature groups are united. This is known as multimodal fusion, in which each module has supplemental material to sustain the ending result. In this framework, dual approaches are used, namely late fusion then early fusion (El-Sappagh et al., 2021).

Figure 3. XAI based predictive model for Alzheimer disease

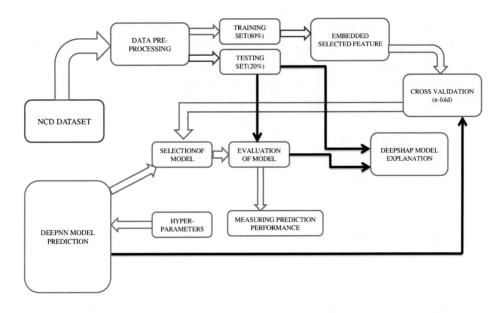

- *Data standardization:* Subsequently splitting data, sharing data records that may have changed the scale order. These derived raw dataset records are not used straight to train under the Random Forest model. To guarantee each feature set of equal significance, dataset records remained consistent with the z-score method (El-Sappagh et al., 2021).
- *Handling absent values:* For taking care of absent values, around 30% of missing values in this data the related feature is removed. Then, the algorithm k-nearest neighbors assign absent values, which are then switched using data from neighbors of similar classes.

We used wrapper means to select automatic, programmed features, attained subgroups of features set, and provided superior model performance than other filter techniques. The most frequent classifiers used in the wrapper are naïve Bayes81, SVM (Maldonado et al., 2014), RF (Rodin et al., 2009), and AdaBoost (Panthong & Srivihok, 2015).

SHAPLEY VALUES

Shapley values are an example of particular perturbation-based methods requiring no hyperparameters, except the baseline. This group comprises techniques that estimate the contribution of input features set by eliminating or changing them, followed by measuring the deviation of the network objective output as the importance of this action (Ribeiro et al., 2016; Zintgraf et al., 2017; Fong & Vedaldi, 2017).

Study a set of N performers P, a function ˆf used to map every subset $S \subseteq P$ to real numbers, modeling the outcome of a game when performers in S join in it. The value is one method to count the total support of every performer to the result as ˆf(P) of the said game when all actors join. For certain actor i, it can be figured as below:

$$R_i = \sum_{S \subseteq P/\{i\}} \frac{|S|!(|P| - |S| - 1)!}{|P|!} [\hat{f}(S \cup \{i\}) - \hat{f}(S)] \tag{1}$$

This value for the actor i defined overhead can be interpreted as the average marginal contribution of performer i to all potential unions S that can be shaped deprived of it.

It has been detected (Lundberg & Lee, 2017) that attributions of Shapley value better agree with the human perception empirically.

In place of definite simple functions f, now it's possible to figure Shapley values accurately in polynomial time. Such as, the inputs values to a max-pooling layer can be figured with $O(N^2)$ function estimates (Lundberg & Lee, 2017). Otherwise, Shapley values sampling (Castro et al., 2009) can be used to estimate approximate its values based on a sampling of Eq. 1. In particular, (Fatima et al., 2008) recommended a polynomial-time estimate for weighted elective games (Osborne & Rubinstein, 1994) constructed on the idea that, as a substitute for counting all combinations, it might be sufficient to guess their predictable aids.

EXPERIMENTAL DESIGN:NON-COMMUNICABLE DISEASES

Experimental background

All tests for the NCD dataset were done on a Personal Computer, with processor Intel Core i5-6600K, and memory 32GB RAM using the operating system Microsoft Windows 10. Python is the programming language used for further coding and analysis.

Dataset

Dataset used were attained from ADNI (https://adni.loni.usc.edu/). The Alzheimer's disease Neuroimaging Initiative Data and Publications Committee (ADNI DPC) take care of patient registration and checks usual exercise on the usage and sharing of the data. The ADNI data were formerly collected through fifty search websites.

Algorithms Classification and its Parameters

Here, models have been compared to the resulting various ML classification-based algorithms for the expectation of NCDs.

- Support Vector Machine (SVM): It is an ML classifier of the supervised ML model for explaining classification and regression problems.
- K-nearest neighbors (KNN): KNN is an ML algorithm able to solve the classification job such as instances classified to the class most often happening between its neighbors calculated by the distance function.
- Random Forest (RF): RF is an ML model to parallel organized ensemble tree-based method that develops bagging to combine multiple ML decision tree classifiers.

Evaluation Metrics

Assessing the NCDs expected model, evaluation ML metrics are determined with values, as follows. The ML evaluation metrics can be defined as:

$$\text{Accuracy} = TP + TN \ /TP + FP + FN + TN \ (4)$$
$$\text{Specificity} = TN \ /TN + FP \ (5)$$
$$\text{Recall} = TP \ /TP + FN \ (6)$$
$$\text{Precision} = TP \ /TP + FP \ (7)$$
$$F - \text{score} = 2 \ \text{Precision.recall/precision} + \text{recall} \ (8)$$

EXPERIMENTAL RESULT AND ANALYSIS

Feature Selection Analysis

Features are extracted by the FreeSurfer tool followed by Data cleaning and transformation, Data fusion, and selection later fusing the raw dataset modalities, for every layer, the complete dataset is stratified and then casually alienated into a model growth feature set name [S1] (90%) and testing feature set name [S2] (10%) that is employed to assess and match the simplification and explain the ability of prototypes.

Table 1. ML models evaluation scale

Model	Accuracy	Specificity	Recall	Precision	F – score
KNN	0.86	0.92	0.82	0.81	0.80
Random Forest	**0.89**	0.86	**0.90**	**0.87**	**0.90**
SVM	0.70	0.68	0.73	0.80	0.76

COMPARISON RESULTS OF PREDICTION MODELS

It is well familiar that the subset data feature selected by Random Forest can enhance the expected performance considerably in most ML classifiers KNN showed the second-highest score.

SVM is quite time-consuming when we used the optimal polynomial kernel function. Even though Random Forest accomplished the fastest compared with others, it worked our purpose.

CONCLUSION

Models of AI resulted in an absence of trust and responsibility. Explainable AI (XAI) is an area in which technologically advanced methods to clarify predictions made by AI-based systems and benefit the healthcare industry. Today in healthcare, non-communicable illness leads to untimely death and turns into a major risk to communal health worldwide. It is required to expose a smarter model to support the timely identification of NCDs in the medicinal field. Here we discussed the XAI-centred DeepSHAP based DNN structure provided with an EN feature selection for prompt prediction of NCDs and discussed briefly a very precise and understandable ML model built on an RF classifier for Alzheimer detection and development estimates.

REFERENCES

Gohel, P., Singh, P., & Mohanty, M. (2017). *Explainable AI: Current status and future directions*. IEEE Access Preprint.

Gunning, D., & Aha, D. (2019). DARPA's Explainable Artificial Intelligence (XAI) Program. *AI Magazine, 40*(2), 44–58. doi:10.1609/aimag.v40i2.2850

Adadi, A., & Berrada, M. (2018). undefined. *IEEE Access: Practical Innovations, Open Solutions, 6*, 52138–52160. doi:10.1109/ACCESS.2018.2870052

Birlasoft. (n.d.). *Demystifying explainable artificial intelligence: Benefits, use cases, and Models*. Retrieved October 23, 2021, from https://www.birlasoft.com/articles/demystifying-explainable-artificial-intelligence

Davagdorj, K., Bae, J., Pham, V., Theera-Umpon, N., & Ryu, K. (2021). Explainable Artificial Intelligence Based Framework for Non-Communicable Diseases Prediction. *IEEE Access: Practical Innovations, Open Solutions, 9*, 123672–123688. doi:10.1109/ACCESS.2021.3110336

The big causes of death from noncommunicable diseases. (2016). Bulletin of the World Health Organization. doi:10.2471/BLT.16.030616

Noncommunicable diseases country profiles 2018. (n.d.). https://apps.who.int/iris/handle/10665/274512

GBD 2015 Risk F Collaborators. (2016). Global, regional, and national comparative risk assessment of 79 behavioural, environmental and occupational, and metabolic risks or clusters of risks, 1990-2015: a systematic analysis for the Global Burden of Disease Study 2015. *Lancet, 388*(10053), 1659–1724. . doi:10.1016/S0140-6736(16)31679-8

Noncommunicable diseases progress monitor 2017. (2017, September 1). *World Health Organization*. https://www.who.int/publications/i/item/9789241513029

Kathirvel, S., & Thakur Rapporteurs, J. (2018). Sustainable development goals and non-communicable diseases: Roadmap till 2030 – A plenary session of world noncommunicable diseases Congress 2017. *International Journal of Noncommunicable Diseases, 3*(1), 3. doi:10.4103/jncd.jncd_1_18

Chen, S., Kuhn, M., Prettner, K., & Bloom, D. E. (2018). The macroeconomic burden of noncommunicable diseases in the United States: Estimates and projections. *PLoS One, 13*(11), e0206702. doi:10.1371/journal.pone.0206702 PMID:30383802

Action plan for the prevention and control of noncommunicable diseases in the WHO European region 2016–2025. (2017, August 15). https://www.euro.who.int/en/health-topics/noncommunicable-diseases/pages/policy/publications/action-plan-for-the-prevention-and-control-of-noncommunicable-diseases-in-the-who-european-region-20162025

Davagdorj, K., Yu, S. H., Kim, S. Y., Huy, P. V., Park, J. H., & Ryu, K. H. (2019). Prediction of 6 months smoking cessation program among women in Korea. *International Journal of Machine Learning and Computing, 9*(1), 83–90. doi:10.18178/ijmlc.2019.9.1.769

Ali, F., El-Sappagh, S., Islam, S. R., Kwak, D., Ali, A., Imran, M., & Kwak, K. (2020). A smart healthcare monitoring system for heart disease prediction based on ensemble deep learning and feature fusion. *Information Fusion*, *63*, 208–222. doi:10.1016/j.inffus.2020.06.008

Panigrahi, R., Borah, S., Bhoi, A. K., Ijaz, M. F., Pramanik, M., Jhaveri, R. H., & Chowdhary, C. L. (2021). Performance assessment of supervised classifiers for designing intrusion detection systems: A comprehensive review and recommendations for future research. *Mathematics*, *9*(6), 690. doi:10.3390/math9060690

El-Sappagh, S., Saleh, H., Sahal, R., Abuhmed, T., Islam, S. R., Ali, F., & Amer, E. (2021). Alzheimer's disease progression detection model based on an early fusion of cost-effective multimodal data. *Future Generation Computer Systems*, *115*, 680–699. doi:10.1016/j.future.2020.10.005

Davagdorj, K., Pham, V. H., Theera-Umpon, N., & Ryu, K. H. (2020). Xgboost-based framework for smoking-induced noncommunicable disease prediction. *International Journal of Environmental Research and Public Health*, *17*(18), 6513. doi:10.3390/ijerph17186513 PMID:32906777

Davagdorj, K., Lee, J. S., Park, K. H., Huy, P. V., & Ryu, K. H. (2020). Synthetic oversampling based decision support framework to solve class imbalance problem in smoking cessation program. *International Journal of Applied Science and Engineering*, *17*, 223–235. doi:10.6703/IJASE.202009_17(3).223

Carvalho, D. V., Pereira, E. M., & Cardoso, J. S. (2019). Machine learning Interpretability: A survey on methods and metrics. *Electronics (Basel)*, *8*(8), 832. doi:10.3390/electronics8080832

Lauritsen, S. M., Kristensen, M., Olsen, M. V., Larsen, M. S., Lauritsen, K. M., Jørgensen, M. J., Lange, J., & Thiesson, B. (2020). undefined. *Nature Communications*, *11*(1). Advance online publication. doi:10.103841467-020-17431-x PMID:32737308

Elshawi, R., Al-Mallah, M. H., & Sakr, S. (2019). On the interpretability of machine learning-based model for predicting hypertension. *BMC Medical Informatics and Decision Making*, *19*(1), 146. Advance online publication. doi:10.118612911-019-0874-0 PMID:31357998

Davagdorj, K., Lee, J. S., Pham, V. H., & Ryu, K. H. (2020). A comparative analysis of machine learning methods for class imbalance in a smoking cessation intervention. *Applied Sciences (Basel, Switzerland)*, *10*(9), 3307. doi:10.3390/app10093307

Chen, H., Lundberg, S., & Lee, S. (2020). Explaining models by propagating Shapley values of local components. *Explainable AI in Healthcare and Medicine*, 261-270. doi:10.1007/978-3-030-53352-6_24

Lundberg, S. M., & Lee, S. I. (2017, December 4). *A unified approach to interpreting model predictions*. ACM DigitalLibrary. https://dl.acm.org/doi/abs/10.5555/3295222.3295230

Shrikumar, A., Greenside, P., & Kundaje, A. (2019). *Learning Important Features Through Propagating Activation Differences*. Opgehaal van. https://arxiv.org/abs/1704.02685

Administrator. (2017, September 11). *Noncommunicable diseases*. WHO. https://www.emro.who.int/annual-report/2016/noncommunicable-diseases.html

Awotunde, J. B., Folorunso, S. O., Bhoi, A. K., Adebayo, P. O., & Ijaz, M. F. (2021). Disease diagnosis system for IoT-based wearable body sensors with machine learning algorithm. *Hybrid Artificial Intelligence and IoT in Healthcare*, 201-222. doi:10.1007/978-981-16-2972-3_10

El-Sappagh, S., Alonso, J. M., Islam, S. M. R., Sultan, A. M., & Kwak, K. S. (2021). A multilayer multimodal detection and prediction model based on explainable artificial intelligence for Alzheimer's disease. *Scientific Reports*, *11*(1), 2660. Advance online publication. doi:10.103841598-021-82098-3 PMID:33514817

Maldonado, S., Weber, R., & Famili, F. (2014). Feature selection for high-dimensional class-imbalanced data sets using Support Vector Machines. *Information Sciences*, *286*, 228–246. doi:10.1016/j.ins.2014.07.015

Rodin, A. S., Litvinenko, A., Klos, K., Morrison, A. C., Woodage, T., Coresh, J., & Boerwinkle, E. (2009). Use of Wrapper Algorithms Coupled with a Random Forests Classifier for Variable Selection in Large-Scale Genomic Association Studies. *Journal of Computational Biology*, *16*(12), 1705–1718. doi:10.1089/cmb.2008.0037 PMID:20047492

Panthong, R., & Srivihok, A. (2015). Wrapper Feature Subset Selection for Dimension Reduction Based on Ensemble Learning Algorithm. *Procedia Computer Science*, *72*, 162–169. doi:10.1016/j.procs.2015.12.117

Ribeiro, M. T., Singh, S., & Guestrin, C. (2016). "Why should i trust you?": Explaining the predictions of any classifier. In *Proceedings of the 22nd ACM SIGKDD International Conference on Knowledge Discovery and Data Mining, KDD '16* (pp. 1135–1144). ACM. doi: .293977810.1145/2939672

Ijaz, M. F., Attique, M., & Son, Y. (2020). Data-driven cervical cancer prediction model with outlier detection and over-sampling methods. *Sensors (Basel)*, *20*(10), 2809. doi:10.339020102809 PMID:32429090

Ijaz, M., Alfian, G., Syafrudin, M., & Rhee, J. (2018). Hybrid Prediction Model for Type 2 Diabetes and Hypertension Using DBSCAN-Based Outlier Detection, Synthetic Minority Over Sampling Technique (SMOTE), and Random Forest. *Applied Sciences (Basel, Switzerland)*, *8*(8), 1325. doi:10.3390/app8081325

Mandal, M., Singh, P., Ijaz, M., Shafi, J., & Sarkar, R. (2021). A Tri-Stage Wrapper-Filter Feature Selection Framework for Disease Classification. *Sensors (Basel)*, *21*(16), 5571. doi:10.339021165571 PMID:34451013

Naga Srinivasu, P., Ahmed, S., Alhumam, A., Bhoi Kumar, A., & Fazal Ijaz, M. (2021). An AW-HARIS Based Automated Segmentation of Human Liver Using CT Images. *Computers. Materials & Continua*, *69*(3), 3303–3319. doi:10.32604/cmc.2021.018472

Zintgraf, L. M., Cohen, T. S., Adel, T., & Welling, M. (2017). *Visualizing deep neural network decisions: Prediction difference analysis*. Academic Press.

Fong, R. C., & Vedaldi, A. (2017). Interpretable explanations of black boxes by meaningful perturbation. *IEEE International Conference on Computer Vision (ICCV)*, 3449–3457.

Lundberg, S. M., & Lee, S.-I. (2017). A unified approach to interpreting model predictions. *Advances in Neural Information Processing Systems*, *30*, 4765–4774.

Castro, J., Gamez, D., & Tejada, J. (2009). Polynomial calculation of the shapley value based on sampling. *Computers & Operations Research*, *36*(5), 1726–1730. doi:10.1016/j.cor.2008.04.004

Fatima, S. S., Wooldridge, M., & Jennings, N. R. (2008). A linear approximation method for the shapley value. *Artificial Intelligence*, *172*(14), 1673 – 1699. doi:10.1016/j.artint.2008.05.003

Osborne, M. J., & Rubinstein, A. (1994). *A course in game theory*. MIT Press.

Chapter 6

Drug Discovery With XAI Using Deep Learning

Iswarya B.
Sri G. V. G. Visalakshi College for Women, India

Manimekalai K.
Sri G. V. G. Visalakshi College for Women, India

ABSTRACT

Deep learning has potential in the process of discovering drug, with enhanced method for analyzing image, structure of molecule and function prediction, along with preset synthesis based on the novel enzymatic structure along tailored features and its applications. Even with expanding quantity based on effective potential approaches, the statistical systems and Machine Learning algorithms that underpin them are sometimes difficult to grasp by the human mind. To meet the required recent paradigm for the automated structure of molecules, for the purpose of 'Explainable Artificial Intelligence' with deep learning approaches. In current era, there is a need for XAI with methods of deep learning to discourse the demand for a developed machine language of the molecular science. This review outlines the important concepts in XAI, possible approaches, and obstacles. It promotes to further development of XAI techniques.

INTRODUCTION

In the area of biomedical environment there is a need for XAI to reach the level of explanation for drugs. Nowadays, Explainable Artificial Intelligence is very popular. XAI plays a vital role to develop "black box" approaches (Bastani O et al. 2017).

DOI: 10.4018/978-1-6684-3791-9.ch006

Figure 1. XAI Approaches

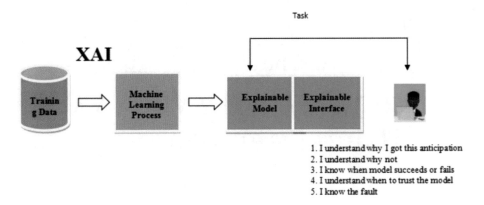

The main goal behind XAI is that Artificial Intelligence programs and technologies are not understandable (Zhaoyi Chen et al. 2020). Origin of XAI comes from a set of techniques, which adds the contextual adaptability and Interpretability to Deep Learning Models. When human not able to do but Artificial Intelligence can achieve and do it, but AI models are complex for black box approaches.

This part attempts to give a complete overview of modern XAI techniques (Guang Yang et al. 2021), Figure.1 provides a review of the approaches and their targets.

The term XAI refers to Explainable Artificial Intelligence. XAI is also referred as Transparent Artificial Intelligence. XAI means how and why the algorithm makes decisions or predictions. XAI explains different cases to reach different conclusions and Strengths/Weakness of the model. XAI solves the black box models in Artificial Intelligence. XAI shows that how machines are performing their procedures and where the problem raises (Dr. Mark Roberts et al. 2019). XAI owns research in various domains, it includes, Antenna design, Algorithmic trading, Medical diagnosis, Autonomous vehicles, Text analytics, Criminal justice. There are three principles in XAI:

1. Transparency addresses how a model works internally.
2. Interpretability has the capability to regulate the purpose, and outcome of Deep learning model.
3. XAI has the perception in representing the nodes along with the performance of model's priority.

In this paper, Section II discusses about the background study of XAI, Drug Discovery, Explainable Artificial Intelligence and Deep learning methods, Section III describes about approaches in XAI with Drug Discovery.

LITERATURE REVIEW

The following table contains several authors' views about the process of drug discovery with XAI.

Table 1. Views on the process of drug discovery using XAI

Author	Year	Inference
Abhay Pandey et al.	2020	Briefed about the drug discovery process in different phases.
Arun Das et al.	2020	XAI algorithms, opportunities, techniques, limitations and future directions are discussed in detail.
Vikas K. Prajapati et al.	2020	This study reviews about the application of Artificial Intelligence in the process of discovering and developing drugs.
Amol B. Deore et al.	2019	Overview about the process of advanced drug discovery and its development.
Connor W coley et al.	2018	Described about the approaches based on Neural Network, and new concept is introduced to validate the chemical reaction of context in CASP.
Kristy A Carpenter et al.	2018	Due to cost and time consuming, author integrates Virtual Screening and Machine Learning in the drug discovery.
Andreas Mayr et al.	2018	Performances of the deep learning methods with drug discovery large datasets are assessed and comparison is made with target prediction and machine learning methods.
Lu Zhang et al.	2017	History of ML and advanced development of deep learning approaches and applications in RDD are summarized.
Himabindu Lakkaraju et al.	2017	BETA is a framework, it explains the behavior of black-box classifier for trustworthiness to the novel model and explained the interpretability.
Hughes JP et al.	2010	This article reviews the key stages in preclinical process of the drug discovery from Target Identification and validation through screening.

BACKGROUND STUDY

Why There Is a Need For XAI

In recent trends there is a need for explainability to do everything, we have moved towards automatic interpretation with human using AI concepts. XAI will interpret, explains and visualize the models with the help of deep learning algorithms. Deep learning methods are well trained to predict the defects with reduced accuracy. XAI has been successfully utilized in the process of drug development which will be demanding technology and time consuming.

XAI involves in each stage in the process of drug development, it includes molecule design, drug quantity identification and effectiveness of drug. There is an biggest challenge to the pharmaceutical industry that they should not communicate about the dosage of drugs until it get approved. We should train the models with testing the safety of drug, effectiveness of drug with specified disease and has to analyse the history of patients after trials. Example - With clinical knowledge, the trained XAI models are utilized to predict the disease. XAI applications provide explanation based on the health care data with AI models to predict the disease using explanations. If there is any inaccurate predictions, the AI model to be enhanced.

The problem can be solved by explainable AI (XAI) which aims to provide area experts with clear justifications.

Drug Discovery

"Hippocrates" is considered as the father of modern medicine, he also resulted in inefficient drugs. Search for drugs is not a new to the real world (Coryandar Gilvary et al. 2019). Traditional methods like ayurveda have thousands of years. Drug refers to a piece of enzymatic which produces a variation in our anatomy. Drugs are used for diagnosis/treatment for selective diseases (Laura Elizabeth Lansdowne et al. 2020).

Complex molecular reactions are carried out by cells in the body. A mistake in one reaction may prevent an important protein from being produced/over-produced, resulting in the body producing insufficient cells, such as Diabetes, or producing too many cells, such as Cancer (Jose Jimenez-Luna et al. 2020). These pathways are influenced by drug molecules interacting with specific molecules along the way, making them more or less active or changing their activity entirely (Vikas K. et al. 2020). Drug Discovery primarily starts in the testing ground with technologists for innumerable activities assists to recognize biological and genomic component for indiscriminate disease.

Rational Drug Discovery

1. Finding new medicines based on target.
2. An organic compound activates the protein.
3. Involves modeling of molecules against phytochemical targets.

Drug Discovery Process

In the last 40 years, drug development has gotten significantly more involved, requiring preclinical investigations, IND submissions, and completed in vivo studies before getting FDA approval. Before being authorized, NDAs and BLAs are normally thoroughly assessed. The drug performance is then again submitted to authorized agencies for marketing research (Martin Drance A et al. 2021). The major aim is to provide is target specific therapies to patients after a complete medical examination.

In US, the drug development process is divided into 5 sections, each having several phases and stages (Abhay Pandey et al. 2020). The drug development process is depicted in Figure 2.

1. New target Discovery and development process
2. Then move to Premedical Research
3. Medical Research
4. Food and Drug Management
5. Food and Drug Management Post-Market Safety Monitoring

Figure 2. Drug progress practice

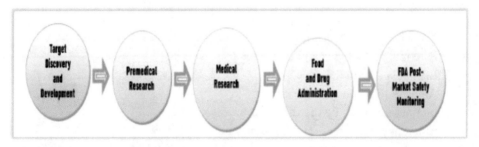

1. **Step 1:** New target Discovery and development process

New drugs are developed through drug discovery. Drugs were previously discovered through the discovery of traditional drugs. Then, pharmacology was employed to identify therapeutic properties in various compounds.

To decrease probable drug adverse effects, drug discovery comprises target screening, clinical chemistry, and target optimization. During drug development process the efficiency was improved.

a. **Finding Target and Validation -** A biomolecular plays a substantial impact in disease is identified as a target. Drug qualities were noted once they have been recognized. Targets must be effective, safe, and drug-like, as well as meet clinical and commercial objectives. To validate targets, scientists utilize photochemical and various pathways.

b. **Hit Discovery Process -** Compound screening assays are created after target validation.

c. **Assay Development and Screening –**These are test systems used to assess the effects of a novel compounds on molecular level.

d. **High Throughput Screening -** HTS reduces scientist's hours of tedious testing. HTS is a technique for detecting active chemicals, genes, or antibodies that alter human molecules.

e. **Hit to Lead -** Ligand from HTS are observed &improved in a restricted way.

f. **Lead Optimization -** Lead optimization designs the drug candidate by conducting trial testing by using ADMET tools.

g. **API -** APIs are physiologically active drugs that have a therapeutic impact. The API or APIs, as well as excipients, make up all medications.

2. **Step 2: Premedical Research**

It is conducted to regulate the drug's efficiency and safety, following steps are used to discover the drug.

- Knowledge on absorption, distribution, metabolization and excretion.
- Potential advantages and mechanisms of action.
- Best dosage and delivery.
- Adverse reactions or side effects.
- Interactions with further medications.
- Efficiency in evaluation to similar meds.

Premedical trials observe the new drug's efficacy, toxicity, and pharmacokinetic (PK) data in nonhuman subjects. Scientists used large dosages of drugs for in vitro and in vivo studies.

3. **Step 3: Medical Research**

Clinical drug development has completed when premedical research is done. It includes medical trials and volunteer studies. Trials must be secure and efficient. It should be completed within the budget, with a system in place to verify that the treatment performs. It will fine-tune the medicine for individual use (Amol B Deore et al. 2019).

4.   **Step 4: Food and Drug Management**

After the successful development of a drug, it is sent to the FDA for an assessment. The FDA evaluates and approves or sometimes it will reject the application. Based on the applications and requirement for patients, the new medication regulatory approval time frame may be differed (Hughes JP et al. 2011).

a.   **IND Application -** Before starting clinical research, IND applications must be submitted to the FDA. The developers may begin the clinical trial, if it is ready and it is not responded by FDA when it is unfavorable.

b.   **NDA / ANDA / BLA Applications -** Medical trials demonstrate pharmaceutical protection and efficiency, and the FDA receives an NDA condensed innovative application for drug named ANDA or BLA.

c.   **Orphan Drug -** When the financial sponsors are unwilling to develop it under standard marketing conditions an orphan drug is intended to treat disease.

d.   **Accelerated Approval -** If there is strong evidence of a positive impact, new drugs may be approved more quickly.

e.   **Reasons for Drug Failure-** New drug applications may fail due to toxicity, efficiency, PH, biological availability and its insufficient drug activity.

  i.   **Toxicity**: If the toxicity of a new drug is too high, the drug may be rejected.

  ii.   **Efficiency**: If a new drug's efficiency is not high the FDA may reject it.

  5.   **Step 5: Food and Drug Management Post-Market Safety Monitoring**

At the time of approval, the complete knowledge on a drug's safety is important. Though the rigorous procedures in the medication development process, there are some limitations. As a result, the true picture of a product is available in the market. When the FDA receives reports of difficulties, it will change the dosage or usage information. In the case of more serious concerns, it will take further steps.

Explainable Artificial Intelligence with Drug discovery

In past few years computer assisted drug discovery has been successfully adopted the concepts of Artificial Intelligence. Deep learning algorithms have the ability to model unstructured I/O relationships, ANN with multiple physical processing layers, pattern recognition and featured extraction from adjunct data representation. In the drug discovery process, the Deep learning approaches are utilized to prove that it works better than the conventional machine learning models and QSAR (Tirthajyoti Sarkar et al. 2019).

Figure 3. XAI in the drug discovery Process

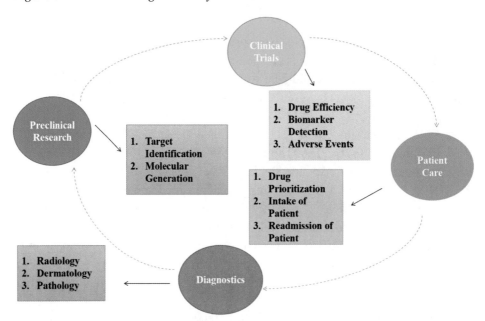

After 1990s, there is a re-growth for Neural Networks in the area of Chemical and Healthcare. The demand has been increased for approached that help to understand and perform the inherent models. Explainability approaches has drawn the attention to mitigate the drawbacks of interpretability to increase human thinking and decision making, and Machine learning approaches (Arun Das et al. 2006). Explainability provides information with statistical systems which directs to

1.   Furnish the explicit decision-making process understandable,
2.   Clever Hans effect –keep away from the exact prognosis for inaccurate rationale,
3.   Prevent unethical favoritism,
4.   Fill the gap within other disciplines and Machine learning models.

XAI applications are categorized into two models 1) global and 2) local model. Global model summarizes the importance of inherent attributes in the model. Local model is based on individual prediction (Mayr A et al. 2016).

The question of whether medical function can be derived from molecular structure and which elements are crucial to the structure is at the heart of the new medicine's paradigm (Zhang L et al. 2017). Clinical techniques seek to reduce the number of syntheses and tests required to discover and optimize a new hit. Explainable AI with drug discovery is supposed to address the aforementioned challenges, allowing for

Figure 4. Layers in deep learning

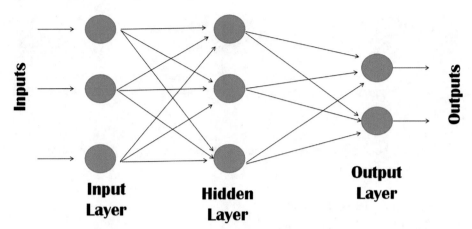

informed decision-making while taking into account medical chemistry knowledge, model logic, and understanding of the system's limitations. Medicinal chemists, chemo informaticians, and data scientists all work together at XAI.

Already XAI enables the interpretation mechanism of drug action and enhanced drug safety. By bypassing the human bias, XAI provides fundamental support in the interpretation and processing of more complex chemical data in the formation of new pharmaceutical hypotheses if there is long-term success. XAI plays an important role by relating human biology and physiologist in the development of applications for coronavirus pandemic.

Deep Learning Method

Deep learning method is used to execute machine learning. Neural network learns the weights in hidden layer, and then it will be multiplied with the input to produce the predicted output which will be closer to the preferred output is depicted in Figure 4. A neural network consists of,

1. Input layer - input is to be pixel(image) or time series data.
2. Hidden layer - it is said to be weights which is gained during the training of neural network.
3. Output layer - it produces the predicted data of the input from the network.

Deep learning methods are used for feature extraction, classification, time series prediction, data prediction, and regression (Sanjoy Dey et al. 2018). Deep learning

Figure 5. Recurrent neural network

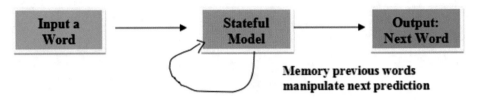

methods can be supervised or unsupervised learning (Eijaz Allibhai et al. 2018), some of them are

1. Recurrent Neural Network
2. Convolution Neural Network
3. Long short- term memory
4. Auto Encoder

Recurrent Neural Network

Recurrent neural network is an old algorithm which was developed in 1980's. RNN become popular due to the extension of RNN as LSTM (Long short-term memory) which will extend the memory. RNN is preferred algorithm for sequential data, it includes time series, voice, textual representation, and audio and video, financial and weather information related data. In RNN, the data moves in unidirectional from the input layer. It passes through hidden layer and finally moves to the output layer. RNN has an inbuilt memory to remember the data what is processed in the past (Niklas Donge et al. 2021).

Example: Drug is a word taken as the input and it will process the word by taking one character at once as a loop. Now it processed 'D', 'r' and it forgotten what data has been previously processed, it is possible in RNN because it has an inbuilt memory to remember the processed characters. RNN produces output, takes the output as input in the loop to process again is depicted in figure 5.

Convolution Neural Network

Convolution Neural network is a scientific operation with couple of functions which produced another function (Manav Mandal et al. 2021). CNN is used to read pin code, zip code in postal sectors. CNN is made up of multilayered artificial neurons is shown in Figure 6. In CNN, the first layer extracts primary features like edges of diagonals. Produced output is passed to the next layer, here it extracts composite

Figure 6. Convolution neural network

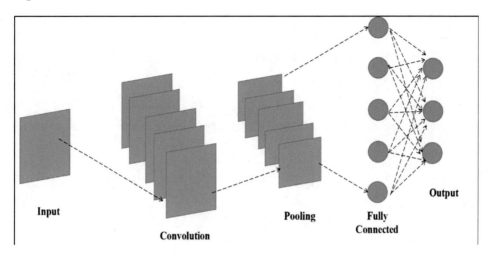

features like corners. If we move into deeper the network can recognize more composite features like face, things and so on.

Long Short-term Memory

Long short-term memory contains information in the memory, it can Read/Write and remove information from the memory (Jason Brownlee et al. 2017). LSTM is an extension of recurrent neural network (Murat Karakaya et al 2020). It permit recurrent neural network to recall input for a long term period. There are 3 gates represented in Figure 7, input (decides to allow new input or not), forget (miscellaneous information can be removed) and output (produces the output through this layer).

Auto Encoder

Auto encoder is also one of the deep learning method, utilized to learn the compressed the raw data representation. Encoder encodes the input and the decoder seeks to regenerate input from the encoder. Once the model is trained encoder model is retained and decoder is dropped.

APPROACHES IN XAI WITH DRUG DISCOVERY

The different approaches in Explainable Artificial Intelligence along with Drug Discovery are discussed below as shown in Figure 8,

Figure 7. Long short-term memory

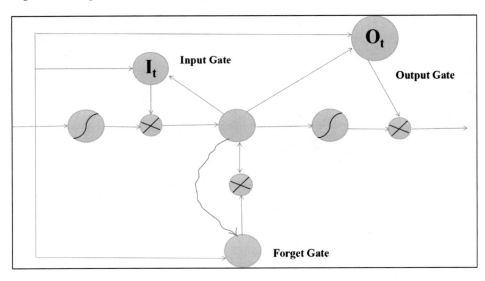

Figure 8. Different approaches of XAI in drug discovery

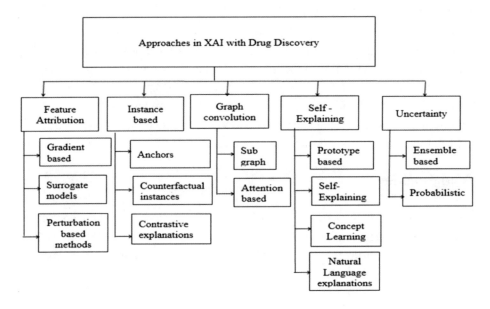

Feature Attribution

Feature Attribution also termed as post-hoc or post-modeling to generate explanation

Figure 9. Feature attribution methods

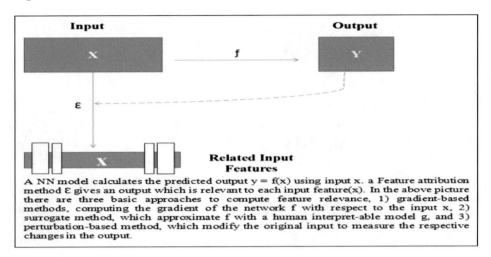

A NN model calculates the predicted output y = f(x) using input x. a Feature attribution method Ɛ gives an output which is relevant to each input feature(x). In the above picture there are three basic approaches to compute feature relevance, 1) gradient-based methods, computing the gradient of the network f with respect to the input x, 2) surrogate method, which approximate f with a human interpret-able model g, and 3) perturbation-based method, which modify the original input to measure the respective changes in the output.

for trained model in XAI. This method accepts model input and highlights the feature contribution based score to the output model. The score results as +ve, zero and -ve value. If the resultant value is positive then it shows that it contribution is towards the prediction of model (Sanjoy Dey et al. 2018). If the resultant value is zero then it shows that there is no contribution, and finally, if the resultant value is negative it shows that to remove the feature which may increase the probability of the prediction. Figure 9 describes about feature attribution methods.

In Equation - 1, Ɛ: x ∈ R^{KR} ® R^{KR} is an model input of feature attribution method, which gives an output based on the relevant value of each input feature for the ultimate prediction calculated with function f: x ∈ R^{KR} ® R (where R is represents the real number and KR represents the K-dimensional set of real number).

$$\mathcal{E}: x \in R^{KR} \rightarrow R^{KR} \qquad \text{Equation - 1}$$

There are two types of feature attribution they are 1) Local Feature Attribution 2) Global Feature Attribution. There are various ways to generate the feature attribution but the basic methods are 1) Gradient based methods, 2) Surrogate methods and 3) Perturbation based methods. Gradient and Surrogate based methods produces the local explanations and perturbation method directly estimate the importance of feature.

In the drug discovery process compared to interpretability, comprehensible molecular descriptors are advisable to choose. Recent research combines the LSTM network and transformers architecture in feature attribution method to find the

Figure 10. Instance-based methods

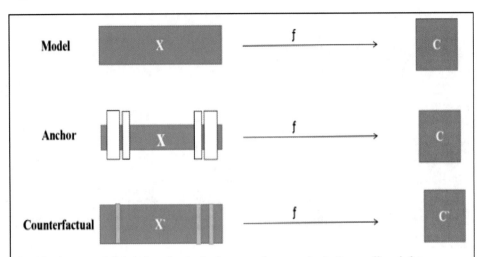

In this given model function f, x is the instance input and c is the predicted class,

1) Anchor algorithm recognizes a minimal subset of features of input x which is adequate to preserve the c predicted class.

2) Counterfactual search produces another instance x`, that recline close in feature space to existing input x, it belongs to the predicted class of c`.

portions of SMILES strings which is pertinent for the bio-activity properties. This approach attempts to connect the gap between deep learning and medical community.

Instance Based Methods

This method calculates a set of related characteristics which may exist or not to bear the anticipation of a stated framework. An instance-based method can be actual or created for on-demand. This approach produces the alternate results to reach the correspondent or various resolutions. There are three instance-based methods shown in Figure 10; they are 1) Anchors algorithm, 2) Counterfactual instances and 3) Contrastive explanations. In XAI with drug discovery, this approach can be valuable to improve the transparency of framework, by highlighting what should be exist or not to bear the anticipation.

During drug discovery process, instance-based method is utilized to improve the transparency of model, by foregrounding what features of molecules should be existing or not to guarantee the prediction of model.

Graph Convolution Method

This method is generally used in Neurological Networks along with the process of analyzing the image is shown in Figure 11. Here, graph convolution method is utilized in drug discovery, to predict the property of molecules. There are two ways to predict the property of molecules they are 1) Sub graph - which identifies the more than one part in the graph to predict the molecular property. 2) Attention - to store the various information to retrieve the hidden representation of level of the node. Graph Convolution method has the direct communication with the chemists to improve the instance and natural connection with drug.

Self-explaining Approaches

Self-explaining approaches can enhance the verification process and error analysis with domain knowledge. In general, XAI can be used only in post model explanations but this method should automatically predict the issues with prior explanations. This approach can be categorized into various methods, namely 1) Prototype based 2) Self-Explaining Neural Network, 3) CL methods and 4) Nature Language Neural Network. This approach has not yet been modeled in drug discovery process.

Uncertainty

This approach has been successfully implemented in the process of drug discovery. Uncertainty approaches are difficult to interpret with algorithms, molecular signifier. There are two methods 1) Ensemble based method and 2) Probabilistic based method is shown in figure 12.

CONCLUSION

This paper delivers the various process of drug development in 5 steps. XAI models need to be developed and applied to enhance the prediction of disease in the better way. There is a biggest challenge to the pharmaceutical industry that they should not communicate about the dosage of drugs until it gets approved. This is a critical difficulty with XAI in the drug development process in terms of improving the system, interpreting the model and training data. Major diseases have been present for a decade, such as COVID-19, and a lack of datasets is the reason why machine learning has not been successful in detecting coronavirus symptoms thus far. Combining the XAI approaches with deep learning methods will improve the models and produces the better solution for explainability.

Figure 11. Graph-based model interpretation

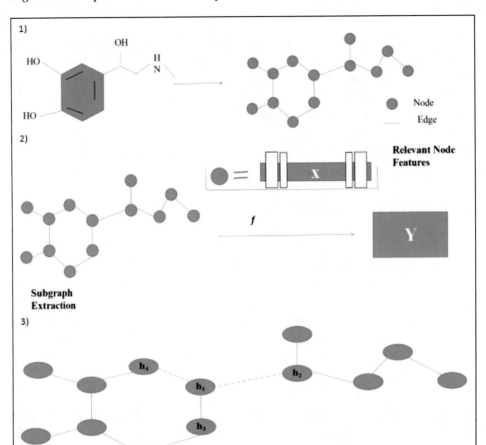

1) Named as Adrenaline structure, it consists of atoms and bonds in a molecular graph as nodes and vertices. 2) Graph Neural Network approach takes input graph to recognize a connected, compact subgraph, features which are relevant to the predicted output y of a graph-neural network model function f. 3) Attention mechanism can be used in conjunction with message-passing algorithms to learn coefficients. Learned coefficients is utilized to feature the predictive relevance of determined edges and nodes.

Figure 12. Uncertainty estimation

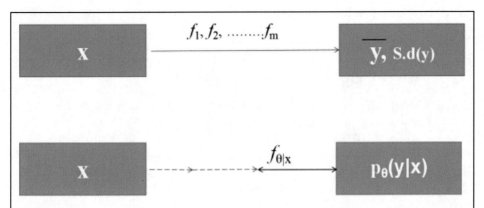

a) Ensemble-based methods accumulate the output of m identical, except differently initialized, models f_i. The final prediction is calculated by accumulating the predictions of all models, while an uncertainty estimate can be obtained from the respective predictive variance such as Standard Deviation.

b) Bayesian probabilistic approaches review a prior $p(\theta)$ over the learnable weights of a NN model f_θ and make use of approximate sampling approaches to learn a posterior distribution over the prediction $p_{\theta(y|x)}$ and the weights $p_{(\theta|x)}$.

REFERENCES

Allibhai, E. (2018). *Building a Deep Learning Model using Keras*. Towards Data Science.

Bastani, O. (2017). *Interpreting Blackbox models via model extraction*. arxiv.org/abs/1705.08504.

Brownlee, J. (2017). *A Gentle Introduction to Long Shor-Term Memory Networks by the experts*. Machine Learning Mastery.

Carpenter, K. A., Cohen, D. S., Jarrell, J. T., & Huang, X. (2018). Deep learning and Virtual drug screening. *Future Medicinal Chemistry*, *10*(21), 2557–2567. doi:10.4155/fmc-2018-0314 PMID:30288997

Chen, Z. (2020). Applications of Artificial Intelligence in drug development using real-world data. *Drug Discovery Today*. Advance online publication. doi:10.1016/j.drudis.2020.12.013 PMID:33358699

Coley, W., Green, W. H., & Jensen, K. F. (2018). Machine Learning in computer-aided synthesis planning. *Accounts of Chemical Research*, *51*(5), 1281–1289. doi:10.1021/acs.accounts.8b00087 PMID:29715002

Das, A. (2006). *Opportunities and challenges in explainable artificial intelligence (XAI): A survey*. IEEE. https://arxiv.org/abs/2006.11371

Deore. (2019). The Stages of Drug Discovery and Development Process. *Asian Journal of Pharmaceutical Research and Development*.

Dey, S. (2018). Predicting adverse drug reactions through interpretable deep learning framework. *International Conference on Intelligent Biology and Medicine (ICIBM): Bioinformatics*. 10.118612859-018-2544-0

Donge. (2021). *Neural Networks and LSTM Networks. Built in expert contributor network*. Academic Press.

Gilvary. (2019). The Missing Pieces of Artificial Intelligence in Medicine. *Rise of Machines in Medicine*. doi: 10.1016/j.tips.2019.06.001

Guang, Y. (2021). Unbox the black-box for the medical Explainable AI via Multi-modal and Multi-center Data Fusion: a mini-review, two showcases and beyond. *Information Fusion*. doi: 1016/j.inffus.2021.07.016

Hughes, J.P. (2011). *Principles of early drug discovery*. Doi: doi:10.1111/j.1476-5381.2010.01127.x

Jimenez-Luna, J. (2020). *Drug Discovery with explainable artificial intelligence*. Nature Machine Language. doi:10.103842256-020-00236-4

Karakaya. (2020). LSTM: Understanding Output Types. *Deep Learning Tutorials with Keras*.

Lakkaraju, H. (2017). Interpretable & Explorable Approximations of Black Box Models. *Workshop on Fairness, Accountability and Transparency in Machine Learning*.

Lansdowne, L. E. (2020). *Exploring the Drug Development*. Technology Networks Drug Discovery.

Mandal, M. (2021). *Introduction to Convolutional Neural Networks (CNN)*. The Startup Medium.

Martin Drance, A. (2021). Neuro symbolic XAI for computational Drug Repurposing. *Proceedings of the International Joint Conference on Knowledge Discovery, Knowledge Engineering and Knowledge Management (IC3K 2021), 2*, 220-225. Doi: 10.5220/0010714100003064

Mayr, A. (2018). *Large-scale comparison of machine learning methods for drug target prediction on ChEMBL*. Royal Society of Chemistry. doi:10.1039/C8SC00148K

Mayr, A., Klambauer, G., Unterthiner, T., & Hochreiter, S. (2016). DeepTox: Toxicity prediction using deep learning. *Frontiers in Environmental Science, 3*. Advance online publication. doi:10.3389/fenvs.2015.00080

Prajapati, V. K. (2020). *AI in drug discovery and development: A brief commentary*. Pharma Tutor. https://www.pharmatutor.org/articles/ai-in-drug-discovery-and-development-a-brief-commentary

Roberts, D. M. (2019). *How Artificial Intelligence is Transforming Drug Design*. Drug Discovery World.

Sarkar. (2019). *Google's New Explainable AI (XAI) Service, towards Data Science*. Academic Press.

Zhang, L., Tan, J., Han, D., & Zhu, H. (2017). From Machine learning to Deep learning: Progress in machine intelligence fir rational drug discovery. *Drug Discovery Today, 22*(11), 1680–1685. doi:10.1016/j.drudis.2017.08.010 PMID:28881183

Chapter 7

Development of Machine Learning Models for Healthcare Systems Using Python:
Machine Learning Models for COVID-19

Hemaraju Pollayi
Department of Civil Engineering, GITAM University (Deemed), Hyderabad, India

Praveena Rao
Department of Civil Engineering, GITAM University (Deemed), Hyderabad, India

ABSTRACT

Machine learning (ML) has been slowly entering every aspect of our lives, and its positive impact has been astonishing. To accelerate embedding ML in more applications and incorporating it in real-world scenarios, automated machine learning (AutoML) is emerging. The main purpose of AutoML is to provide seamless integration of ML in various industries, which will facilitate better outcomes in everyday tasks. After a violent disaster, the supply of medical services may fall short of the rising demand, leading to overcrowding in hospitals and, consequently, a collapse in the healthcare system. In the chapter, the authors created learning models for COVID-19 to understand how to design a proper ML workflow, which results in an organized, efficient product that produces desired results in terms of diagnosis, prediction, and recommendations. Large amounts of labeled training data are processed and analyzed to identify correlations, patterns, and make predictions using these patterns about future trends.

DOI: 10.4018/978-1-6684-3791-9.ch007

Table 1. Machine learning in healthcare

S. No.	Healthcare systems
1	Prediction of diseases and appropriate treatments
2	Forecasting health risks for different populations
3	Distinguish tumors from healthy organs
4	Aiding discovery of targeted drugs with lowered cost of production
5	Assists pathologists to make faster and more accurate diagnosis
6	Determine possible opportunities for clinical trials
7	Facilitating management of healthcare data base and workflow
8	Detects gaps in healthcare

INTRODUCTION

The most perpetual concerning issues of human beings has been good health and well-being. The healthcare sector has been fast evolving with remarkable technological advances for the benefit of human society. Presently, artificial intelligence and machine learning plays a vital role in many healthcare industry, including invention of latest diagnostic procedures, treatment of chronic diseases, formulation of breakthrough drugs for high risk diseases, recording and managing of patient hospitalization records. Machine learning can be applied to different healthcare systems as shown in Table 1. Machine learning is finding a wide range of healthcare applications, ranging from handling of prevalent chronic diseases to leveraging patient medical history data, in conjunction with external factors like pollution exposure and weather factors (Venkatramanana, 2018). ML technology has the capacity to transcend the dynamics of healthcare sector altogether by analyzing and interpreting valuable insights from large volumes of data, thus facilitating professionals to generate problem specific medicine solutions (Escobar, 2021).

According to the reports given by IBM TJ Watson Research Center, there is a multi-universe of data in healthcare. In the year 2012 the amount of digital data generated globally in healthcare sector was estimated to be approximately 500 petabytes and it was expected to shoot up to 25,000 petabytes in 2020. Data plies with large amounts of noise can be preprocessed and analyzed for desired outcomes from the accumulated continuum data. With recent innovations in ML, cloud computing, robotics and automation; which have continually impacted the health sector emphasis on accessible structured and unstructured healthcare data has been increasingly evident. Designing a proper machine learning model tailored for typical data and problem at hand is vital for achieving desired efficiency and accuracy. The supervised learning approach for diagnosis of patients from a set of visible symptoms reported by them (in the form of tabular data, medical images, text, or signals) using binary and multi-class classification (Muhammad, 2021).

Figure 1. Output of the supervised learning approach for a patient. [image by ScienceSoft]

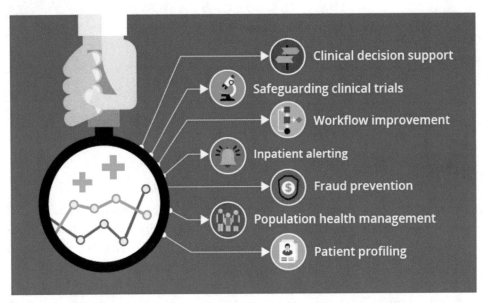

Development and deployment of a machine learning model in the healthcare sector for data processing and effective manipulation is a cumbersome process. Proper deployment of a machine learning system requires considering the healthcare regulations and controls to ensure quality with standardized model environment. When condition of a patient is assessed, the physician gathers and records information in the Electronic Health Record (EHR) (Prabhu, 2020). Which includes personal data such as occupation, date of birth, gender, age, contacts, marital status, insurance, as well as health data regarding vitals, symptoms, allergies, chief complaint, lifestyle choices, co morbidities, traumas, lab test results, family diseases, diagnosis, treatment, childhood diseases, and transaction data (med claims, billing receipts). The output is shown in Figure 1 after analyzing the Python-based machine learning models.

The expenditures generated by healthcare sector on the global front is nearly 10.3% of the gross domestic product which sums to about $9 trillion worldwide and is expected to grow at the rate of 3.9% annually over the next few years. With the advent of newer technologies encompassing large scale digitalization, the landscape of the healthcare business has been changing dynamically. A wide range of wearable smart devices with IoT based sensors for health monitoring are becoming increasingly popular in the consumer technologies. The users are capable of tracking, analyzing and transmitting data pertaining to individual health vitals such as body temperature, heart rate, levels of blood pressure, sleep patterns, etc. A worldwide market of $93 billion is foreseen for wearable smart devices in 2022 and the number is estimated to be one billion. Virtual consulting and telemedicine is on high demand amongst the patients since the pandemic begun. AI integrated medical equipments with advanced surgical facilities are supporting doctors and physicians globally (Luz, 2020). For enhanced customer services and improvised service providers, end-to-end data encrypted ecosystems are being developed. Subsequently, the model of healthcare and wellness has evolved into data-drive entirely.

The healthcare industry in the present times may be classified into the following sectors:

1. Healthcare providers and facilities (such as hospitals, nursing homes, surgery centers, or general physicians and doctors),
2. Medical equipment and devices (such as orthopedic treatment devices, diagnostic equipment, or medical instrumentations),
3. Distributors and wholesalers (such as pharmacies or drug distributors and healthcare equipment for providers),
4. Health insurance and managed care, and
5. Pharma, biotechnology, and life sciences.

Figure 2. Various applications of ML in healthcare industry

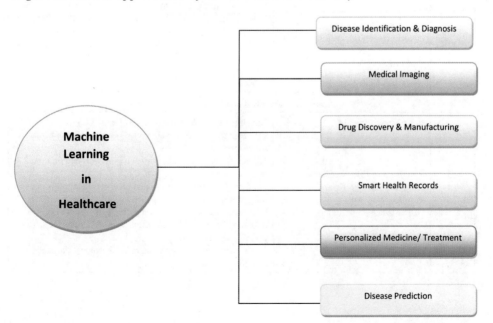

Table 2. Ongoing applications of machine learning techniques in healthcare industry with companies (Mike Thomas, 2021)

S. No.	Company	Machine learning in healthcare
\multicolumn{3}{c}{**Application 1: Smart Records**}		
1 2 3	Quotient Health (Denver, Colorado) KenSci (Seattle, Washington) Ciox Health (Georgia)	Reduced management cost of EMR (Electronic Medical Records) systems with the help of software applications development Machine learning based illness and treatment prediction for helping physicians and payers Effective exchange, handling and utilization of health information with the implementation of machine learning
\multicolumn{3}{c}{Application 2: Medical Imaging data and Diagnostics}		
4 5 6	PathAI (Massachusetts) Quantitative Insights (Chicago, Illinois) Microsoft (Redmond, Washington)	Increased diagnosis efficacy and accuracy in pathology with the deployment of machine learning Computer aided breast MRI workstation Quantx for improved interpretation and accuracy of breast cancer diagnosis using 3D radiological image interpretation with machine learning for distinguishing between tumors and healthy anatomy
\multicolumn{3}{c}{Application 3: Drug Discovery and Development}		
7 8 9	Pfizer (New York, New York) Insitro (San Francisco, California) BioSymetrics (Boston, Massachusetts)	Machine learning based immuno-oncology research Developing lower cost drugs with the goal of faster recovery rate in patients Data pre-processing via Augusta -ML platform, which enables customers to utilize automated ML
\multicolumn{3}{c}{Application 4: Medical Data}		
10 11 12	ConcertAI (New York) Orderly Health (Denver, Colorado) MD Insider (Santa Monica, California)	Employed machine learning for analyzing oncology data and drawing insights, aids pharmaceutical companies to practice precision in medicine and healthcare service providers Concierge services in healthcare via attendant text messages, email, video-conferencing for a24/7 automated helpdesk Uses machine learning for best suited doctors profiles with patient health problems
\multicolumn{3}{c}{Application 5: Treatment and Prediction of Disease}		
13 14 15 16	Beta Bionics (Massachusetts) Tempus (Chicago, IL) Prognos (New York) BERG (Massachusetts)	Develop wearable bionic pancreas (calls iLet) for patients suffering from Type 1 diabetes for better control of blood sugar levels on 24/7 basis Aiming to create breakthroughs in diagnosis and treatment in cancer research Platform for disease detection at early stages, appropriate therapy suggestion, utilizes registry data containing 19 billion records for 185 million patients in order to provide best care facilities, identification of opportunities for possible clinical trials Mapping disease with treatments in neurology, oncology, and other conditions

There are five major machine learning applications in healthcare industry, (1) Smart Records, (2) Medical Imaging and Diagnostics, (3) Drug Discovery and Development, (4) Medical Data, and (5) Treatment and Prediction of Disease. Some of the companies in USA that are harnessing benefits from its power for the betterment of patients are given in Table 2.

Data science is growing with leaps and bounds in the domain of Information Technology at present times. Companies across the globe have been continually adopting machine learning and data science implementations into their operational systems.

EXPLORING HOW DATA SCIENCE AND MACHINE LEARNING ARE USED IN DIFFERENT AREAS OF THE MEDICAL INDUSTRY

Revolutionary breakthroughs in the field of healthcare and medicine is foreseen with the integration of data science solutions. A whole new level in medical science is envisaged with technological advancements and computerization of post-surgery/treatment monitoring, patients medical records maintenance and drug discovery. It is anticipated that with Artificial Intelligence very soon it may be possible for the doctors to assess and predict which disease a patient has by just running a mathematical formula over the medical history records. For good diagnostic abilities acquiring large set of disease labels may be essential for physicians. Each of these label sets are bound with illness idea and its consequent symptoms, antecedents and possible cure for the illness.

AutoML in Healthcare Industry

Studies on implementation of AutoML models in the healthcare systems focus on two generalized approaches, which include (a) building new tools with AutoML for healthcare datasets; and (b) performing predictive classification on existing platforms available in AutoML modeling libraries. These datasets are generally available in structured or unstructured forms.

Structured Dataset

Datasets that are presented in tabular formats i.e., rows and columns within in large database systems and can be processed facilely by computers are called structured datasets. These databases contain large spreadsheets with continuum data collected on daily basis such as lab results with particulars of patients. For example lab reports for blood tests on hemoglobin, thyroid, cholesterol, etc. contain information about the patients such as name, sex/gender and age.

Un-Structured Dataset

Whereas, unstructured datasets are characterized by data in an unformatted manner. It may contain images, documents, text, and videos which are not arranged in tables or rows and columns. Linear regression, SVM (support vector machines) and some other machine learning algorithms conventionally follow a transitional process where all unstructured data are converted into structured data formats. Over 90% data in the industry available for processing are unstructured of which 90% is yet to be harnessed for extracting valuable insights in medicine and healthcare sectors. Most commonly available examples of unstructured datasets are medical imaging data and clinical notes with patient descriptions such as symptoms of illness, treatment provided, observed outcomes of given treatment, etc. Listed in Table 2 are several

Table 3. AutoML platforms used for different datasets in the medicine research (Mustafa, 2021)

S. No.	Format of Dataset	Type of Dataset	Specialty\Disease	AutoML Platform		
				Commercial	Open Source	Health-Related
1	Unstructured	Audio	Hearing Aid	√	×	×
		Images	Covid-19	√	×	×
		Images	Liver Injury	√	×	×
			Generic	×	×	√
				×	×	√
				√	×	×
			Cancer	√	×	×
			Pachychoroid	√	×	×
2	Structured	Tabular	BioSignature	×	×	√
			Brain Age	×	√	√
			Alzheimer	×	√	×
			Brain Tumor	×	√	×
			Cardiac	×	√	√
			Metabolic	×	√	×
			Generic	×	√	√
			Diabetes	×	√	×

previous related work accomplishments of AutoML platforms for wide varieties of applications in medicine industry. According to the type of dataset, two general categorizes are shown in the table, which comprise structured data (tabular format) and unstructured data (such as audio or images).

Algorithms Selection and Optimization

Firstly, preparation or preprocessing of datasets is carried out, followed by extraction of features and subsequently selection of features. Thereby a suitable machine learning algorithm is selected and trained for datasets available for features extraction and selection. The accuracy and performance of the adopted model is evaluated for the required datasets in the assessment. Not only does the performance indicate how well the model is trained, but also predicts how will it shall perform on new datasets in future analytic studies (Akbulut, 2018). Ideally, 80% of is chosen for training clinical datasets while 20% of datasets are required for testing the adopted model (Chatterjee, 2020).

The process of feature extraction typically involves construction of the number of variables or resources required to describe a large dataset for solving high precision problems. Performance is the major concern involved with handling large number of variables in complex data analysis which requires large amounts of memory space configurations and high end computational power (Sustersic, 2021).

Targets and Evaluations

Based on the metrics defined for evaluation the adopted machine learning algorithm is designed and optimized soon after feature extraction and selection processes.

In this chapter, the authors highlighted the following characteristics of the selected model:

- Why to choose a particular epidemiological model ?
- How to optimize critical parameters in the epidemiological model ?
- Will the epidemiological model allow to fit training data, to forecast accurately and to validate the performance ?
- Can the epidemiological model applicable to multiple variants across the world ?

COVID-19

World Health Organization (WHO)

The United Nations established an international health agency on 7 April 1948 called the world health organization (who) which aims at attaining best possible health and well being for people globally (who, 2019). Its head office is seated at Geneva, Switzerland with field offices operational from 150 locations and regional offices at six different locations across the world. The who's major objectives constitute monitoring risks and potential threats posed to public health and well being of people worldwide, coordinating immediate healthcare facilities during emergencies, promoting health care as well as advocating for hygiene, sanitation, malnutrition issues, clean drinking water facilities, immunization and many more issues concerning health hazards. Providing countries with assistance in technical issues, setting international standards for good healthcare provisions and facilities, collecting and reporting data pertaining health risks or issues at global levels are some of its key functions. The world health report is published which addresses worldwide topics on healthcare systems, drawbacks, provisions and essentially acts as a forum for discussions related to issues in public healthcare. Eradication of fatal diseases like small pox, polio, tuberculosis, vaccine discovery for Ebola virus, cure communicable diseases like HIV/Aids are some of the most remarkable achievements of the who. It has been currently working mainstream for dealing with present covid-19 pandemic and disseminating vaccines to the remote locations worldwide. The agency is governed by world health assembly constituting specialists in healthcare and a director-general. It plays a vital role in goal setting, prioritizing tasks undertaken, decision-making, regulating/monitoring activities in all sub-offices, approval of budgets and financing.

Covid-19 (The Problem)

Corona virus 2019 (COVID-19) is a disease causing critical respiratory condition due to the invasion of Severe Acute Respiratory Syndrome Corona Virus 2 (SARS-CoV-2), first case was identified in China in the year 2019. This virus has spread exponentially all over the world due to its high transmissibility and mutating capacity as a result of adapting to hosts through genetic evolution. This virus lead to complete crash down of healthcare systems in most of the countries due to overwhelming of facilities and insufficient supplies. The pandemic has had catastrophic consequences on the global demographics with worldwide deaths above 2.9 million in past two years and collapse of global economy.

Figure 3. Spreading of COVID-19 virus

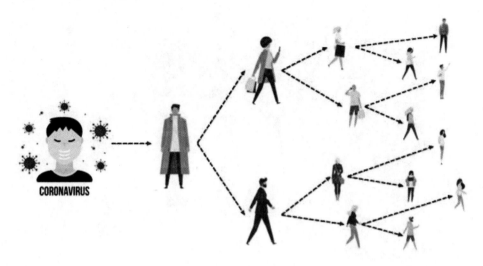

As shown in Figure 3, the COVID-19 virus spreads primarily through droplets of saliva or discharge from the nose when an infected person coughs or sneezes. The most common symptoms of COVID-19 virus include illness due to light, moderate to severe respiratory disorders and serious health risks for people with co-morbidities such as cardiac problems, lung disorders, severe diabetic medical history and undergoing cancer treatment.

Worldwide, there have been 267,865,289 confirmed cases of COVID-19 as per WHO reports of 10 December 202, 4:48pm CET, including 5,285,888 deaths. Totally, 8,158,815,265 vaccine doses were administered globally as of 8 December 2021. The WHO Corona virus (COVID-19) Dashboard is shown in Figure 4 and the weekly global situation of COVID-19 is shown in Figure 5. The weekly cases and deaths registered by WHO region is shown in Figure 6 and Figure 7, respectively. Figure 8 shows the data table for Global and WHO Region-wise situation of COVID-19.

The outbreak of novel corona virus has resulted in devastating repercussions on health, economy and demographics globally. Despite a high survival rate, the number of cases with risk of fatality resulting in deaths is growing every day. Patients survival rates are projected to improve and fatality rates might decrease if high-risk patients are identified and given preventative measures with timely predictions (Maher, 2021).

Figure 4. WHO Corona virus (COVID-19) dashboard [image by WHO]

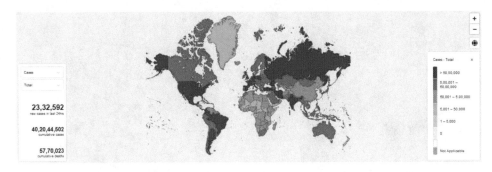

Figure 5. Weekly global situation of COVID-19 [image by WHO]

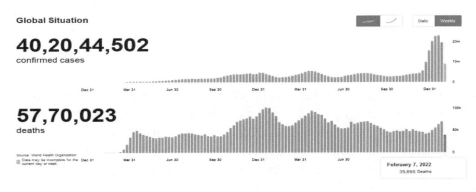

Figure 6. Cases: Weekly global situation of COVID-19 [image by WHO]

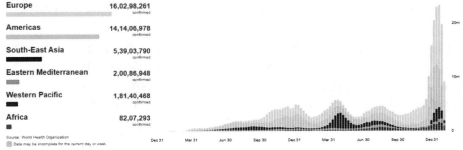

Figure 7. Deaths: weekly global situation of COVID-19 [image by WHO]

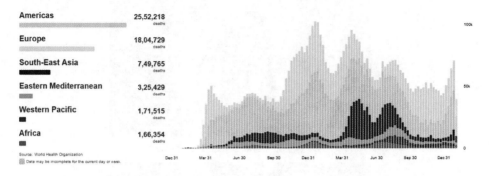

Figure 8. Data table: global and WHO region-wise situation of COVID-19 [image by WHO]

Name	Cases - cumulative total	Cases - newly reported in last 7 days	Deaths - cumulative total	Deaths - newly reported in last 7 days	Total vaccine doses administered per 100 population	Persons fully vaccinated per 100 population
Global	402,044,502	17,711,497	5,770,023	71,701	129.52	53.36
+ By WHO Region						
Africa	82,07,293	74,745	1,66,354	1,537	19.47	8.26
Western Pacific	1,81,40,468	14,63,485	1,71,515	3,036	194.51	80.82
Eastern Mediterranean	2,00,86,948	7,81,656	3,25,429	2,980	84.31	35
South-East Asia	5,39,03,790	10,99,665	7,49,765	8,640	117.74	49.69
Americas	14,14,06,978	38,88,549	25,52,218	30,918	157.29	64.3
Europe	16,02,98,261	1,04,03,397	18,04,729	24,590	155.52	60.08

Covid-19 (The Solution)

COVID-19 is quite imperceptible initially yet grows rapidly to its maximum value soon after it acquires a significant level. The virus will ultimately run out of people to infect, causing the count to slow down. This is known as logistic growth, and the curve is termed a sigmoid. At any given time during the curve peak healthcare facilities get jam-packed and running out of medical supplies or resources for the cure of afflicted people. The most effective solution for this problem can be achieved by flattening of the curve at any given point of time to bring down the count of affected cases such that it comes closer to or in line with the existing health care facilities. The process can be illustrated as shown in Figure 9.

Figure 9. Beginning to solution of COVID-19

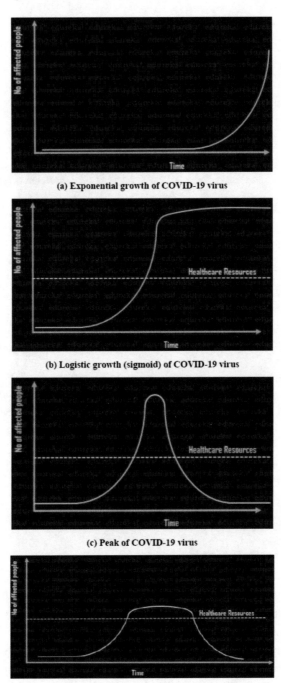

(a) Exponential growth of COVID-19 virus

(b) Logistic growth (sigmoid) of COVID-19 virus

(c) Peak of COVID-19 virus

(d) Best solution: Flatten curve of COVID-19 virus

MACHINE LEARNING MODELS FOR COVID-19 USING PYTHON

Machine Learning (ML) provides a wide variety of visualization and prediction tools, which are being utilized worldwide to examine the pattern of COVID-19 spread considering the confirmed infections, recoveries, and fatalities (Guleria P, 2022). Other parameters impacting the COVID-19 forecast include factors such as age group, gender, quarantining, medical history of patients, co-morbidities, environmental factors, etc. The accuracy of the prediction analysis largely depends on the database which forms the basis for achieving best results. The datasets have yet to be standardized, also statistical anomalies have not been accounted, thus making it extremely challenging for implementation of ML techniques in COVID-19 (Xu, 2020). Other obstacles in training a model include choosing the right set of parameters and choosing the most optimal machine learning model for prediction (Hassantabar, 2020).

DIAGNOSIS BASED ON SYMPTOMS

Effective virus screening allows for rapid detection and accurate diagnosis of COVID-19, thereby reducing the excessive pressure imposed on healthcare systems (Qureshi, 2020). Development of prediction models that combine all possible factors are required to reckon the risk posed due to infection. This will assist medical staff worldwide in triaging patients, especially due to limited healthcare resources. In

Figure 10. The most prevalent symptoms of COVID-19

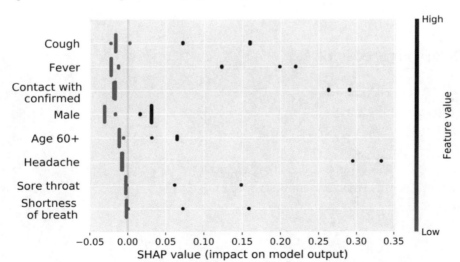

order to deal the present scenario of resource constraints, this framework shall work best for prioritizing testing of COVID-19. The ranking of the most important features of the model are summarized in Figure 10.

SPREAD VISUALIZATION AND PREDICTION

In this chapter, linear regression, support vector machine, multilayer perceptron, ensemble methods on the Johns Hopkins University's COVID-19 data to anticipate the future effects of COVID-19 pandemic in the world are performed. The impact of parameters such as geographic conditions, economic statistics, population statistics, and life expectancy in prediction of COVID-19 spread are examined. The following libraries are imported for the present work:

Python Code for SEIRD Model

Main Program

```
SEIRDmodel = BarebonesSEIR()
SEIRDmodel.parameters = SEIRDmodel.get_fit_parameters()
train_initial_conditions = SEIRDmodel.get_initial_
conditions(train_subset)
train_t = np.arange(len(train_subset))
  (S,E,I,R,D) = SEIRDmodel.predict(train_t, train_initial_
conditions)
```

Definitions used in Class

```
classBarebonesSEIR:
def__init__(self,parameters=None):
defget_fit_parameters(self):
defget_initial_conditions(self,data):
defstep(self,initial_conditions,t):
defpredict(self,t_range,initial_conditions):
```

Definitions used for Qaurantine Measures:

```
defsigmoid(x,xmin,xmax,a,b,c,r):
defstepwise_soft(t,coefficients,r=20,c=0.5):
```

Python Code for Modified SEIRD Model

```
train_initial_conditions=model.get_initial_conditions(train_df)
train_t=np.arange(len(train_df))
  (S,E,I,Iv,R,Rv,D,Dv),history=model.predict(train_t,train_
initial_conditions)
(new_exposed,
new_infected_invisible,new_infected_visible,
new_recovered_invisible,
new_recovered_visible,
new_dead_invisible,new_dead_visible=model.compute_daily_
values(S,E,I,Iv,R,Rv,D,Dv)
```

Python Code for Finding Future Strains using Modified SEIRD Model

```
defmake_two_strain_forecast(model,beta2_mult=1.5,new_strain_
ratio=0.01,**kwargs):
strain2_model=SEIRHiddenTwoStrains.from_strain_one_model(model)
strain2_model.params['beta2_mult'].value=beta2_mult
forkey,valueinkwargs.items():
strain2_model.params[key].value=value
E2_0=E[-1]*new_strain_ratio
E1_0=E[-1]*(1-new_strain_ratio)
Iv2_0=Iv[-1]*new_strain_ratio
Iv1_0=Iv[-1]*(1-new_strain_ratio)
I2_0=I[-1]*new_strain_ratio
I1_0=I[-1]*(1-new_strain_ratio)
future_initial_conds_two_strain=(S[-1],
E1_0,
```

Figure 11. Present status of COVID-19 cases across the world

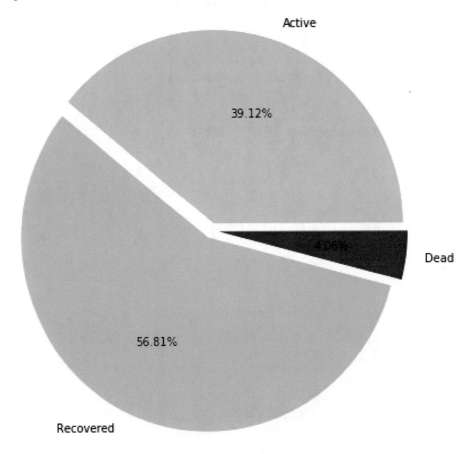

```
I1_0,
Iv1_0,
E2_0,
I2_0,
Iv2_0,
R[-1],
Rv[-1],
D[-1],
Dv[-1])
print('new strain I, Iv',I2_0,Iv2_0)
future_states,future_history=strain2_model.predict(future_t,
future_initial_conds_two_strain)
future_daylies=strain2_model.compute_daily_values(*future_
```

Figure 12. Present status of COVID-19 cases across the world

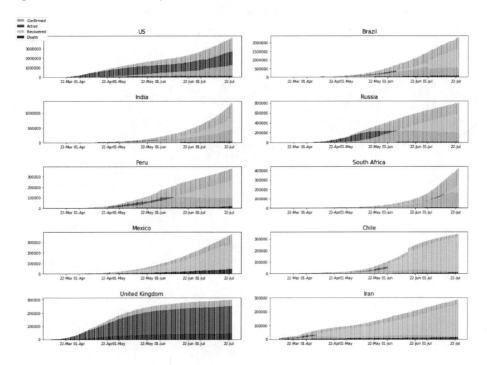

```
states)
returnstrain2_model,future_states,future_history,future_daylies
```

The present status of the COVID-19 cases of the world is shown in the Figure 11.

Figure 13 shows recorded active cases, confirmed cases, recovered and death cases in ten most-affected countries including Brazil, USA, India, United Kingdom, Russia, Peru, Mexico, South Africa, Iran and Chile.

SIR

SIR model is termed as the father of epidemic models, that simulates the progression of an epidemic over time. The population under consideration is distinguished into three categories including: susceptible, infected, and recovered in this model. It is an epidemiological model used to determine the theoretical number for infected people with any contagious illness over a period of time in a closed population environment (gordio, 2020). Coupling equations that relate the following parameters including the numbers of people susceptible $S(t)$, number of infected people $I(t)$,

Figure 13. (a) Confirmed cases, (b) Death cases, and (c) Recovered cases in ten most-affected countries such as Brazil, Peru, USA, India, Chile, Russia, South Africa, United Kingdom, Iran, and Mexico

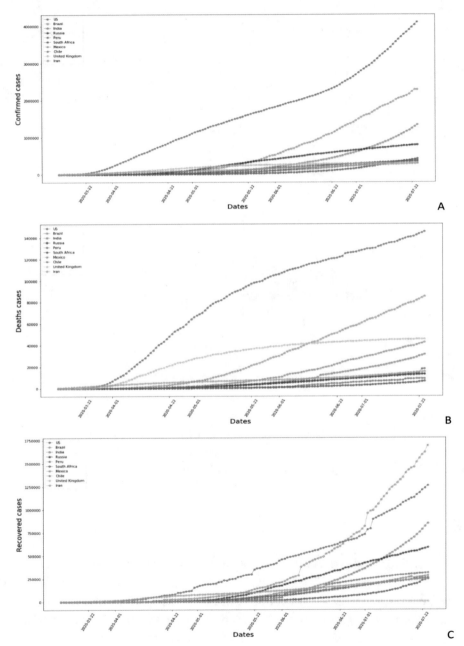

and number of people who have recovered $R(t)$ are used to derive this model class. SIR models are very simple models; one such model is the Kermack-Mckendrick model.

Epidemic Modeling of Multiple Virus Strains: SARS-Cov-2 B.1.1.7

Multiple highly dangerous strains have mutated from the SARS-CoV-2 virus ever since the onset of the worldwide pandemic. Some of these strains were listed as Variants of Concern (VOC) which possess alarming potential to transcend the course of pandemic. The list of most life threatening variants red-flagged by the WHO includes strain termed as B.1.1.7 originating from the regions of United Kingdom, another strain called B.1.351 which was initially found in South Africa and also strain called B.1.1.28.1. Out of these strains, the basic reproduction number of B.1.1.7 strain was reportedly found to be 40% - 90% larger than the base virus SARS-CoV-2 which has rapidly spread worldwide across 130 countries. In combined mutation with the base virus makes B.1.1.7 the most fatal and it is crucial to assess the hazards in advance for developing response strategy. Epidemic modeling has the capacity to provide tools which facilitate planning for optimal response strategies in advance and used to successfully estimate the spread of virus. Particularly, modified SEIR (Susceptible-Exposed-Infectious-Removed) model was found to be simple, effective and capable of performing simulations for complex epidemic situations (Godio, 2020). Several attempts were made for COVID-19 forecasting by applying more advanced machine learning techniques. Lack of sufficient training data and an over-fitting model are some of the reasons for not achieving significant improvements when working with advanced machine learning models. A closed population with N size is used to simulate the implications of an epidemic with the original SEIR model.

The SEIRD (Susceptible-Exposed -Infected - Recovered-Death) model is an extension of SEIR with addition of number of fatalities due to infection (Bae, 2020). The SEIRD model is used in the present chapter as it is more relevant. Results of studies performed with SEIRD model show accurate predictions with nearly negligible (RMSE) root mean square error for several peaks in different countries (Aliyeva, 2021). Researchers have found that the behavior of the model depends largely on the factor R_0 indicator which indicates the average number of people infected by one infected person (Purushotham, 2018). The model has the ability to analyze the real-time input data and also provide with confidence intervals on long-to-short-term predictions (Gupta, 2021). By employing the modified SEIRD model, predictions about the spread of COVID-19 can be made by considering both symptomatic as well as asymptomatic infectious population. Mathematical epidemiologic models can predict the trends and patterns in epidemic trajectory and the potential COVID-19 peak for various scenarios worldwide (Tiwari, 2020). The predictions of SEIRD model regarding infection patterns was observed to be considerably influenced by parameters which dominantly affect the actual trend of infection spread, which include incubation period and transmission rate (Piccolomini, 2020).

The SEIRD epidemic model comprises partitioning the population into five compartments including: Susceptible (S), Exposed (E), Infections (I), Recovered (R) and Deceased (D). Susceptible individuals are the ones most likely to be infected. Exposed are those individuals that have contracted the infection, but are not yet spreading infection causing pathogens. While Infectious ones are already spreading the virus to other individuals. Recovered individuals are considered to be permanently immune to the pathogens. The compartment sizes at time (t) is denoted by the following terms S(t), E(t), I(t), R(t), D(t) combined into ordinary differential equations (ODE) system that explains the population transfer amongst compartments:

$$\frac{dS}{dt} = -\frac{\beta S(t) I(t)}{N}$$

$$\frac{dE}{dt} = \frac{\beta S(t) I(t)}{N} - E(t)$$

$$\frac{dI}{dt} = \delta E(t) - \gamma(1-\alpha) I(t) - \gamma \alpha I(t)$$

$$\frac{dR}{dt} = \gamma(1-\alpha) I(t)$$

$$\frac{dD}{dt} = \gamma \alpha I(t)$$

Subject to initial conditions $\mathbf{S}_0, \mathbf{E}_0, \mathbf{I}_0, \mathbf{R}_0, \mathbf{D}_0$ and the constraint

$$\mathbf{N} = \mathbf{S}(t) + \mathbf{E}(t) + \mathbf{I}(t) + \mathbf{R}(t) + \mathbf{D}(t).$$

The parameters considered for the model are: α, which is the infection fatality rate, β is the number of cases generated in one day due to one infected individual,

$$\delta = \frac{1}{d_{incubation}}$$

Where $d_{incubation}$ is the length of incubation period,

$$\gamma = \frac{1}{d_{inf\ ectious}}$$

Where $d_{infectious}$ is the time in days till recovery or death. The defining characteristic of a pandemic is given by the basic reproduction number $\mathbf{R}_0$. It equals the expected number of people infected by one infectious individual during the course of their sickness and can be computed as follows:

$$R_0 = \frac{\beta}{\gamma}$$

Figure 14. Five compartments for SEIRD epidemic model

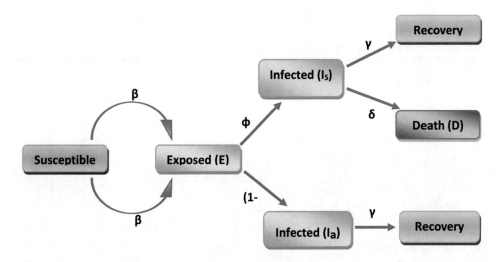

For each date the following statistics are necessary for ML model: new confirmed cases reported, new recoveries recorded, new deaths, all over total confirmed cases, total recoveries, and total deaths. The model is optimized such that predicted new daily infections, deaths and recoveries are brought to be as far as possible closest

Table 4. Parameters of the one-strain model obtained by optimization

Parameter	Values range	Estimated value
R_0	$[3, 5]$	4.782
α	$[5 \times 10^{-3}, 7.9 \times 10^{-3}]$	6.4×10^{-3}
δ	$\left[\dfrac{1}{14}, \dfrac{1}{2}\right]$	$\dfrac{1}{2}$
γ	$\left[\dfrac{1}{14}, \dfrac{1}{7}\right]$	$\dfrac{1}{9}$
p_i	$\left[0.15, 0.3\right]$	0.25
p_d	$\left[0.15, 0.9\right]$	0.35
q_{60}	$\left[0, 1\right]$	0.692
q_{120}	$\left[0, 1\right]$	0.869
q_{180}	$\left[0, 1\right]$	0.715
q_{240}	$\left[0, 1\right]$	0.713
q_{300}	$\left[0, 1\right]$	0.765
q_{360}	$\left[0, 1\right]$	0.761

to recorded statistical data. The Levenberg-Marquardt method (via lmfit library) is used for all optimization tasks in the model. The ranges of possible parameter values are really constrained when using information from COVID-19 studies. The optimized parameters of the one-strain model are tabulated in Table 4.

The resulting training is presented on figure 20. Consider the scenarios for different R_0 values of **B**.1.1.7 as shown in figure 21. For these scenarios we assume that by 2021.01.10, 0.1% of infectious are carrying the **B**.1.1.7 strain the simulation

Figure 15. Various Python libraries used in the present framework

```
In [1]: import numpy as np
        import pandas as pd
        import seaborn as sns
        from matplotlib import pyplot as plt
        from scipy.integrate import odeint
        from sklearn.metrics import mean_absolute_error
        import lmfit
        from tqdm.auto import tqdm
        import pickle
        import joblib
        import matplotlib.dates as mdates
```

Figure 16. Total population infected and population infected per day by COVID-19

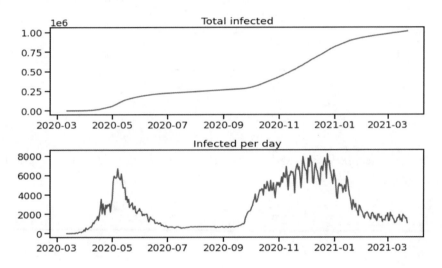

Figure 17. Cumulative deaths as predicted by the classic SEIRD model for COVID-19

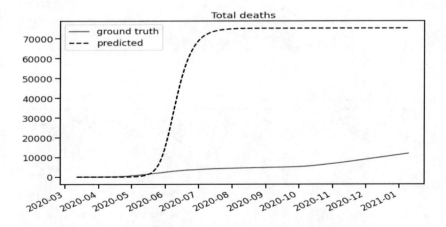

Figure 18. Cumulative death predictions on training data by SEIRD model for COVID-19

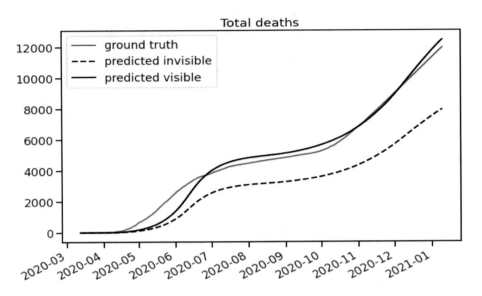

Figure 19. Susceptible-Exposed-Infected-Recovered-Death predictions on training data by SEIRD model for COVID-19

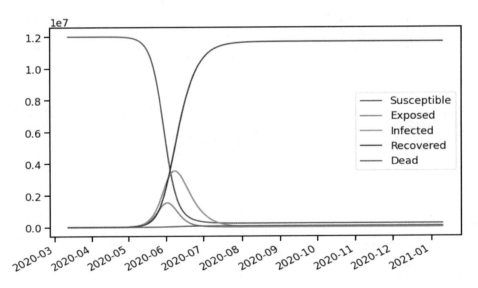

Figure 20. One-strain SEIRD versus the ground truth on training data for COVID-19

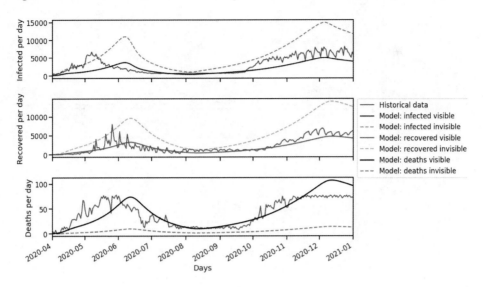

Figure 21. Forecasted scenarios depending on the R_0 of B.1.1.7

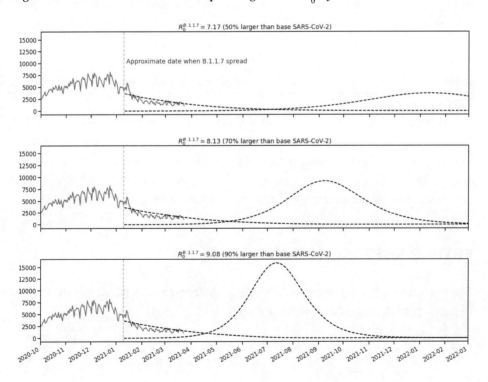

Figure 22. Forecasted scenarios depending on the ratio of new strain

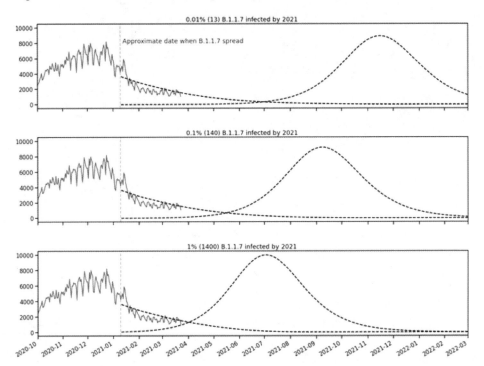

indicates that for any possible $R_0^{B.1.1.7}$ an impending new wave is most likely to happen.

Figure 22 indicates the scenarios for B.1.1.7 strain carriers at 2021.01.10. It is assumed that $R_0^{B.1.1.7} = 8.13$ (which is about 70% greater than the base R_0) for all the scenarios. In the best case, if new case carriers are only 0.01% (13), then new wave peak can be expected in November-December 2021, whereas for 1%(1400) new case carriers, the new wave peak may be expected to occur in July 2021.

FUTURE RESEARCH DIRECTIONS

The Python Program implemented for this chapter can be extended to the healthcare industry considering other critical parameters.

CONCLUSION

This chapter deals with ML- and AutoML implementation in the healthcare industry. It helps researchers for development of a powerful tool in order to enhance the quality of life for humanity. Significant breakthrough technical advancements to augment patient outcomes in the prospects of reduced costs of treatment, high-end diagnoses techniques, shortened duration with effective treatment methods. Python-based models are developed to assess the risk of a new virus strains. Johns Hopkins University's databases for COVID-19 are used in the present work to predict the trends of COVID-19 pandemic for future strains across the world. The proposed SEIRD model has been verified by cross-validation applied to historical data and has found to outperform in comparison with the baselines. The strains of COVID-19 are simulated and forecasted the impact of B.1.1.7strain.

ACKNOWLEDGMENT

This research received no specific grant from any funding agency in the public, commercial, or not-for-profit sectors.

REFERENCES

Akbulut, A., Ertugrul, E., & Topcu, V. (2018). Fetal health status prediction based on maternal clinical history using machine learning techniques. *Computer Methods and Programs in Biomedicine*, *163*, 87–100. doi:10.1016/j.cmpb.2018.06.010 PMID:30119860

Aliyeva, T., Rzayeva, U., & Azizova, R. (2021). SEIRD Model for Control of COVID-19: Case of Azerbaijan. *SHS Web of Conference, Volume 92. The 20th International Scientific Conference Globalization and its Socio-Economic Consequences 2020.*

Bae, T. W., Kwon, K. K., & Kim, K. H. (2020). Mass Infection Analysis of COVID-19 Using the SEIRD Model in Daegu-Gyeongbuk of Korea from April to May 2020. *Journal of Korean Medical Science*, *3*(34), e317. doi:10.3346/jkms.2020.35.e317

Chatterjee, S., Sarkar, A., Karmakar, M., Chatterjee, S., & Paul, R. (2020). SEIRD model to study the asymptomatic growth during COVID-19 pandemic in India. *Indian Journal of Physics.* . doi:10.1007/s12648-020-01928-8

Cheng, V.C., Lau, S.K., Woo, P.C., & Yuen, K.Y. (2007). Severe acute respiratory syndrome coronavirus as an agent of emerging and reemerging infection. *Clinical Microbiology Reviews*, *20*(4), 660–694.

Escobar, J. D., Guillén, N. E. O., Reyes, S. V., Mosqueda, A. G., Kober, V., Rodriguez, R. R., & Rizk, J. E. L. (2021). Deep-learning based detection of COVID-19 using lung ultrasound imagery. *PLOS global. Public Health*, *16*(8), e0255886. Advance online publication. doi:10.1371/journal.pone.0255886

Godio, A., Pace, F., & Vergnano, A. (2020). SEIR Modeling of the Italian Epidemic of SARS-CoV-2 Using Computational Swarm Intelligence. *International Journal of Environmental Research and Public Health*, *2020*(17), 3535. doi:10.3390/ijerph17103535 PMID:32443640

Guleria, P., Ahmed, S., Alhumam, A., & Srinivasu, P. N. (2022). Empirical Study on Classifiers for Earlier Prediction of COVID-19 Infection Cure and Death Rate in the Indian States. *Health Care*, *10*(1), 85. https://doi.org/10.3390/healthcare10010085

Gupta,, A., Gupta, S., & Katarya, R. (2021). InstaCovNet-19: A deep learning classification model for the detection of COVID-19 patients using Chest X-ray. *Applied Soft Computing*, *99*, 106859.

Hassantabar, S., Ahmadi, M., & Sharifi, A. (2020). Diagnosis and detection of infected tissue of COVID-19 patients based on lung x-ray image using convolution neural network approaches. *Chaos, Solitons and Fractals-Nonlinear Science, and Non-equilibrium and Complex Phenomena*, *140*, 110170. PMID:32834651

Luz, C. F., Vollmer, M., Decruyenaere, J., Nijsten, M. W., Glasner, C., & Sinha, B. (2020). Machine learning in infection management using routine electronic health records: Tools, techniques, and reporting of future technologies. *Clinical Microbiology and Infection*, *26*(10), 1291–1299. doi:10.1016/j.cmi.2020.02.003 PMID:32061798

Maher, A., Majdalawieh, M., & Nizamuddin, N. (2021). Modeling and forecasting of COVID-19 using a hybrid dynamic model based on SEIRD with ARIMA corrections. *Infectious Disease Modelling*, *6*, 98–111.

Muhammad, L. J., Algehyne, E. A., Usman, S. S., Ahmad, A., Chakraborty, C., & Mohammed, I. A. (2021). Supervised Machine Learning Models for Prediction of COVID-19 Infection using Epidemiology Dataset. *SN Computer Science*, *2*, 11.

Mustafa, A., & Azghadi, M.R. (2021). *Automated Machine Learning for Healthcare and Clinical Analysis*. Academic Press.

Piccolomini, E. L., & Zama, F. (2020). Monitoring Italian COVID-19 spread by a forced SEIRD model. *PLOS One, Global Health*. doi:10.1371/journal.pone.0237417

Prabhu, A. J., Sengan, S., Kamalam, G. K., Vellingiri, J., Jagadeesh, G., Velayutham, P., & Subramaniyaswamy, V. (2020, October). Medical information retrieval systems for e-Health care records using fuzzy based machine learning model. *Microprocessors and Microsystems*, *17*, 103344.

Purushotham, S., Meng, C., Chea, Z., & Liua, Y. (2018). Benchmarking deep learning models on large healthcare datasets. *Journal of Biomedical Informatics*, *83*, 112–134.

Qureshi, K. N., Din, S., Jeon, G., & Piccialli, F. (2020). An accurate and dynamic predictive model for a smart M-Health system using machine learning. *Information Sciences*, *538*, 486–502. doi:10.1016/j.ins.2020.06.025

Sustersic, T., Blagojevic, A., Cvetkovic, D., Cvetkovic, A., Lorencin, I., Segota, S. B., Milovanovic, D., Baskic, D., Car, Z., & Filipovic, N. (2021, October). Epidemiological Predictive Modeling of COVID-19 Infection: Development, Testing, and Implementation on the Population of the Benelux Union. *Frontiers in Public Health*, *28*, 727274. Advance online publication. doi:10.3389/fpubh.2021.727274 PMID:34778171

Thomas, M. (2021). *Machine Learning in Healthcare*. https://builtin.com/artificial-intelligence/machine-learning-healthcare

Tiwari, V., Deyal, N., & Bish, T. N. S. (2020). Mathematical Modeling Based Study and Prediction of COVID-19 Epidemic Dissemination Under the Impact of Lockdown in India. *Frontiers Physics*. doi:10.3389/fphy.2020.586899

Venkatramanana, S., Lewis, B., Chen, J., Higdon, D., Vullikanti, A., & Marathe, M. (2018). Using data-driven agent-based models for forecasting emerging infectious diseases. *Epidemics*, *22*, 43–49.

WHO. (2019). *WHO's Country Office in the People's Republic of China picked up a media statement by the Wuhan Municipal Health Commission from their website on cases of 'viral pneumonia' in Wuhan, People's Republic of China*. https://www.who.int/

Xu, X., Jiang, X., Mac, C., Dud, P., Li, X., Lv, S., Yu, L., Ni, Q., Chen, Y., Su, J., Lang, G., Li, Y., Zhao, H., Liu, J., Xu, K., Ruan, L., Sheng, J., Qiu, Y., Wua, W., ... Li, L. (2020). A Deep Learning System to Screen Novel Coronavirus Disease 2019 Pneumonia. *Engineering*, *6*, 1122–1129.

Chapter 8

Topical Repute on Artificial Intelligence–Based Approaches in COVID–19 Supervision:
Distinct Kingpin on Drug Re-Purposing Blueprint

Shamayita Basu
University of Kalyani, India

Jana Shafi
ⓘ https://orcid.org/0000-0001-6859-670X
Prince Sattam bin Abdul University, Saudi Arabia

ABSTRACT

The ongoing COVID-19 pandemic has led to a major oppression of worldwide healthcare infrastructure. In current times, artificial intelligence (AI) and network medicine provide groundbreaking implementation of information science in defining diseases, therapeutics, medicines, and in associating targets with the minimum fallacy. In this big data era, artificial intelligence (AI) has immensely reduced the time and investment of novel targeted drug discovery. As there is continual unfolding of the results of the possible drug combinations, exploitation of artificial intelligence is of utmost necessity so as to hone combination therapy plan. Drug repositioning or repurposing is a methodology by means of which subsisting drugs are being manipulated to handle challenging and emerging diseases, including COVID-19. In this chapter, the authors present the regulations on how to use AI to expedite drug repurposing or repositioning, for which AI propositions are not only intimidating but are also inevitable.

DOI: 10.4018/978-1-6684-3791-9.ch008

INTRODUCTION

Currently, Coronavirus Disease 2019 (COVID-19) outbreak, engendered by severe acute respiratory syndrome coronavirus 2 (SARS-CoV-2), has eventually ushered to major oppression of global healthcare infrastructure. The emergence of this novel coronavirus SARS-CoV-2, also known as the 2019-nCoV, has brought about 2.81 million established infection victims. Even more than 193,825 patients succumbed to the coronavirus disease 2019 (COVID-19), which affected 210 countries and territories, while the death tally is sharply climbing up till now. The SARS-CoV-2 was for the first time reported in Wuhan, China, and, very soon afterward, human-to-human communication was reported accompanied by a worldwide pandemic, declared by WHO on Marc 11, 202020. A large proportion of Corona-affected persons reportedly showed respiratory manifestations and fever, and even death in some severe, complicated cases (Hui et al., 2020). Many clinical study reports continue to manage COVID-19 with prospective elderly drugs and explore novel drugs. In fast rectifying the present pandemic situation with some more medicinal restores, remodeling old drugs are among the hugely appreciated strategies.

An Artificial Intelligence (AI) system may be a potential means of quickly screening the huge number of substances with allotted learning datasets and identifying drugs for discrete impetus like therapy of COVID-19 infected patients showing desirable efficacy. The confirmed AI system scrutinized the utmost key signifiers, gave rise to significant predictive models, carried out identification and testing of the commercialized drugs to promptly pinpoint those drugs that can inhibit SARS-CoV-2. A cell model (in-vitro) presenting the replication of this cunning coronavirus was instituted to assess the drugs identified by AI for authentication of antiviral activity. Some present studies recognized that Machine Learning and Artificial Intelligence are optimistic technologies preferred by healthcare providers because they are trustworthy and guarantee improved scale-up, acceleration of processing power, and even surpassing humans in some particular healthcare tasks (Phillips-Wren et al., 2008). Henceforth, various clinicians and healthcare industries hired many ML and AI technology to get hold of this outrageous pandemic and address the various difficulties and challenges that are an integral part of the outbreak. In the medical industries, AI is mostly applied not to supplement human interactions but to inform clinicians about what they are geared for (M. Tayarani-N et al., 2015). During the coronavirus outbreak, a group of actions was pioneered by China to combat the spread of COVID-19 y endorsing a few AI-based technologies. Due to this process, they traversed the implementation of various ideas, such as using specialized cameras that can carry out recognition via the face to track the infected patient's drones for disinfecting places exposed to the virus (Browning et al., 2021). These robots can deliver food, medications, necessary items, and many more. There have been many different fields for applications of these recent and new AI approaches to tackle and reduce the adverse effects of this deadly disease.

Such applications include clinical applications, processing the images regarding covid-19, and epidemiological and pharmaceutical studies. Besides, we have also tried to organize and present the study rooted in various Artificial Intelligence techniques adopted. The most important categorization is centered around the applications; however, the research is subdivided for the same application, depending on the various AI approaches they have applied. The most common examples of AI approaches are machine learning, deep learning, evolutionary algorithms, and Artificial Neural Networks. Employment of AI-based ideas and techniques for developing novel drugs has allured the heed since the initial phase of this outbreak. The abilities and potentials of AI to discover newer molecules have been immensely executed in research. For a long time, AI approaches have been implemented with the aim of the development of treatment and diagnostic systems. In the current scenario, the pandemic has given rise to a whole new obstacle for this area of science. The development of intelligent methodologies and systems that may assist practitioners in monitoring, diagnosing, and forecasting patient parameters and propounding treatment protocols may be very useful for the healthcare system, which is already under immense pressure amidst this global pandemic.

AI AND ML EXPLOITED TO STABILISE HEALTH CARE SYSTEM AMIDST COVID-19 OUTBREAK

Recently, AI and ML technology have been implemented to improve the prediction accuracy for screening of infectious(COVID-19) and non-infectious diseases (Ruiz Estrada et al., 2020; Guleria P et al., 2022). The relationship between AI and health care begins with developing the first-ever maestro set up called MYCIN in 1976 (Agrebi et al., 2020). MYCIN is designed to utilize 450 rules obtained from an expert in the medical field to treat and cure bacterial infections by giving antibiotics to affected patients. The expert system serves as the clinical resolution bear for the medical experts and the clinicians (Shortliffe et al., 1976). Recent findings that are apparent on the scopes of ML and AI technologies for various previous pandemic outbreaks suggest that these AI aspects support the worldwide healthcare experts in different communicable disease manifestations like EBOLA, SARS, COVID-19, HIV (Peiffer-Smadja et al., 2019, Barbat et al., 2019, Li et al., 2020, Shang et al., 2014, Gao et al., 2017, Colibri et al., 2019, Choi et al., 2017, Nápoles et al., 2014, Chockanathan et al., 2019, Toğaçar et al., 2020, Vaka et al., 2020); also, non-communicable disorders (Stroke, Cancer, Heart disease, Diabetes) (Saxena et al.,

2020, Nazir et al., 2019, Kavakiotis et al., 2017, Sharma et al., 2020, Lalmuanawma et al., 2020, Liu et al., 2019) outbreak too.

Treatment

One of the most important areas of AI applications to deal with pandemic problems is the procedures being put forward to treat COVID-19 disease. A method that measures and analyzes the differences and similarities between the treatment protocols has been proposed (Dourado Jr et al., 2019). It is very useful for predicting the patients' recovery and cure since it can guide choice makers to align the resources. Three machine learning techniques are being used (Pu et al., 2020) to predict and survey the patients' recovery. SVM, ANN, and regression models are being implemented to set up and organize the intelligent system (Naga, S.P. et al., 2020). The ability of AI to forecast the progression and course of any disease is investigated. Scientists are using three ML algorithms and one deep learning model to effectively build an algorithm that can predict whether a particular patient may show fatal symptoms that require oxygen. An AI-related multi-strategic decision-analysis algorithm has been put forward to process the patients on their health parameters (Hassanien et al., 2020). The methodology utilizes a group of information that includes laboratory procedures. Patients recently exposed to the virus and subsequently recovered are already harboring antibodies to fight against the virus that is transmitting throughout their bloodstream., In the selection of. One ML algorithm has been used in the election-making method to select the most suitable plasma donor and prioritize patients (Obinata et al., 2020).

Diagnosis

RT-PCR, together with the sequencing of DNA and its identification being the current testing method, takes a long time (mostly more than 24hours) to be available and is an expensive method (roughly around 3000 INR per patient sample). Some of the rapid tests based on IgM/IgG antibody levels in the patients' serum have also been used. Still, they reportedly have low sensitivity and specificity, which often leads to unwanted false-positive results and are not trustworthy. In some research, without using these RT-PCR techniques or the CT scan images, Artificial Intelligence methodologies are being used to diagnose this disease. To construct an even more precise diagnostic paradigm for covid-19, related to various signs among the patients and the routine laboratory test results, ML algorithms are implemented with the data from approximately 151 published findings (Albahri et al., 2020). Besides, various machine learning algorithms are being implemented to successfully undertake the clinical data collected from patients to perform the diagnosis (O. S et al., 2020). For improving the accuracy of diagnostics for clinical impetus, recently, an AI-dependent mainstream diagnosis intimates being initiated (Li et al., 2020).

On the other hand, a new machine learning algorithm has been proposed that aggregates data obtained from patients currently undergoing hemodialysis because of renal failure and speculates the probability of patients suffering from undetected cases of covid-19 disease (Feng et al. 2021). An AI algorithm (Peng et al., 2020) that utilizes clinical symptoms, CT scan images, laboratory testing, and history of exposure and detects and diagnoses suspected covid-19 cases have been reported. Relevant data were collected from about 905 patients, amongst which data of 419 patients indicated only laboratory-confirmed positive instances. For applications and CRISPER-based nucleic acid detection, experimental resources and assay designs may be hired for prevailing surveillance (Monaghan et al., 2020). The scientists have exploited machine learning algorithms intending to contribute assay designs for detecting approximately 67 viral species and subspecies of the SARS-CoV-2. Contingent forest units are also being utilized to consign covid-19 patients (Mei et al., 2020). ML algorithms may be effectively used for processing the patients' signs and symptoms to diagnose patients affected with Covid-19 (Metsky et al., 2020). The signs are evaluated by asking some of the basic questions to the patients. Mobile phones may effectively serve as a potential platform to develop AI methodologies for diagnosis. They are available on a large scale. They can also gather a major proportion of facts and figures from people, starting right from symptoms to behavior and travel. Besides, they also may apprise people from the face of any kind of risk that they might face. An AI-related algorithm that functions on the cloud has been administered in a mobile phone app (Chen et al., 2020) that surveys people's coughs to identify corona cases.

Monitoring COVID-19 Patients

Due to various limitations on the resources, most hospitals have not successfully contributed tracking, analysis, and treatment services that are needed for every patient showcasing fatal and severe signs and symptoms. Concerning this, the prediction of mortality or recovery rate of the patients is of utmost importance since this information can help the hospitals distribute the medical amenities more effectively. For the classification of data collected from the patients of South Korea, a neural network methodology is being used (Zoabi et al., 2020). This algorithm successfully predicts the recovered and the death cases found in hospitals. A randomized forest codification algorithm has been employed (Imran et al., 2020) to recognize the important soothsayers and their influence on the mortality rate among hospitals. An indistinct classifier is suggested to assess disease and predict the mortality rate among the covid-19 patients as obtained from their biomarkers (Al-Najjar et al.,

2020). Data obtained from approximately 117,000 patients worldwide are being extensively used for generating an AI methodology to predict the mortality chance of the patients affected with covid-19 (de Moraes Batista et al., 2020). In totality, five ML algorithms, including support vector machine, logistic regression, random forest, KNN, and gradient boosting algorithms, have been exploited to anticipate the mortality toll of the confirmed covid-19 affected patients of South Korea (Gemmar et al., 2020). A machine learning perspective is presented to effectively predict a patient's recovery (Pourhomayoun et al., 2020). Support vector machine (SVM) algorithm, regression model, and ANN are utilized to finally build this model. A refined and randomized Forest model uplifted by the AdaBoost algorithm has been dispensed (DAS et al., 2,020), wielding the patients' geographical, demographic, travel, and health data for predicting the lethality of cases and also the possible consequences, death or recovery.

Some researchers used five ML algorithms- elastic net, logistic regression, partial lowest square regression, bagged flexible discriminant analysis, and random forest to exercise the patients' details findings and speculate mortality chances for patients (S et al., 2020). Some machine learning techniques, including KNN, SVM, and Random Forest, are implemented to construct an accurate model that effectively predicts patient mortality (Iwendi et al., 2020, Hu et al., 2020). On the other hand, in another similar venture (Thorsen-Meyer et al., 2020), a different machine learning algorithm has been presented to forecast mortality and most of the critical events in New York. A multi-dimensional logistic regression incorporated with a facet selection algorithm may be used to diagnose and identify patients at risk to develop lethal covid-19 (An et al., 2020). A proper chassis is being accorded for some fresh edge traits in the Graph Neural Networks through an amalgamation of self-inspected and uninspected learning, which is exploited for node classification tasks (Vaid et al., 2020). This system predicts the infection and fatality of this viral disease among the patients. A deep learning algorithm and a multivariate logistic regression are used to predict the chances of any patient having mild symptoms of developing future malignant infection (Yao et al., 2021). For anticipating the survival analysis and the time of discharge rooted in the clinical statistics, some of the ML algorithms are being utilized by scientists (Sehanobish et al., 2020). Such data includes different features such as symptoms, gender, travel history, and chronic disease history. The researchers have used Support Vector Machines, Component-wise Gradient Boosting, and Stage-wise Gradient Boosting. An XG Boost ML algorithm to predict the severity of patients is used (Bai et al., 2020). This model exploits mainly three clinical features, lactic dehydrogenase dyspnea, Highly sensitive C-reactive protein (CRP), lymphocyte, from the basin of above 300 features.

EMPLOYING AI FOR X-RAY IMAGE PROCESSING AND CHEST COMPUTED TOMOGRAPHY

For treatment of the COVID-19 patients and also to isolate them, early identification is crucial alongside control of the virus spread. Hence, many researchers have put immense effort into developing techniques and methods that may potentially identify the patients even more promptly and are costly to a lesser extent. The system for standardized testing, i.e., Reverse transcription (RT) - polymerase chain reaction (RT-PCR) technique, is not only time taking but also gives quite a limited supply. The X-Ray images and chest Computed Tomography (CT) scan in corona-affected persons are some alternative screening methods that bestow valuable information regarding patients' status. But, virus-caused pneumonia, a common complication of COVID-19, frequently exhibits various visual pretensions such as reports and images. In such scenarios, AI may be of considerable help in these image processing protocols (Goh et al., 2020, Zhu et al., 2020, Ke et al., 2020).

CONTROLLING AND MONITORING THE PANDEMIC THROUGH THE WORLD OF AI AND MI

The AI world can contribute in many different ways in monitoring the pandemic and its effect on various sectors of human society. Cross-breed cellular automata have been reportedly proposed that may predict effects of the pandemic concerning the number of deaths, count of people affected, and recovered (Pyzer-Knapp et al., 2020). An ML algorithm is also proposed to study and analyze the effects of humidity, temperature, and wind speed on several infected people (Ge et al., 2021). It has been suggested that a modest contrary link between the daily count and temperature of the infections has taken place. The impending effect of this outrageous pandemic in tourism has also been researched (Mohanty et al., 2020). In this concern, the neural network of Prolonged Short Term Memory has been calibrated for gears of this pandemic.

For tackling and keeping this pandemic under control, it has been an absolute necessity to retain the reproduction rate at a minimum. Machine learning techniques are increasingly being used to develop an application to trace the contacts (Nemanti et al., 2020). This exercise automatically records communications between people and shows a self-evaluation device to scan and analyze the symptoms. An ML simulating algorithm is proposed to detect and prevent further spread of this pandemic and foretell the upcoming epidemic of our future, and for constructive contact tracing (Yan et al., 2020). It is of utmost importance to inspect and monitor society to tackle the transmission of this gruesome disease. A call-rooted dialog proxy is hired for active monitoring (Sharma et al., 2020). An AI-rooted idea for the sake of enhanced mobilization blueprint for mobile computation envoys for these outbreaks is demonstrated (Kundu et al., 2020). This blueprint is skilled by utilizing data obtained from ancient mobile crowdsensing campaigns. A cheaper blockchain and Artificial Intelligence-related self-diagnostics tracing machinery for this disease have been put forward (Neri et al., 2020).

SIGNIFICANT ROLE OF AI IN MANAGEMENT OF THE OUTCOMES OF COVID-19 PANDEMIC

This outrageous COVID-19 pandemic has caused some unprecedented challenges and obstacles for the value and operators in the grid. Due to prolonged lockdowns and several curtailments, shifting the power expenditure profiles worldwide has occurred in pattern and magnitude. This eventually led to strains in load prophesy. Contemporary and conventional algorithms hire timing and weather details and the magnitude of the old intake as input variables; because of this pandemic, all such quantifications have failed to explain these upcoming new patterns. Portability is used to apprehend this brand behavior (Kolozsvari et al., 2021) as means of economic functions. This work utilizes ML algorithms to manufacture the predictive system. An ANN model and a comparative regressive model have been developed to inspect the adverse consequences of covid-19 on petroleum and electricity in China (Zheng et al., 2020). AI aids are being used to help the welfare trusts deal with the problems faced during this ongoing pandemic (Khan et al., 2020). An AI algorithm has been proposed that effectively optimizes all the library services and resource allocation amid this pandemic (Kumar et al., 2020). This pandemic has also made our legal system suffer and face difficulty delivering the required service (justice to the victims on time). Many different AI approaches like the Ross intelligence, natural language processing, and machine learning are being widely used to produce techniques such as stilted lawyers. These emerged difficulties have immensely elevated pressure to bring intelligent institutions to assist our country's justice system. Many different ways have been implemented, like using AI to assist and manage the obstacles produced by this pandemic (Moftakhar et al., 2020). A repetitive neural network has been put forward (Pokkuluri et al., 2020) for detecting swindling transactions throughout this pandemic. An AI-based methodology is being proposed to analyze the current increase in the price of crude oil as a result of the impact of this pandemic (Abdollahi et al., 2020). Besides this, the demand for fuel also plunged amidst this pandemic, and in several cases, oil prices went fatalistic.

An ML-based replica is recently showcased, which utilizes instructions such as trip and travel ventures and fuel and constructs a dummy to extrapolate the

USA medium period command for gasoline and the impact of many government interventions (Polyzos et al., 2021). Again, this pandemic caused immense upshot on the psychological aggravations that include under and unemployment, fear of being unmasked to the virus and thereby becoming infected, helplessness, hopelessness, physical and social isolation from near ones, and insufficient psychological support. The immense adverse effects of covid-19 on people's mental health from almost all over the world are explored (Pandey et al., 2022) to abet the policymakers in creating various actionable policies. Another set of AI-based methodologists is projected to manage these psychological effects post this pandemic (Hashem et al., 2020). To understand the regular lifestyle, mental health, and learning styles, different activities of the younger students of our country, India, the course of this pandemic, an ML algorithm is employed (Lee et al., 2020). ML algorithms are utilized to detect all parameters having a plausible effect on people's mental health during this outbreak (Simsek et al., 2020). For example, some of the key factors known to affect mental health are identified using a Bayesian Network deduction.

On the other hand, the decision regarding the transplant of kidneys amidst this scenario is arguably known to be an enigma. In this regard, a machine learning algorithm has been proposed (Mashamba-Thompson et al., 2020), which reportedly accomplishes the decision-making procedure between the instantaneous transplant versus the hindrance of the end of the pandemic. Pathways that dispatch instruments and appliances for stroke patients are also absolutely pressurized because of this pandemic. As a result, the already existing pathways must be realigned both within and between the hospitals. An AI-rooted algorithm has been put forward to the Royal Berkshire Hospital to manage this hitch (Chen et al., 2020).

CORRELATING AI WITH PHARMACEUTICAL STUDIES

Innovation of an effective drug may help significantly diminish the mortality toll of COVID-19. Protocols for treatment of this disease constitute mainly three investigational methods, repurposing therapies generally remdesivir and vaccine development. Repurposing those drugs that have already been reported to show several side effects in treating this disease is a promising and important aspect in developing these new therapeutic strategies. In some ongoing research, AI approaches are being used in pharmaceutical studies to battle against covid-19. As the COVID-19 pandemic continues to grow vigorously, it is claimed that the capabilities of AI may be earnestly harnessed in this process of drug repurposing and screening (Norouzi et al., 2020, Johnstone et al., 2020).

Repurposing the Drugs

The entire process of drug revelation is high-peril, tedious, costly, and lengthy. (Nawaz et al., 2020). As per the ERG (Eastern Research Group) report, the success rate is roughly 2.01% only, while it requires approximately 10-15 long years to generate a novel molecular unit (Chandra et al., 2020). The entire concept behind drug redesigning re-employs the older drugs to treat a first-time ever-contemplated therapeutic manifestation. It is nothing but a theoretical approach to recognize an already shelved, approved, discontinued, and inspectional therapeutics for approved reiteration to treat various other manifestations of the disease. Traditional development of drugs generally includes mainly five phases: (i) innovation; growth, (ii) before clinical research, (iii) major aspects of clinical research, (iv) FDA's critique, and (v) monitoring of commercial welfare and production by FDA.

Nonetheless, four such steps are in practice in case of repurposing of the drug: (i) identifying compound (ii) compound accretion, (iii) clinical research (iv) monitoring and developing post-market security by FDA (Bildirici et al., 2020). A repositioned drug jumps directly to the stage of preclinical phase testing and clinical trials, thereby excluding early phase steps, hence tailing down many dangers and considerably reducing costs. Elementary principles in the process of drug repurposing lie in a familiar molecular alley that is correlated and also amenable for many different disease manifestations as well as a horde of crystal clear information, hospitable on the articulation, pharmacology, dose, drug toxicity, and also data of clinical tribunal of approved, authorized, delayed or ceased drugs (Ou et al., 2020).

Artificial intelligence (AI) is the general ability of machines to perform tasks that generally require human intelligence, such as to perceive, recognize, reason, plan, or take action. ML is a subset of AI that involves the capabilities of machines to learn from data without explicit programming. Further, a subset of ML methods called DL uses artificial neural networks to determine more complex structures and pattern data. These AI systems are employed for drug repurposing of already approved drugs, novel drug discovery, and vaccine development for COVID-19 therapeutics (Li et al., 2020).

COVID-19 Drug Repurposing

"Repurposing" of drugs in this chapter raises usage of already existing ratified drugs treatment of a first-ever contemplated therapeutic manifestation – which, herein, is Coronavirus. The revelation and expansion of the advanced molecular structures are getting protracted, lingering, and highly expensive for the clinical litigations to receive auditing authorizations or retributions. The brief passage to successful and effective treatment is the repositioning or repurposing of induced and approved

Figure 1. Artificial intelligence

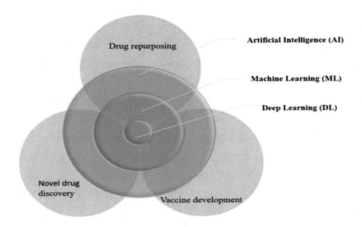

drugs only for Corona infection treatment. In this regard, Chloroquine (CQ) and its structural analog-Hydroxychloroquine (HCQ), are reportedly utilized for treating viral infections. All such drugs also have anti-malarial properties and are known to be an effective treatment of COVID-19 in-vitro (Hossain et al., 2020). Likewise, Remdesivir (antiviral drug), predominantly utilized to treat Ebola viral infection, has also been exposed to fruitful effects in-vitro against COVID-19. An adenosine congener integrates into the incipient viral RNA chains, subsequently showing in early conclusion (Khattar et al., 2020). Ritonavir, along with Lopinavir, is being used for therapeutic assistance of COVID-19 sufferers. These agents are mainly reported to affect the process of proteolysis in the replicative cycle of the coronavirus (Jha et al., 2020). Ribavirin is a counterpart of ribonucleic acid and acts as a force of hindrance for RNA polymerization. This drug has been announced in preclinical studies to show activity in vitro against this SARS-CoV-2 virus (Massie et al., 2020).

Moreover, Tocilizumab, a known immunosuppressant, also is being used in China for the in-vivo treatment and superintendence of COVID-19 patients. Tocilizumab is solely recruited to guide rheumatoid arthritis detected among corona patients. Tocilizumab contentedly attenuates mostly clinical symptoms and signs of this infection. Still, the total number of patients scrutinized for the study came out to be a handful (Nagaratnam et al., 2020). In Japan, a drug having anti-flu characteristics has reportedly revealed significant and evident outcomes in the clinical trials of about 340 patients (Ho et al., 2020). Again, this same drug in China has been considered to treat Influenza virus infection and proved to be well organized against many types of viruses together with COVID-19. Correspondingly, Vitamin C or ascorbic acid coalescence with the antiviral compound has reportedly proved to be benevolent in treating patients positive for COVID-19.

AI Procedures Proposed for Repurposing Drugs

Major encumbrance in drug repositioning strategy has been verifying identifying the idiosyncratic drug-disease alliance. To inscribe such concern, various procedures are expanded, comprising computational propositions, hypothetical biological protocols, and variegated propositions. Accordingly, probabilities are there that implementation of AI methods in the drug invention is attainable (Sonntag et al., 2020). Scientists found various analogies among COVID-19 and 2003 SARS viruses. Depending on these data, which led to SARS, various models for AI research may be generated to apprehend drug structures that may potentially treat COVID-19 (DiMasi et al., 2011). Despite effectively pronounced repurposed drugs, a requirement for acknowledging an increasing number of repurposed drugs is required (Carter et al., 2016). AI and ML may succour this stratagem by briskly discerning drugs with sufficiency against this virus and hence conquer any barricade between huge figures of the drugs that are repurposed, laboratory or scientific appraising; also eventual approbation of a drug. Ejected by various health organizations and companies, a considerable volume of information is approachable on many open platforms (Xue et al., 2018). AI contains a subset called ML that uses a factual plan of action and the ability to grasp with or even without getting amended via an extraneous customer. ML is fractionated into unconquered, reinforcement, and supervised training (Ngo et al., 2016).

AI Models (Algorithms) used in Drug Repurposing Blueprint

Deep Learning Architecture

Deep learning is a subunit of machine learning(ML,) referring to the paragon of data exploration with different layers of non-linear and linear transformations assembled in a hierarchical pattern (Rolain et al., 2007). The most commonly employed deep learning version is artificial neural networks(ANNs). The building wodge is an artificial neuron responsible for non-linearly transforming the encumbered sum of input facet variables. Another architecture is a Fully connected feedforward neural network (FNN), wherein artificial neurons have been associated layer after layer starting from the input facets up to the output targets. There is a correlation of weight with each interconnection. Optimization is done by cutting down prognostic forfeiture of the output targets on coaching specimens via backpropagation. (Gautret et al., 2020) FNNs are peculiarly used to motivate data specimens that are constituted as vectors. Scientists (Guida et al., 2020) employed FNN to classify the drugs in various pharmaceutical and therapeutic groups hinged on the courses of transcriptome profile of the drugs. Lenselink and colleagues (Jagtap et al., 2020) collated the presentation of a unique algorithmic set based on the molecule's divination and target functioning in connection with the ChEMBL database. FNN may execute even better execution when compared to ordinary ML techniques, viz logistic deterioration. (Onder et al., 2020)

In those cases, where images are being captured, and each element becomes a trademark variable, the FNNs have emerged as impracticable since the symbol of weights reportedly is way too huge. Nevertheless, the intricacy neural network (the CNN team) is exceptionally acceptable for image processing. Instead of fully bridging neurons in abutting layers, CNN utilizes strainers (tiny spreadsheets of weights) that register contortion operation on the local specks of images, which immensely diminishes the number of weights. CNN is being utilized to study chemical images and attain intuition into therapeutic drug tasks. (Chan et al., 2013, Chan et al., 2015)

Graph Representation Learning

A superior way of repurposing drugs is via network medicine, which involves building up medical knowledge histograms and relationships between various medical bodies (e.g., diseases, proteins, and drugs) and comes up with novel links between the already existing ones sanctioned diseases like COVID-19 and drugs. Methodologies grounded on a graph submerging are procuring notice for predicting links within graphs (Mohs et al., 2017), which put forward edges and nodes in the form of low-dimensional facet points. Utilizing these facet vectors of diseases and drugs, their similarities can be easily measured, and hence identification of these effective drugs may be made for any particular disease. A limitation of this embedding method for the graphs is that of scalability. Knowledge of real-world histograms is generally huge. The figure of units in a knowledge graph in a medical context could even be up to millions. Some already existing ML networks like Py-Torch and TensorFlow are predominantly sketched for data and general construction but not meant for huge-spectrum histograms. Henceforth, various networks that focus on learning from huge-scale graphs are generated. Scientist Zhu and colleagues (Gns et al., 2019, Chenthamarakshan et al., 2020, Paul et al., 2010, Mak et al., 2019) generated a high-concert system named GraphVite that has the potential to be promising for repurposing of the drugs for future purposes, because this system may effectively undertake up to approximately hundreds and millions of the nodes.

Abbreviations are as below:

- AI=artificial intelligence.
- PARP1=poly-ADP-ribose polymerase

Figure 2. Overviewing use of algorithms of AI-associated repurposing of the drug for COVID-19, for drug remodification, which is cost-effective and rapid for discovering novel therapy procedures for various emerging diseases

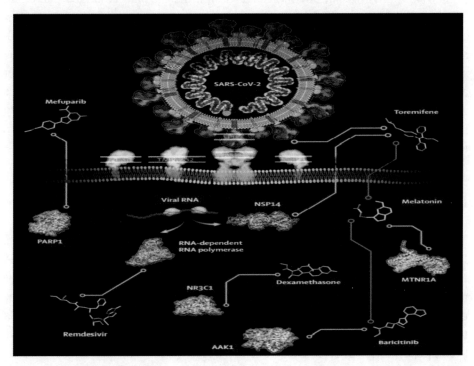

- NR3C1=nuclear receptor subfamily 3 group C member
- AAK1=AP2-associated protein kinase
- MTNR1A=melatonin receptor
- TMPRSS2=transmembrane serine protease
- ACE2=angiotensin I converting enzyme
- NRP1=neuropilin
- NSP14=non-structural protein 14. (Zhou et al., 2020)

STUDYING DRUG DISCOVERY TECHNIQUES USING AI

It has been discussed in a few find how an AI-aided prognostication may help come about new drugs against the disease. In one of the studies (Mohanty et al., 2020), an LSTM framework is skilled to peruse a SMILES thumbprint of a particular molecule and anticipate IC50 of that very molecule while getting bound to RdRp. The replica is instructed to utilize the binding facts and figures of IC50 from the PDB database of about 310,000 chemical compounds having drug-like properties from the ZINC database. The methodology is applied to perceive a contender therapeutic molecule to manage this virus. An Aw molecular design master plan is lodged (Ke et al., 2020), utilizing the AI algorithm to come across therapeutic biological molecules against covid19. The system manipulates the Monte Carlo Tree hunt algorithm with a syndicate ANN substitute model. A substructure is submitted that merges the adjustable pre-preparatory phase of a minuscule SMILES Differential Autoencoder and a multi-accredit superintended sampling venture (Beck et al., 2020). The procedure utilizes information from ascribing diviners trained on quiescent properties. A protein binding rapport prognosticator is being utilized in this project to gene optimal and novel therapeutic compounds for obscured viral-specific targets.

DISCOVERING POTENTIAL DRUGS

To locate and find prospective therapeutic drugs against this disease (Ekins et al., 2020), an athenaeum of 1,670 different compounds was pressed via deep learning. A DNN was utilized (Arora et al., 2020) to forage for host-target intervening antivirals among the approved and experimental drugs with inherent activity to combat the disease. The algorithm explores the designation of gene expression of molecular trepidations close to the SARS-CoV virus. AI methodologies are manipulated to accomplish transcriptional inspection to connect latent antiviral drugs from the FDA-approved and natural products (Schultz et al., 2020). An AI manifesto has been entrenched (Patankar et al., 2020) to pin down plausible old drugs having antiviral attributes against coronavirus. Then, the authors have tested all the AI envisaged drugs at odds with the slinky covid-19 virus cell-based assessment, in-vitro. After that, the AI network interpreted the assessment results to relearn and initiate a redesigned AI mold to again search remote drugs. To combat this pandemic, the puissant most supercomputer, namely SUMMIT, emerged to help in the hard battle against this deadly virus. It was exploited to spot the existing tiny-sized pharmaceutical molecules, which possibly have some plausible repercussions against the COVID-19 virus.

Further, to upgrade the execution (Srinivasan et al., 2021), it is illustrated how Bayesian enhancement may help set out calculations paramount to hastened recognition of the candidates having the same computational capacity. A data-operated drug transposing framework is generated (Srilok et al., 2020), which registers ML to consolidate and excavate large-scale perception graphs to come across plausible drug contenders against coronavirus. An AI-rooted drug-repositioning scheme has been proposed (Srilok et al., 2020) to construct a learning prognostic predictive and locate the drugs that possess the capability to treat this viral disease.

Table 1. AI-based studies for COVID-19 therapeutics (Ekins et al., 2014)

Author Country	AI Tool	Protocol	No. of drugs and database screened	Target(s)	Top-ranked promising candidate drug(s)
Beck et al.(2020) Korea	Molecule transformer-drug target interaction(MT-DTI)	Binding affinity values prediction based on chemical sequences (SMILES) and amino acid sequences (FASTA) of target proteins	3410 binding DB, (FDA approved drugs)	3CL pro, Helicase, EndoRNAse,RdRp, 3'-exonuclease, EndoRNAse, 2'-O-Ribose methyltransferase	Atazanavir, Remdesivir, Ritonavir, Lopinavir, Darunavir, Asunaprevir, Daclatasvir, Simeprevir, Dolutegravir
Hu et al.(2020) China	Multi-task neural network	Homology modelling, estimation of binding affinity(pK_a) between drug and target	4895 commercial drugs, Global Health Drug Discovery Institute(GHDDI)	RdRp, 3CL pro, PLpro, helicase, S protein, E protein, 3'-exonuclease, EndoRNAse, 2'-O-Ribose methyltransferase	Abacavir, Darunavir, Itraconazole, Daclatasvir, Metoprolol tartrate
Zhang et al.(2020) China	DFCNN(dense fully conventional neural network	Homology modelling identification and ranking of protein ligand interactions by virtual drug screening	Chimdiv, PDBbind, Targetmol approved, Natural compound and bioactive compound libraries	3CL pro	Meglumine, Ganciclovir, Mannitol, Dulcitol, D-Sorbitol, D-Mannitol, Sodium Gluconate
Kim et al.(2020) USA	Fluency(AI platform) Disease Cancelling Technology Platform	Binding prediction analysis Gene expression analysis	657 drugs, Selleckchem, FDA approved drug library	ACE2, TMPRSS2	Fosamprenavir, Emricasan, Piperacillin, Glutathione, Glutamine, Elbasvir, Bictegravir
Ke et al.(2020) Taiwan	Deep-neural network(DNN)		2684 drugs, DrugBank	3CL pro	Bedaquiline, Brequinar, Celecoxib, Clofazimine, Comivaptan
Zhu et al.(2020) China	Infinity phenotype(Deep-neural network)	Analysis of transcriptional changes induced by various compunds	3682 (FDA approved drugs and natural products library)	Negative regulation of viral genome	Liquirtin, Procaterol, Pibrentasvir, Carbocisteine
Richardson et al.(2020) United Kingdom	Benevolent AI	Medical knowledge graph	378 AAK1 inhibitors in benevolent AI knowledge graph	AP2 -associated protein kinase 1(AAK1)	Baricitinib
Bung et al.(2020) India	Deep-neural network based generative and predictive models	Smiles representation, Generative model using transfer learning, reinforcement learning, virtual screening analysis	1.6 million drug-like small molecules from the ChEMBL database	3CL pro	31 novel drug like small molecules including 2 structurally similar compound to natural compound "Aurantiamide"
Zhavoronkov et al.(2020) China	Generative deep learning pipeline	Homology modelling, protease database assembly, co-crystallized fragment	5891, Integrity, ChEMBL, Experimental Pharmacology Module and Protegen database	3CL pro	Most recent data package available at insilico.com/n cov-sprint

CONCLUSION & FUTURE DIRECTIONS

Artificial Intelligence (AI) is an imminent and beneficial tool for identifying premature infections caused by the coronavirus and assists in surveillance of the patients' condition. It can remarkably ameliorate treatment uniformity and decision-making, developing beneficial algorithms. Apart from being cooperative in treating Coronavirus virus infections, AI also monitors their regular health. It can keep an eye on the cataclysm of COVID-19 at many different spectrums like medical, epidemiological, and molecular applications. Again, it is valuable to expedite the study findings regarding this virus by looking over the data available. AI can be of immense assistance in producing ideal treatment rules, thwarting plans, vaccine and drug generation. The drug repurposing based on AI is cheaper, faster, and more effective and can also minimize failure rates in clinical trials. Currently, there is no direct entry into the advanced trial stage without the initial trial phases and the toxicity tests. It is in its nascent phase. This initiative is an auspicious elucidation for developing plausible drugs against COVID-19. The repositioning of the drug molecules and computational intelligence-aided designing of drug compounds may be of immense help in the prognosis of outstanding antiviral therapy. Whatsoever, the divination efficacy may immensely magnify along with a systematic grounding database as well as developing apposite swotting algorithms. Alongside industrial furtherance in AI conjoined with escalating computational capacity, drug repurposing based on AI may benefit this current COVID-19 scenario.

This article traverses the contemporary cultivation of AI-sanctioned repurposing of drugs regarding the COVID virus. In this era of macro data, repurposing the drugs may be accomplished expeditiously via employing deep learning methods.

REFERENCES

Agrebi, S., & Larbi, A. (2020). Use of artificial intelligence in infectious diseases. In *Artificial intelligence in precision health* (pp. 415–438). Academic Press. doi:10.1016/B978-0-12-817133-2.00018-5

Albahri, A. S., Al-Obaidi, J. R., Zaidan, A. A., Albahri, O. S., Hamid, R. A., Zaidan, B. B., Alamoodi, A. H., & Hashim, M. (2020). Multi-biological laboratory examination framework for the prioritization of patients with COVID-19 based on integrated AHP and group VIKOR methods. *International Journal of Information Technology & Decision Making, 19*(05), 1247–1269. doi:10.1142/S0219622020500285

Albahri, O. S., Al-Obaidi, J. R., Zaidan, A. A., Albahri, A. S., Zaidan, B. B., Salih, M. M., Qays, A., Dawood, K. A., Mohammed, R. T., Abdulkareem, K. H., Aleesa, A. M., Alamoodi, A. H., Chyad, M. A., & Zulkifli, C. Z. (2020). Helping doctors hasten COVID-19 treatment: Towards a rescue framework for the transfusion of best convalescent plasma to the most critical patients based on biological requirements via ml and novel MCDM methods. *Computer Methods and Programs in Biomedicine*, *196*, 105617. doi:10.1016/j.cmpb.2020.105617 PMID:32593060

Al-Najjar, H., & Al-Rousan, N. (2020). A classifier prediction model to predict the status of Coronavirus COVID-19 patients in South Korea. *European Review for Medical and Pharmacological Sciences*. Advance online publication. doi:10.26355/eurrev_202003_20709 PMID:32271458

An, C., Lim, H., Kim, D. W., Chang, J. H., Choi, Y. J., & Kim, S. W. (2020). Machine learning prediction for mortality of patients diagnosed with COVID-19: A nationwide Korean cohort study. *Scientific Reports*, *10*(1), 1–11. doi:10.103841598-020-75767-2 PMID:33127965

Abdollahi, A., & Rahbaralam, M. (2020). Effect of temperature on the transmission of COVID-19: A machine learning case study in Spain. MedRxiv. Doi:10.1101/2020.05.01.20087759

Arora, K., & Bist, A. S. (2020). Artificial intelligence based drug discovery techniques for covid-19 detection. *Aptisi Transactions on Technopreneurship*, *2*(2), 120–126. doi:10.34306/att.v2i2.88

Browning, L., Colling, R., Rakha, E., Rajpoot, N., Rittscher, J., James, J. A., Salto-Tellez, M., Snead, D. R. J., & Verrill, C. (2021). Digital pathology and artificial intelligence will be key to supporting clinical and academic cellular pathology through COVID-19 and future crises: The PathLAKE consortium perspective. *Journal of Clinical Pathology*, *74*(7), 443–447. doi:10.1136/jclinpath-2020-206854 PMID:32620678

Barbat, M. M., Wesche, C., Werhli, A. V., & Mata, M. M. (2019). An adaptive machine learning approach to improve automatic iceberg detection from SAR images. *ISPRS Journal of Photogrammetry and Remote Sensing*, *156*, 247–259. doi:10.1016/j.isprsjprs.2019.08.015

Bai, X., Fang, C., Zhou, Y., Bai, S., Liu, Z., Xia, L., . . . Chen, W. (2020). Predicting COVID-19 malignant progression with AI techniques. doi:10.1101/2020.03.20.20037325

Bildirici, M., Guler Bayazit, N., & Ucan, Y. (2020). Analyzing crude oil prices under the impact of covid-19 by using lstargarchlstm. *Energies*, *13*(11), 2980. doi:10.3390/en13112980

Beck, B. R., Shin, B., Choi, Y., Park, S., & Kang, K. (2020). Predicting commercially available antiviral drugs that may act on the novel coronavirus (SARS-CoV-2) through a drug-target interaction deep learning model. *Computational and Structural Biotechnology Journal*, *18*, 784–790. doi:10.1016/j.csbj.2020.03.025 PMID:32280433

Colubri, A., Hartley, M. A., Siakor, M., Wolfman, V., Felix, A., Sesay, T., Shaffer, J. G., Garry, R. F., Grant, D. S., Levine, A. C., & Sabeti, P. C. (2019). Machine-learning prognostic models from the 2014–16 Ebola outbreak: Data-harmonization challenges, validation strategies, and mHealth applications. *EClinicalMedicine*, *11*, 54–64. doi:10.1016/j.eclinm.2019.06.003 PMID:31312805

Choi, S., Lee, J., Kang, M. G., Min, H., Chang, Y. S., & Yoon, S. (2017). Large-scale machine learning of media outlets for understanding public reactions to nation-wide viral infection outbreaks. *Methods (San Diego, Calif.)*, *129*, 50–59. doi:10.1016/j.ymeth.2017.07.027 PMID:28813689

Chockanathan, U., DSouza, A. M., Abidin, A. Z., Schifitto, G., & Wismüller, A. (2019). Automated diagnosis of HIV-associated neurocognitive disorders using large-scale Granger causality analysis of resting-state functional MRI. *Computers in Biology and Medicine*, *106*, 24–30. doi:10.1016/j.compbiomed.2019.01.006 PMID:30665138

Chen, Y., Ouyang, L., Bao, F. S., Li, Q., Han, L., Zhu, B., . . . Chen, S. (2020). *An interpretable machine learning framework for accurate severe vs non-severe covid-19 clinical type classification.* doi:10.1101/2020.05.18.20105841

Chen, Y., Yang, W., & Zhang, B. (2020). *Using mobility for electrical load forecasting during the covid-19 pandemic.* arXiv preprint arXiv:2006.08826.

Chandra, G., Gupta, R., & Agarwal, N. (2020). *Role of artificial intelligence in transforming the justice delivery system in covid-19 pandemic.* . doi:10.1038/nrd.2016.104

Chan, J. F., Chan, K. H., Kao, R. Y., To, K. K., Zheng, B. J., Li, C. P., Li, P. T. W., Dai, J., Mok, F. K. Y., Chen, H., Hayden, F. G., & Yuen, K. Y. (2013). Broad-spectrum antivirals for the emerging Middle East respiratory syndrome coronavirus. *The Journal of Infection*, *67*(6), 606–616. doi:10.1016/j.jinf.2013.09.029 PMID:24096239

Chan, J. F. W., Yao, Y., Yeung, M. L., Deng, W., Bao, L., Jia, L., Li, F., Xiao, C., Gao, H., Yu, P., Cai, J.-P., Chu, H., Zhou, J., Chen, H., Qin, C., & Yuen, K. Y. (2015). Treatment with lopinavir/ritonavir or interferon-β1b improves outcome of MERS-CoV infection in a nonhuman primate model of common marmoset. *The Journal of Infectious Diseases*, *212*(12), 1904–1913. doi:10.1093/infdis/jiv392 PMID:26198719

Chenthamarakshan, V., Das, P., Hoffman, S., Strobelt, H., Padhi, I., Lim, K. W., ... Mojsilovic, A. (2020). Cogmol: Target-specific and selective drug design for covid-19 using deep generative models. *Advances in Neural Information Processing Systems*, *33*, 4320–4332.

Dourado Jr, C. M., da Silva, S. P. P., da Nobrega, R. V. M., Barros, A. C. D. S., Reboucas Filho, P. P., & de Albuquerque, V. H. C. (2019). Deep learning IoT system for online stroke detection in skull computed tomography images. *Computer Networks*, *152*, 25–39. doi:10.1016/j.comnet.2019.01.019

de Moraes Batista, A. F., Miraglia, J. L., Donato, T. H. R., & Chiavegatto Filho, A. D. P. (2020). COVID-19 diagnosis prediction in emergency care patients: a machine learning approach. MedRxiv. doi:10.1101/2020.04.04.20052092

Das, A., Mishra, S., Hassanien, A. E., Salam, A., & Darwish, A. (2020). Artificial intelligence approach to predict the covid-19 patient's recovery. *EasyChair Preprint*, *3223*. Advance online publication. doi:10.1007/978-3-030-63307-3_8

DiMasi, J. A., & Faden, L. B. (2011). Competitiveness in follow-on drug R&D: A race or imitation? *Nature Reviews. Drug Discovery*, *10*(1), 23–27. doi:10.1038/nrd3296 PMID:21151030

Ekins, S., Freundlich, J. S., & Coffee, M. (2014). A common feature pharmacophore for FDA-approved drugs inhibiting the Ebola virus. *F1000 Research*, *3*, 277. Advance online publication. doi:10.12688/f1000research.5741.1 PMID:25653841

Ekins, S., Mottin, M., Ramos, P. R., Sousa, B. K., Neves, B. J., Foil, D. H., Zorn, K. M., Braga, R. C., Coffee, M., Southan, C., Puhl, A. C., & Andrade, C. H. (2020). Déjà vu: Stimulating open drug discovery for SARS-CoV-2. *Drug Discovery Today*, *25*(5), 928–941. doi:10.1016/j.drudis.2020.03.019 PMID:32320852

Feng, C., Wang, L., Chen, X., Zhai, Y., Zhu, F., Chen, H., . . . Li, T. (2021). A Novel Triage Tool of Artificial Intelligence-Assisted Diagnosis Aid System for Suspected COVID-19 Pneumonia in Fever Clinics. MedRxiv, 2020-03. doi:10.1101/2020.03.19.20039099

Gao, F., You, J., Wang, J., Sun, J., Yang, E., & Zhou, H. (2017). A novel target detection method for SAR images based on shadow proposal and saliency analysis. *Neurocomputing*, *267*, 220–231. doi:10.1016/j.neucom.2017.06.004

Gemmar, P. (2020). An interpretable mortality prediction model for COVID-19 patients–alternative approach. MedRxiv. doi:10.1101/2020.06.14.20130732

Goh, G. K. M., Dunker, A. K., Foster, J. A., & Uversky, V. N. (2020). A novel strategy for the development of vaccines for SARS-CoV-2 (COVID-19) and other viruses using AI and viral shell disorder. *Journal of Proteome Research*, *19*(11), 4355–4363. doi:10.1021/acs.jproteome.0c00672 PMID:33006287

Ge, Y., Tian, T., Huang, S., Wan, F., Li, J., Li, S., Wang, X., Yang, H., Hong, L., Wu, N., Yuan, E., Luo, Y., Cheng, L., Hu, C., Lei, Y., Shu, H., Feng, X., Jiang, Z., Wu, Y., ... Zeng, J. (2021). An integrative drug repositioning framework discovered a potential therapeutic agent targeting COVID-19. *Signal Transduction and Targeted Therapy*, *6*(1), 1–16. doi:10.103841392-021-00568-6 PMID:33895786

Gautret, P., Lagier, J. C., Parola, P., Meddeb, L., Mailhe, M., Doudier, B., ... Raoult, D. (2020). Hydroxychloroquine and azithromycin as a treatment of COVID-19: Results of an open-label non-randomized clinical trial. *International Journal of Antimicrobial Agents*, *56*(1), 105949. doi:10.1016/j.ijantimicag.2020.105949 PMID:32205204

Guida, J. P. (2020). Chloroquine, Hydroxychloroquine and Covid-19: A systematic review of literature. *InterAmerican Journal of Medicine and Health*, *3*, 1–10. doi:10.31005/iajmh.v3i0.79

Guleria, P., Ahmed, S., Alhumam, A., & Srinivasu, P. N. (2022). Empirical Study on Classifiers for Earlier Prediction of COVID-19 Infection Cure and Death Rate in the Indian States. *Health Care*, *10*(1), 85. doi:10.3390/healthcare10010085 PMID:35052249

Gns, H. S., Saraswathy, G. R., Murahari, M., & Krishnamurthy, M. (2019). An update on Drug Repurposing: Re-written saga of the drug's fate. *Biomedicine and Pharmacotherapy*, *110*, 700–716. doi:10.1016/j.biopha.2018.11.127 PMID:30553197

Hui, D. S., Azhar, E. I., Madani, T. A., Ntoumi, F., Kock, R., Dar, O., ... Petersen, E. (2020). The continuing 2019-nCoV epidemic threat of novel coronaviruses to global health—The latest 2019 novel coronavirus outbreak in Wuhan, China. *International Journal of Infectious Diseases*, *91*, 264–266. doi:10.1016/j.ijid.2020.01.009 PMID:31953166

Hassanien, A. E., Salam, A., & Darwish, A. (2020). Artificial intelligence approach to predict the covid-19 patient's recovery. *EasyChair Preprint*, *3223*. Advance online publication. doi:10.1007/978-3-030-63307-3_8

Hu, C., Liu, Z., Jiang, Y., Zhang, X., Shi, O., Xu, K., . . . Chen, X. (2020). Early prediction of mortality risk among severe COVID-19 patients using machine learning. MedRxiv. doi:10.1101/2020.04.13.20064329

Hashem, I. A. T., Ezugwu, A. E., Al-Garadi, M. A., Abdullahi, I. N., Otegbeye, O., Ahman, Q. O., . . . Chiroma, H. (2020). *A machine learning solution framework for combatting covid-19 in smart cities from multiple dimensions*. doi:. 05.18.20105577 doi:10.1101/2020

Hossain, M. M., McKyer, E. L. J., & Ma, P. (2020). Applications of artificial intelligence technologies on mental health research during COVID-19. doi:10.31235/osf.io/w6c9bosf.io/w6c9b

Ho, D. (2020). Addressing COVID-19 drug development with artificial intelligence. *Advanced Intelligent Systems*, *2*(5), 2000070. doi:10.1002/aisy.202000070 PMID:32838299

Iwendi, C., Bashir, A. K., Peshkar, A., Sujatha, R., Chatterjee, J. M., Pasupuleti, S., Mishra, R., Pillai, S., & Jo, O. (2020). COVID-19 patient health prediction using boosted random forest algorithm. *Frontiers in Public Health*, *8*, 357. doi:10.3389/fpubh.2020.00357 PMID:32719767

Imran, A., Posokhova, I., Qureshi, H. N., Masood, U., Riaz, M. S., Ali, K., John, C. N., Hussain, M. D. I., & Nabeel, M. (2020). AI4COVID-19: AI enabled preliminary diagnosis for COVID-19 from cough samples via an app. *Informatics in Medicine Unlocked*, *20*, 100378. doi:10.1016/j.imu.2020.100378 PMID:32839734

Johnstone, S. (2020). *A viral warning for change. COVID-19 versus the red cross: Better solutions via blockchain and artificial intelligence. COVID-19 Versus the Red Cross: Better Solutions Via Blockchain and Artificial Intelligence*. University of Hong Kong Faculty of Law Research Paper, (2020/005). doi:10.2139/ssrn.3530756

Jha, I. P., Awasthi, R., Kumar, A., Kumar, V., & Sethi, T. (2020). *Explainable-machine-learning to discover drivers and to predict mental illness during covid-19*. . doi:10.2196/25097

Jagtap, V. S., More, P., & Jha, U. (2020). *A review of the 2019 novel coronavirus (COVID-19) based on current evidence*. . doi:10.1016/j.ijantimicag.2020.105948

Kavakiotis, I., Tsave, O., Salifoglou, A., Maglaveras, N., Vlahavas, I., & Chouvarda, I. (2017). Machine learning and data mining methods in diabetes research. *Computational and Structural Biotechnology Journal*, *15*, 104–116. doi:10.1016/j. csbj.2016.12.005 PMID:28138367

Ke, Y. Y., Peng, T. T., Yeh, T. K., Huang, W. Z., Chang, S. E., Wu, S. H., Hung, H.-C., Hsu, T.-A., Lee, S.-J., Song, J.-S., Lin, W.-H., Chiang, T.-J., Lin, J.-H., Sytwu, H.-K., & Chen, C. T. (2020). Artificial intelligence approach fighting COVID-19 with repurposing drugs. *Biomedical Journal*, *43*(4), 355–362. doi:10.1016/j. bj.2020.05.001 PMID:32426387

Kundu, S., Elhalawani, H., Gichoya, J. W., & Kahn, C. E. Jr. (2020). How might AI and chest imaging help unravel COVID-19's mysteries? *Radiology. Artificial Intelligence*, *2*(3), e200053. doi:10.1148/ryai.2020200053 PMID:33928254

Kolozsvari, L. R., Bérczes, T., Hajdu, A., Gesztelyi, R., Tiba, A., Varga, I., . . . Zsuga, J. (2021). Predicting the epidemic curve of the coronavirus (SARS-CoV-2) disease (COVID-19) using artificial intelligence. MedRxiv, 2020-04. doi:10.1101/2020.04.17.20069666

Khan, F. M., & Gupta, R. (2020). ARIMA and NAR based prediction model for time series analysis of COVID-19 cases in India. *Journal of Safety Science and Resilience*, *1*(1), 12–18. doi:10.1016/j.jnlssr.2020.06.007

Kumar, P., Kalita, H., Patairiya, S., Sharma, Y. D., Nanda, C., Rani, M., . . . Bhagavathula, A. S. (2020). Forecasting the dynamics of COVID-19 pandemic in top 15 countries in April 2020: ARIMA model with machine learning approach. MedRxiv. doi:10.1101/2020.03.30.20046227

Khattar, A., Jain, P. R., & Quadri, S. M. K. (2020, May). Effects of the disastrous pandemic COVID 19 on learning styles, activities and mental health of young Indian students-a machine learning approach. In *2020 4th International Conference on Intelligent Computing and Control Systems (ICICCS)* (pp. 1190-1195). IEEE. 10.1109/ICICCS48265.2020.9120955

Ke, Y. Y., Peng, T. T., Yeh, T. K., Huang, W. Z., Chang, S. E., Wu, S. H., Hung, H.-C., Hsu, T.-A., Lee, S.-J., Song, J.-S., Lin, W.-H., Chiang, T.-J., Lin, J.-H., Sytwu, H.-K., & Chen, C. T. (2020). Artificial intelligence approach fighting COVID-19 with repurposing drugs. *Biomedical Journal*, *43*(4), 355–362. doi:10.1016/j. bj.2020.05.001 PMID:32426387

Li, H. C., Yang, G., Yang, W., Du, Q., & Emery, W. J. (2020). Deep nonsmooth nonnegative matrix factorization network with semi-supervised learning for SAR image change detection. *ISPRS Journal of Photogrammetry and Remote Sensing*, *160*, 167–179. doi:10.1016/j.isprsjprs.2019.12.002

Lalmuanawma, S., Hussain, J., & Chhakchhuak, L. (2020). Applications of machine learning and artificial intelligence for Covid-19 (SARS-CoV-2) pandemic: A review. *Chaos, Solitons, and Fractals*, *139*, 110059. doi:10.1016/j.chaos.2020.110059 PMID:32834612

Liu, T., Fan, W., & Wu, C. (2019). A hybrid machine learning approach to cerebral stroke prediction based on imbalanced medical dataset. *Artificial Intelligence in Medicine*, *101*, 101723. doi:10.1016/j.artmed.2019.101723 PMID:31813482

Li, W. T., Ma, J., Shende, N., Castaneda, G., Chakladar, J., Tsai, J. C., Apostol, L., Honda, C. O., Xu, J., Wong, L. M., Zhang, T., Lee, A., Gnanasekar, A., Honda, T. K., Kuo, S. Z., Yu, M. A., Chang, E. Y., Rajasekaran, M. R., & Ongkeko, W. M. (2020). Using machine learning of clinical data to diagnose COVID-19: A systematic review and meta-analysis. *BMC Medical Informatics and Decision Making*, *20*(1), 1–13. doi:10.118612911-020-01266-z PMID:32993652

Lee, S. W., Jung, H., Ko, S., Kim, S., Kim, H., Doh, K., . . . Ha, J. W. (2020). *Carecall: a call-based active monitoring dialog agent for managing covid-19 pandemic*. doi:10.1016%2Fj.chaos.2020.110338

Li, S., Wang, Y., Xue, J., Zhao, N., & Zhu, T. (2020). The impact of COVID-19 epidemic declaration on psychological consequences: A study on active Weibo users. *International Journal of Environmental Research and Public Health*, *17*(6), 2032. doi:10.3390/ijerph17062032 PMID:32204411

Monaghan, C., Larkin, J. W., Chaudhuri, S., Han, H., Jiao, Y., Bermudez, K. M., . . . Maddux, F. W. (2020). Artificial intelligence for covid-19 risk classification in kidney disease: can technology unmask an unseen disease? medRxiv. doi:10.1101/2020.06.15.20131680

Mei, X., Lee, H. C., Diao, K. Y., Huang, M., Lin, B., Liu, C., ... Yang, Y. (2020). Artificial intelligence–enabled rapid diagnosis of patients with COVID-19. *Nature Medicine, 26*(8), 1224-1228. doi:.04.12.20062661 doi:10.1101/2020

Metsky, H. C., Freije, C. A., Kosoko-Thoroddsen, T. S. F., Sabeti, P. C., & Myhrvold, C. (2020). CRISPR-based COVID-19 surveillance using a genomically-comprehensive machine learning approach. BioRxiv. doi:10.1101/2020.02.26.967026

Mohanty, S., Rashid, M. H. A., Mridul, M., Mohanty, C., & Swayamsiddha, S. (2020). Application of Artificial Intelligence in COVID-19 drug repurposing. *Diabetes & Metabolic Syndrome, 14*(5), 1027–1031. doi:10.1016/j.dsx.2020.06.068 PMID:32634717

Moftakhar, L., Mozhgan, S. E. I. F., & Safe, M. S. (2020). Exponentially increasing trend of infected patients with COVID-19 in Iran: a comparison of neural network and ARIMA forecasting models. *Iranian Journal of Public Health, 49*(Suppl 1), 92. 10.18502%2Fijph.v49iS1.3675

Mashamba-Thompson, T. P., & Crayton, E. D. (2020). Blockchain and artificial intelligence technology for novel coronavirus disease 2019 self-testing. *Diagnostics (Basel), 10*(4), 198. doi:10.3390/diagnostics10040198 PMID:32244841

Massie, A. B., Boyarsky, B. J., Werbel, W. A., Bae, S., Chow, E. K., Avery, R. K., Durand, C. M., Desai, N., Brennan, D., Garonzik-Wang, J. M., & Segev, D. L. (2020). Identifying scenarios of benefit or harm from kidney transplantation during the COVID-19 pandemic: A stochastic simulation and machine learning study. *American Journal of Transplantation, 20*(11), 2997–3007. doi:10.1111/ajt.16117 PMID:32515544

Mohs, R. C., & Greig, N. H. (2017). Drug discovery and development: Role of basic biological research. *Alzheimer's & Dementia: Translational Research & Clinical Interventions, 3*(4), 651–657. doi:10.1016/j.trci.2017.10.005 PMID:29255791

Mak, K. K., & Pichika, M. R. (2019). Artificial intelligence in drug development: Present status and future prospects. *Drug Discovery Today, 24*(3), 773–780. doi:10.1016/j.drudis.2018.11.014 PMID:30472429

Mohanty, S., Harun Ai Rashid, M., Mridul, M., Mohanty, C., & Swayamsiddha, S. (2020). Application of Artificial Intelligence in COVID-19 drug repurposing. *Diabetes & Metabolic Syndrome, 14*(5), 1027–1031. doi:10.1016/j.dsx.2020.06.068 PMID:32634717

Naga, S. P., Rao, T., & Dicu, A. (2020). Mihaela & Mnerie, Corina & Olariu, Iustin: A comparative review of optimisation techniques in segmentation of brain MR images. *Journal of Intelligent & Fuzzy Systems, 38*, 1–12.

Nápoles, G., Grau, I., Bello, R., & Grau, R. (2014). Two-steps learning of Fuzzy Cognitive Maps for prediction and knowledge discovery on the HIV-1 drug resistance. *Expert Systems with Applications, 41*(3), 821–830. doi:10.1016/j.eswa.2013.08.012

Nazir, T., Irtaza, A., Shabbir, Z., Javed, A., Akram, U., & Mahmood, M. T. (2019). Diabetic retinopathy detection through novel tetragonal local octa patterns and extreme learning machines. *Artificial Intelligence in Medicine*, *99*, 101695. doi:10.1016/j.artmed.2019.07.003 PMID:31606114

Nemati, M., Ansary, J., & Nemati, N. (2020). Machine-learning approaches in COVID-19 survival analysis and discharge-time likelihood prediction using clinical data. *Patterns*, *1*(5), 100074. doi:10.1016/j.patter.2020.100074 PMID:32835314

Neri, E., Miele, V., Coppola, F., & Grassi, R. (2020). Use of CT and artificial intelligence in suspected or COVID-19 positive patients: Statement of the Italian Society of Medical and Interventional Radiology. *La Radiologia Medica*, *125*(5), 505–508. doi:10.100711547-020-01197-9 PMID:32350794

Norouzi, N., de Rubens, G. Z., Choupanpiesheh, S., & Enevoldsen, P. (2020). When pandemics impact economies and climate change: Exploring the impacts of COVID-19 on oil and electricity demand in China. *Energy Research & Social Science*, *68*, 101654. doi:10.1016/j.erss.2020.101654 PMID:32839693

Nawaz, N., Gomes, A. M., & Saldeen, M. A. (2020). Artificial intelligence (AI) applications for library services and resources in COVID-19 pandemic. *Artificial Intelligence (AI)*, *7*(18), 1951-1955. . doi:10.1016/j.dsx.2020.04.012

Nagaratnam, K., Harston, G., Flossmann, E., Canavan, C., Geraldes, R. C., & Edwards, C. (2020). Innovative use of artificial intelligence and digital communication in acute stroke pathway in response to COVID-19. *Future Healthcare Journal*, *7*(2), 169–173. doi:10.7861/fhj.2020-0034 PMID:32550287

Ngo, H. X., Garneau-Tsodikova, S., & Green, K. D. (2016). A complex game of hide and seek: The search for new antifungals. *MedChemComm*, *7*(7), 1285–1306. doi:10.1039/C6MD00222F PMID:27766140

Obinata, H., Ruan, P., Mori, H., Zhu, W., Sasaki, H., Tatsuya, K., . . . Yokobori, S. (2020). Can artificial intelligence predict the need for oxygen therapy in early stage COVID-19 pneumonia? doi:10.21203/rs.3.rs-33150/v1

Ou, S., He, X., Ji, W., Chen, W., Sui, L., Gan, Y., Lu, Z., Lin, Z., Deng, S., Przesmitzki, S., & Bouchard, J. (2020). Machine learning model to project the impact of COVID-19 on US motor gasoline demand. *Nature Energy*, *5*(9), 666–673. doi:10.103841560-020-0662-1 PMID:33052987

Onder, G., Rezza, G., & Brusaferro, S. (2020). Case-fatality rate and characteristics of patients dying in relation to COVID-19 in Italy. *Journal of the American Medical Association*, *323*(18), 1775–1776. doi:10.1001/jama.2020.4683 PMID:32203977

Phillips-Wren, G., & Ichalkaranje, N. (Eds.). (2008). *Intelligent decision making: An AI-based approach* (Vol. 97). Springer Science & Business Media. doi:10.1007/978-3-540-76829-6

Peiffer-Smadja, N., Maatoug, R., Lescure, F. X., D'ortenzio, E., Pineau, J., & King, J. R. (2020). Machine learning for COVID-19 needs global collaboration and data-sharing. *Nature Machine Intelligence, 2*(6), 293–294. doi:10.103842256-020-0181-6

Pu, X., Chen, K., Liu, J., Wen, J., Zhneng, S., & Li, H. (2020). Machine learning-based method for interpreting the guidelines of the diagnosis and treatment of COVID-19. *Sheng Wu Yi Xue Gong Cheng Xue Za Zhi= Journal of Biomedical Engineering= Shengwu Yixue Gongchengxue Zazhi, 37*(3), 365-372. . doi:10.7507/1001-5515.202003045

Paul, S. M., Mytelka, D. S., Dunwiddie, C. T., Persinger, C. C., Munos, B. H., Lindborg, S. R., & Schacht, A. L. (2010). How to improve R&D productivity: The pharmaceutical industry's grand challenge. *Nature Reviews. Drug Discovery, 9*(3), 203–214. doi:10.1038/nrd3078 PMID:20168317

Peng, M., Yang, J., Shi, Q., Ying, L., Zhu, H., Zhu, G., ... Li, J. (2020). *Artificial intelligence application in COVID-19 diagnosis and prediction.* Academic Press.

Pourhomayoun, M., & Shakibi, M. (2020). Predicting mortality risk in patients with COVID-19 using artificial intelligence to help medical decision-making. MedRxiv. doi:10.1101/2020.03.30.20047308

Pyzer-Knapp, E. O. (2020). *Using bayesian optimization to accelerate virtual screening for the discovery of therapeutics appropriate for repurposing for covid-19.* arXiv preprint arXiv:2005.07121.

Pokkuluri, K. S., & Nedunuri, S. U. D. (2020). A novel cellular automata classifier for covid-19 prediction. *Journal of Health Sciences, 10*(1), 34–38. doi:10.17532/jhsci.2020.907

Polyzos, S., Samitas, A., & Spyridou, A. E. (2021). Tourism demand and the COVID-19 pandemic: An LSTM approach. *Tourism Recreation Research, 46*(2), 175–187. doi:10.1080/02508281.2020.1777053

Pandey, R., Gautam, V., Pal, R., Bandhey, H., Dhingra, L. S., Misra, V., Sharma, H., Jain, C., Bhagat, K., Arushi, Patel, L., Agarwal, M., Agrawal, S., Jalan, R., Wadhwa, A., Garg, A., Agrawal, Y., Rana, B., Kumaraguru, P., & Sethi, T. (2022). A machine learning application for raising wash awareness in the times of covid-19 pandemic. *Scientific Reports, 12*(1), 1–10. doi:10.103841598-021-03869-6 PMID:35039533

Patankar, S. (2020). Deep learning-based computational drug discovery to inhibit the RNA Dependent RNA Polymerase: application to SARS-CoV and COVID-19. doi:10.31219/osf.io/6kpbgosf.io/6kpbg

Ruiz Estrada M. A. (2020). *The uses of drones in case of massive epidemics contagious diseases relief humanitarian aid: Wuhan-COVID-19 crisis.* doi:10.2139/ssrn.3546547

Rolain, J. M., Colson, P., & Raoult, D. (2007). Recycling of chloroquine and its hydroxyl analogue to face bacterial, fungal and viral infections in the 21st century. *International Journal of Antimicrobial Agents*, *30*(4), 297–308. doi:10.1016/j.ijantimicag.2007.05.015 PMID:17629679

Shortliffe, E. H. (1976). Books: Computer-Based Medical Consultations: MYCIN. *Journal of Clinical Engineering*, *1*(1), 69. doi:10.1097/00004669-197610000-00011

Shang, R., Qi, L., Jiao, L., Stolkin, R., & Li, Y. (2014). Change detection in SAR images by artificial immune multi-objective clustering. *Engineering Applications of Artificial Intelligence*, *31*, 53–67. doi:10.1016/j.engappai.2014.02.004

Saxena, S., & Gyanchandani, M. (2020). Machine learning methods for computer-aided breast cancer diagnosis using histopathology: A narrative review. *Journal of Medical Imaging and Radiation Sciences*, *51*(1), 182–193. doi:10.1016/j.jmir.2019.11.001 PMID:31884065

Sharma, P., Choudhary, K., Gupta, K., Chawla, R., Gupta, D., & Sharma, A. (2020). Artificial plant optimization algorithm to detect heart rate & presence of heart disease using machine learning. *Artificial Intelligence in Medicine*, *102*, 101752. doi:10.1016/j.artmed.2019.101752 PMID:31980091

S. (2020). Predicting community mortality risk due to CoVID-19 using machine learning and development of a prediction tool. medRxiv. doi:10.1101/2020.04.27.20081794

Sehanobish, A., Ravindra, N. G., & van Dijk, D. (2020). *Gaining insight into sars-cov-2 infection and covid-19 severity using self-supervised edge features and graph neural networks.* arXiv preprint arXiv:2006.12971. doi:10.1016%2Fj.chaos.2020.110338

Sharma, S. (2020). *Drawing Insights from COVID-19 Infected Patients With no Past Medical History Using CT Scan Images and Machine Learning Techniques: A Study on 200 Patients.* . doi:10.3390/ijerph17103437

Simsek, M., & Kantarci, B. (2020). Artificial intelligence-empowered mobilization of assessments in COVID-19-like pandemics: A case study for early flattening of the curve. *International Journal of Environmental Research and Public Health*, *17*(10), 3437. doi:10.3390/ijerph17103437 PMID:32423150

Sonntag, D. (2020). AI in Medicine, Covid-19 and Springer Nature's Open Access Agreement. *KI-Künstliche Intelligenz, 34*(2), 123–125. doi:10.100713218-020-00661-y PMID:32518472

Schultz, M. B., Vera, D., & Sinclair, D. A. (2020). Can artificial intelligence identify effective COVID-19 therapies? *EMBO Molecular Medicine, 12*(8), e12817. doi:10.15252/emmm.202012817 PMID:32569446

Srinivasan, S., Batra, R., Chan, H., Kamath, G., Cherukara, M. J., & Sankaranarayanan, S. K. (2021). Artificial intelligence-guided De novo molecular design targeting COVID-19. *ACS Omega, 6*(19), 12557–12566. doi:10.1021/acsomega.1c00477 PMID:34056406

Srilok, S., Rohit, B., Henry, C., Ganesh, K., Mathew, J., & Cherukara, S. (2020). *Artificial Intelligence Guided De Novo Molecular Design Targeting*. Advance online publication. doi:10.1021/acsomega.1c00477

Tayarani-N, M. H., Yao, X., & Xu, H. (2014). Meta-heuristic algorithms in car engine design: A literature survey. *IEEE Transactions on Evolutionary Computation, 19*(5), 609–629. doi:10.1109/TEVC.2014.2355174

Toğaçar, M., Ergen, B., & Cömert, Z. (2020). COVID-19 detection using deep learning models to exploit Social Mimic Optimization and structured chest X-ray images using fuzzy color and stacking approaches. *Computers in Biology and Medicine, 121*, 103805. doi:10.1016/j.compbiomed.2020.103805 PMID:32568679

Thorsen-Meyer, H. C., Nielsen, A. B., Nielsen, A. P., Kaas-Hansen, B. S., Toft, P., Schierbeck, J., Strøm, T., Chmura, P. J., Heimann, M., Dybdahl, L., Spangsege, L., Hulsen, P., Belling, K., Brunak, S., & Perner, A. (2020). Dynamic and explainable machine learning prediction of mortality in patients in the intensive care unit: A retrospective study of high-frequency data in electronic patient records. *The Lancet. Digital Health, 2*(4), e179–e191. doi:10.1016/S2589-7500(20)30018-2 PMID:33328078

Vaka, A. R., Soni, B., & Reddy, S. (2020). Breast cancer detection by leveraging Machine Learning. *ICT Express, 6*(4), 320–324. doi:10.1016/j.icte.2020.04.009

Vaid, A., Somani, S., Russak, A. J., De Freitas, J. K., Chaudhry, F. F., Paranjpe, I., . . . Glicksberg, B. S. (2020). Machine learning to predict mortality and critical events in covid-19 positive new york city patients. medRxiv. doi:10.1101/2020.04.26.20073411

Xue, H., Li, J., Xie, H., & Wang, Y. (2018). Review of drug repositioning approaches and resources. *International Journal of Biological Sciences, 14*(10), 1232–1244. doi:10.7150/ijbs.24612 PMID:30123072

Yan, L., Zhang, H. T., Xiao, Y., Wang, M., Sun, C., Liang, J., . . . Yuan, Y. (2020). Prediction of survival for severe Covid-19 patients with three clinical features: development of a machine learning-based prognostic model with clinical data in Wuhan. medRxiv. doi:10.1101/2020.10.09.20165431

Yao, Z., Zheng, X., Zheng, Z., Wu, K., & Zheng, J. (2021). Construction and validation of a machine learning-based nomogram: A tool to predict the risk of getting severe coronavirus disease 2019 (COVID-19). *Immunity, Inflammation and Disease*, 9(2), 595–607. doi:10.1002/iid3.421 PMID:33713584

Zoabi, Y., & Shomron, N. (2020). COVID-19 diagnosis prediction by symptoms of tested individuals: a machine learning approach. MedRxiv. doi:10.1101/2020.05.07.20093948

Zhu, J., Deng, Y. Q., Wang, X., Li, X. F., Zhang, N. N., Liu, Z., . . . Xie, Z. (2020). An artificial intelligence system reveals liquiritin inhibits SARS-CoV-2 by mimicking type I interferon. BioRxiv. doi:10.1101/2020.05.02.074021

Zheng, Y., Li, Z., Xin, J., & Zhou, G. (2020). *A spatial-temporal graph based hybrid infectious disease model with application to COVID-19*. arXiv preprint arXiv:2010.09077. doi:10.1101/2020.07.20.20158568

Zhou, Y., Hou, Y., Shen, J., Huang, Y., Martin, W., & Cheng, F. (2020). Network-based drug repurposing for novel coronavirus 2019-nCoV/SARS-CoV-2. *Cell Discovery*, 6(1), 1–18. doi:10.103841421-020-0153-3 PMID:32194980

KEY TERMS AND DEFINITIONS

Algorithms: Set of rules followed by a computer for problem-solving operations.

Computational Tools: Methods executed in computers to solve problems by repeated solution methods.

FDA: The Food and Drug Administration (FDA), a government agency (1906) responsible for protecting public health worldwide.

In-Vitro: Procedure performed in a test tube or culture plates under controlled laboratory conditions outside any living body.

Machine Learning: Utilisation of computer systems to learn, adapt and draw inferences from data patterns.

Pharmacophore: A molecular structural part responsible for any particular biological or pharmacological interaction that it undergoes.

Vaccine: Obtained from the causative agent of a disease or from its products or a synthetic substitute, which elicits an immune response by acting as an antigen without inducing the disease in the recipient.

Chapter 9

An Efficient Multi–Layer Perceptron Neural Network– Based Breast Cancer Prediction

Saravana Kumar N. M.
M. Kumarasamy College of Engineering, India

Tamilselvi S.
Bannari Amman Institute of Technology, India

Hariprasath K.
Vivekanandha College of Engineering for Women, India

Kaviyavarshini N.
Anna University, Chennai, India

Kavinya A.
Anna University, Chennai, India

ABSTRACT

Cancer is the most deadly disease for human beings across the world due to the adoption of new food habits and pollution. Breast cancer is becoming a common disease for women. After years of research a better analysis and possessing a higher prediction of any kind of cancer, it is still a very imperative contribution in healthcare. In the literature, several attempts were made deploying machine learning methods yielding a significant prediction of cancer. The goal of this study is on machine learning techniques that can enable prediction of breast cancer from the attributes with more accuracy. In this study, Wisconsin Breast Cancer (WBC) dataset has been used to compute machine and deep learning algorithm. This research focuses on logistic regression, decision tree, and random forest and a novel deep learning adoption, multi-layer perceptron. The performances of these algorithms have been correlated with each other using accuracy percentage. Also, sensitivity and specificity are computed as evaluation metrics. The multi-layer perceptron (MLP) gives 97% accuracy.

DOI: 10.4018/978-1-6684-3791-9.ch009

INTRODUCTION

Breast cancer is the particular type of cancer that induces death among women globally Y. Wang et al., (2020). If the disease is predicted at its earlier stages, several medication diagnoses cure cancer, and it greatly decreases the percentage of death for a curable disease. Breast cancer is treatable and curable by taking preventive measures and advanced inventive methods. So, it is convenient for the prediction of breast cancer in the earliest with increased efficiency because sufferers could get early analysis at the right moment and can recover from cancer. First, observing the importance of feature methods on the breast cancer dataset to make important features Naveen, R et al., (2019). The detection of breast cancer in the conventional human-centric way will take a long time. There is always a shortage of skilled specialists to diagnose, especially in developing countries. So, detecting cancer over different automated diagnosis methods is indispensable N. Khuriwal and N. Mishra, (2018). Carcinoma analysis is performed by segregating tumors. A tumor may be benign or malignant. Physicians will prefer a stable recognition to identify among tumors. Yet it is complicated to distinguish tumors even with expert physicians and by a non-automatic approach. Thus, computerization of recognition system is important for distinctive tumors M. S. Yarabarla et al., (2019). This research is regulated to classify the accomplishment of machine learning techniques in endorsement to be capable of detecting breast cancer C. Easttom et al., (2020).

Very fast production of abnormal tissues that spread behind the regular barriers in the breast induces tumor. This tumor can be categorized as Malignant (uncontrolled growth) and Benign (benignant). A single person on stroke can feel a specific tumor. Later it becomes enhanced into lemon shape. This is known as self-examination. This examination recognizes cancer at the last minute noticeably by A. Kajala and V. K. Jain (2020).

In computer technology, machine learning can be categorized into three types. The first is supervised machine learning, the second is unsupervised learning, and the third is reinforcement learning. In supervised machine learning, the data is labeled, and the system/machine forecasts the label of the non-labeled input attributes. In unsupervised learning, the entire attributes are feasible but externally, no labels or any output label. In reinforcement learning, learning is a method of allowing the prototype to learn by itself. Through this type, the system/machine achieves a particular task. It will get one of two (reward and penalty), which is completely based upon a firm of known standards and targets to increase the entire reward T. Thomas (2020).

Formally Machine Learning techniques establish the data analysis and relation among the extorting the major attributes and knowledge about the dataset. Further, it constructs a computation model for better characterization of data. Notably, researchers suggested that machine learning methods will be useful to handle the initial detection and diagnosis of cancer E. A. Bayrak et al., (2019). The main endeavor implemented an analysis in machine learning methods, predicting the outcomes when validated with data set, analyzing some methods studied earlier by practicing various advancements in training the data. Iqbal (2019) Furthermore, a neural network model was included that has not been analyzed for the particular data set. Some researchers investigated this method in various image datasets F. Teixeira et al., (2019). The conclusion was figured out by evaluation metrics in machine learning techniques when related to various techniques.

The goal of this study is on a few Machine Learning techniques that can enable pre-prediction of breast cancer from the cancer attributes with more accuracy. In this study, Wisconsin Breast Cancer (WBC) dataset has been used to compute Machine and Deep learning algorithms. This research focuses on Logistic Regression, Decision Trees, Random Forests, and a novel deep learning adoption as Multi-Layer Perceptron.

RELATED WORKS

E. A. Bayrak et al., (2019) here Machine learning was used to categorize breast cancer. The implementation of the two most prominent machine Learning for classification in the Wisconsin Breast Cancer (WBC) dataset and performing the classification of the two methods then comparing another by using evaluation metrics like accuracy, ROC, precision, and recall. The utmost performance is achieved by SVM (Support Vector Machine) algorithm with high accuracy. Support vector machine is used to classify tumors (benign or malignant) depending upon the sufferer's age and size of the tumor. The ANN (Artificial Neural Network) is described as the system of a biological neuron. Specifically, it is the same as the processing of the individual brain. It comprises more nodes that are linked or connected to every other node. Artificial Neural Network has the quality to model advanced and influential definite functions. Discussion of these two algorithms for WBC dataset classification, ANN and SVM algorithms are used for machine learning approach executed in WEKA tool. The efficiency of applying the machine learning approach is evaluated using performance metrics. Depending on these metrics, sequential minimal optimization algorithms had utmost performance in predicting the accuracy (96%) for analysis. The application of SVM and ANN procedures to forecast the characterization of malignant breast growth to find which AI strategies execution is better. Vladimir Vapnik first clarified SVM, and the great exhibitions of SVMs have been seen in many theme acknowledgment issues. SVMs can show better characterization execution when contrasted and numerous other grouping procedures.SVM is one of the most famous AI order methods utilized to anticipate and conclude malignancy.

As per SVM, the classes are isolated with a hyperplane comprised of help vectors that are basic examples from all classes. The hyperplane is a separator recognized as a choice limit among the two example bunches. SVM can be utilized to arrange growths as harmless or dangerous depending on persistent age and cancer size.

Artificial Neural Network (ANN) can be communicated through the biological neuron framework. Particularly, it is like the human mind process framework. It is comprised of a ton of nodes that interface every node. ANN has the capacity of demonstrating normal and incredible non-direct capacities. It is comprised of an organization of loads of Artificial neurons. Every one of these blends is contained information/yield qualities that play out a nearby numerical capacity. The capacity could be a calculation of weighted amounts of information sources, which yields if it goes past the given limit esteem. The yield could be a contribution to different neurons in the organization. This exchange repeats until the most recent yield are created. The creators likewise distributed a few near outcomes around here. SVM and ANN are applied with the WEKA AI device as AI procedures. The conclusion of the applied AI procedures application on the WBC dataset is accounted for. K=10-fold cross-validation is applied and rate split (% 66 and % 33 parts), which are preparing choices that split the dataset into a preparation set to prepare the model and a testing set to assess it. In WEKA programming, SVM and ANN procedures are applied to the breast disease dataset. The test results are illustrated. In the outcomes, execution measurements of exactness, accuracy, review, and ROC Area are considered.

A. Kajala and V. K. Jain (2020) proposed the efficiency of various machine learning techniques as Logistic Regression, support vector machines, naïve Bayes, artificial neural networks, and decision tree algorithms were used by many analysts. The attributes in mammograms are considered as an input to predict. It is noticed that the utilization of ML techniques needs a large quantity of data to predict better accuracy. The accessibility of adequate data is also a challenging issue for machine learning applications. These mammogram images are handled using CNN (Convolutional Neural Networks) for the automation selection of features. It is a deep learning technique that is one of the neural networks. The Convolutional neural networks can be used to extract the significant attributes necessarily, as stated by Deepalakshmi et al. (2021). Though Artificial Neural Network is not the best method to predict, using the number of layers and neurons did not give the best accurate result.

N. Khuriwal and N. Mishra (2018) suggested an ensemble learning technique for analyzing breast cancer. The results show that their proposed techniques were produced 98% of accuracy. They are considering 16 attributes for the analysis of breast cancer. The future enhancement is to work with the remaining attributes in the UCI dataset to produce better accuracy results. The authors confirmed that for a medical problem, the neural network has also been used for significant data analysis and can start to do analysis previously beyond more appropriate therapeutic intelligence. First Wisconsin Breast Cancer Database from the UCI site is gathered, pre-handled the dataset, and selected 16 significant elements. For include choice Recursive element Elimination Algorithm utilizing Chi2 strategy and get 16 top attributes. After that, applied ANN and Logistic calculation exclusively and figured the precision. At long last, the proposed Ensemble Voting technique was utilized and processed best strategy for conclusion breast malignancy illness. The gathering technique for conclusion breast disease with neural organization and have calculated calculation. All cycles comprise principle three sections: Pre-handling information, features selection, and voting models. In this work, the BCI dataset having 569 lines and 30 sections of the dataset has been used. In the test part, the components from the default dataset have first assessed. The Univariate Features determination technique and Recursive Features Selection strategy with Cross-Validation Method has been used for features selection.

Data pre-handling utilizes raw information for handling. For pre-handling normalization strategy is used. The data is a typical prerequisite for some AI estimators in this technique. There are various information perceptions for information pre-handling. Counting harmful and harmless from all datasets and plotting in graph format is done. In the second stage, the Violin plot is made for data compression. It shows the conveyance of quantitative information across a few degrees of one absolute factor with the end goal of measuring dissemination. In the proposed worktop, 16 features violin plot for correlation is used. In AI and statistics, feature selection, otherwise called variable choice, The numerous feature selection techniques are univariate, including feature selection. In the proposed work, the Univariate feature selection technique is used to analyze every element independently to decide the power of the element's connection with the dependent parameter. Overall, this technique is easy to run and comprehend and is especially useful for acquiring a superior understanding of information. After running this strategy, 16 top features are selected for breast disease findings. Univariate highlight choice calculation utilized the chi2 strategy for figuring chi-square details.

S. Niticaet al. (2020) has compared the analysis of three machine learning unsupervised techniques to detect breast cancer. T distributed stochastic neighbor embedding algorithm (t-SNE), self-organizing maps (SOM), and autoencoder (AE) had been used. All these 3 unsupervised learning techniques achieve a dimensional non-linearity reduction for input cases by perpetuating the data holds in the initial one. Observations are executed by using two freely accessible breast cancer datasets. They are picked from the UCI machine learning repository and Surface-enhanced Raman spectroscopy. The performance of unsupervised learning techniques is correlated, adjacent to the supervised classifier. The performance of the unsupervised learning process is estimated in terms of specificity, the area under the ROC curve, and sensitivity.

T. Thomas et al. (2020) proposed that breast cancer is critical and must be detected earlier before it spreads to a high level. This year, the expectation of 2 lakhs women will be analyzed intrusively for breast cancer in the US. Also, an estimation of around two thousand men will be diagnosed with breast cancer in the US. Thus the predicting method is needed to attain breast cancer detection. For the prediction at the progressive level, the authors used 6 various ML methods. Decision trees, support vector machines, k – nearest neighbor, artificial neural network, naïve Bayes, and k-means. WBC (Wisconsin Breast Cancer) dataset had been used that is freely accessible. The authors compared all six algorithms and concluded that ANN performs best and produced 97% of accuracy when compared with the remaining algorithms. Wisconsin Diagnostic dataset for breast malignant growth forecast makes them missing esteems. Information pre-handling was likewise utilized on the referenced dataset to deal with these missing qualities.

M. S. Yarabarla, L. K. Ravi and et al. (2019) propose the detection of breast cancer and prediction using the RF (Random Forest) algorithm. It is used for the two methods. One is classification, and another one is Regression. This gives the utmost accuracy. This staging is previously trained using different datasets. It is very useful when someone gives inputs; the algorithm validates the attributes and produces the conclusion. This algorithm predicts the utmost accuracy because it performs two processes (Regression and classification). KNN implies that there is no need for explicit preparing segment before order. This technique makes it simpler rather than the rehashed endeavors to sum up and unique the information orders. This implies that begin characterizing when the information gets summed up, i.e., there will be a square proportion of some inborn issues with this kind of algorithmic program. The dataset should be put away safely in memory until some kind of strategy is applied for the decrease. Not many arrangements might be pricy to play out its computational work as the algorithmic program separates through the information focuses in the dataset for each characterization. Because of these reasons, KNN appears to give its best on little datasets with few choices. The value of k is not settled, which will be utilized. The value perhaps set of unpredictable focuses or endeavor of cross-validation to search out neighbor should be possible. Next comes the most confounded, which is to find the distance metric. The square measure might have numerous elective manners by which distance can be found. As distance is the main measurement, it is still up in the air by the dataset and characterization. The two most normally utilized strategies for finding distance here are Euclidean distance and Cosine likeness.Hiba Asriaet al. (2016) analyzed medical data through different machine learning algorithms, and data mining algorithms are necessary for prediction. A challenging task in ML and data mining is building the accurate and effective classifier computation for applications in medicine. This work is concentrated on four techniques as C4.5, support vector machine, k-nearest neighbor. These algorithms are implemented using WBC (Wisconsin Breast Cancer) original datasets. The authors compared the performance and computational efficiency through algorithms' accuracy, specificity, precision, and sensitivity. Thesupport vector machine algorithm reaches an accurate value of 97% by comparing all other algorithms. To conclude, the support vector machine proved an efficient model for diagnosing and predicting breast cancer disease and achieved utmost efficiency as described in low error rate and precision.

J. Sivapriya et al., (2019) the four prominent methods inference, naive Bayes, support vector machine, logistic regression, and random forest on cancer dataset. The primary motive of this work is to introduce the best method that accomplishes accurate, efficient, and quick results. Random Forest achieved the best accuracy compared with all remaining techniques with 99%. Thus, the Random forest algorithm concludes that it has a low error value and high precision for appropriate prediction and analysis of breast cancer disease. Ch. Shravya et al. 2019) concentrates on improving prediction methods to accomplish better accuracy in validating accurate cancer disease using (SML) Supervised Machine Learning techniques. The analysis of the result that proclaims the assimilation of data in multi-dimensions and a selection of features, reduction methods in dimension, and classification implements the appropriate tool for the conclusion. The breast disease dataset from the UCI store is collected and utilized Anaconda spyder to code. The system includes utilization of order methods like Support Vector Machine (SVM), Logistic Regression, K-Nearest Neighbor (K-NN) with Reduction in Dimensionality procedure, for example, Principal Component Analysis (PCA). Dimensionality Reduction is utilized to get two different dimensional information, so better representation of AI models should be possible by plotting the expectation areas and the forecast limit for each model. Anything that might be the number of autonomous factors which regularly ends up with two free factors by applying an appropriate dimensionality decrease strategy.

METHODOLOGY

The main theme of this chapter is the process of predicting breast cancer by computing and analyzing the cancer dataset using machine and deep learning approaches. The algorithms studied in developing these learning models are Logistic Regression, Decision Tree, Random Forest, and a deep learning algorithm built on a novel Multi-layer Perceptron. The evaluation metrics are accuracy, sensitivity, and specificity. The attributes in the dataset are used to compute the prediction of cancer.

Data Collection

The Breast Cancer Wisconsin (diagnostic) dataset is obtained from a repository called UCI Machine Learning. The dataset has 32 attributes that hold both numerical and categorical variables. The dataset contains 569 instances. This dataset has multivariate and real characteristics.

Table 1. Some of the attributes that is present in the dataset

S.No	Attribute Name
1	Id
2	concave points_worst
3	Diagnosis
4	Perimeter_mean
5	fractal_dimension_mean
6	Texture_mean
7	symmetry_se
8	Area_mean
9	Radius_meanRadius_mean
10	fractal_dimension_worst
11	Smoothness_mean
12	compactness_worst

Implementation Environment

Anaconda IDE is the implementation environment used in this study. It supports Python Programming language. It is mainly used for machine learning, deep learning applications like predictive analytics, large-scale data processing, etc... It mainly focuses on data-driven projects.

Data Pre-Processing

Data pre-processing is indispensable in the machine learning technique, which transfers raw data into known data. The real data is incomplete, inconsistent, and lacks some features. It also contains at least minimal errors. The data set was maintained in a CSV file containing 32 attributes. The first step is to handle the missing value, which must be removed. Next is to compute the number of rows and columns and count the empty values. Then, the column with missing values has to be dropped. After missing values are dropped, the train and test set is split into 75 and 25, respectively, in percentage.

Figure 1. Architecture of the proposed model

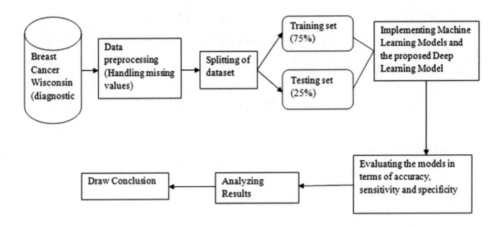

ALGORITHM USED

Cross-Validation: 10-Fold Cross-Validation

Cross-Validation is used to train several models based on a subset of data. PIMA dataset is split into 10 gatherings. The dataset is prepared for the prototype of 10-1 folds. The prototype is iterated for the m intervals. On every fold, data argumentation is utilized for validation.

$$Cross\,Validation\left(cv_{(m)}\right) = \frac{1}{m}\sum_{l=1}^{m}MSE_{l} \qquad (1)$$

Logistic Regression

The utilization of this regression prototype has been recommended, particularly in various fields like the medical discipline. This algorithm aims to analyze or segregate numerous data into categorical data. Generally, the target variable of Logistic Regression is binary; it specifies the data as zero or one. Here is the problem, it invokes positive and negative disease(prediction) in patients. The function of this algorithm is to evaluate the best model, which is reasonable to outline the relation among the targeted variable and the selected predicted variables. It mainly depends on the linear regression algorithm. S. Mojrian et al., (2020)

$$y = h_\theta\left(x\right) = \theta^T x \tag{2}$$

This equation is immensely ineffectual for predicting binary variables $\left(y^i \in \{0,1\}\right)$, accordingly proposing a new function for predicting probability for a patient feature which resides zero for negative class against the probability for the patient feature which resides one for positive class. Heidari et al., (2018)

$$P\left(y = 1 \mid x\right) = h_\theta\left(x\right) = \frac{1}{1 + exp\left(-\theta^T x\right)} \equiv \sigma\left(\theta^T x\right) \tag{3}$$

$$P\left(y = 0 \mid x\right) = 1 - P\left(y = 1 \mid x\right) = 1 - h_\theta\left(x\right) \tag{4}$$

Implementing equation (3), called sigmoid function, there is a need to hold the rate of $\theta^T x$ inside 0 to 1 range. Further inspecting a value of θ so that the probability $P\left(y = 1 \mid x\right) = h_\theta\left(x\right)$ is immense when x tends to class 1 and short when x tends to class 0.

The main objective function:

$$f\left(y\right) = \alpha + \beta * M \tag{5}$$

Here, y is the predicted variable, and M is the independent variable. α, β are the regression beta coefficients or parameters

Pseudocode

Training the data set
Step 1:   Set the threshold, epoch, weight, and cost function
Step 2:   Mapping function selected.
Step 3:   Weight of augmentation matrix θ is updated using

Table 2. Proposed mapping functions

Function 1 (F1)	[1 M0 M1 M2 …M5]
Function 2 (F2)	[1 M0^{2}M1^{2}M2^2 … M5^2]
Function 3 (F3)	[1 M0^{3}M1^{3}M2^3…..M5^3]
Function 4 (F4)	[1 M0 M1 M2 …M5 M0.M1 M2.M3M4.M5]
Function 5 (F5)	[1 M0^{2}M1^{2}M2^2 …M5^{2}M0.M1 M2.M3M4.M5]

$$\theta_j\left(n\right) = \theta_j\left(n-1\right) + \alpha.v_j \tag{6}$$

Step 4:   Cost function is found using

$$J\left(\theta\right) = J\left(\theta\right) + \left(-\frac{1}{m}\right)\left(\sum_{i=1}^{m} y^{(i)} log\left(h_\theta\left(x^{(i)}\right)\right) + \left(1 - y^{(i)}\right) log\left(1 - h_\theta\left(x^i\right)\right)\right) \tag{7}$$

Step 5:   If $\left|J\left(\theta\right)\right| \leq \in \left(or\right) N = N_{max}$ Go to Step 6

Step 6:   Obtain optimum weight

Testing the data set

Output is found using,

$$y = sgn\left(\theta^T x\right) \tag{8}$$

Mapping Functions Proposed for Evaluation

Logistic Regression meets when the entire dataset is separated in linear. This Regression is little inclined to overfitting, but it must over fit in immense or large dimensional datasets. There is a need to deal with Regularization methods to avoid overfitting in such situations. This algorithm is not meant only to accord to certain limits of how suitable the predictor is. It also focused on finding the direction of cooperation (both positive and negative). It is simple for implementation interpretation and extremely adequate for training. Logistic Regression is the hypothesis of magnitude between dependent and independent variables. In the current scenario, data is unlikely to separate in linearity. Remarkably, data would be tangled. If the count of the observations is lower than the number of attributes, this type of Regression is not applicable; otherwise, it leads to overfitting. Only the discrete functions can be predicted by using this Regression. Accordingly, dependent variables are limited to the set of discrete numbers. This limitation is problematic, as it is excessive continuous data for prediction.

Decision Tree

A Decision Tree (DT) is an effective learning technique utilized for Regression and classification. It is a tree framework where every private node is a valid precondition for measuring the magnitude, and the last node denotes the grade or target variable for prediction. The decision tree is better for classifying fewer classes' labels and will not execute appropriate conclusions in case there are various classes and low training investigations. Decision Tree is extravagant for training the classes Thomas et al. (2020)

A decision tree algorithm is developed to replace classification and regression work. This algorithm framework can comprise a fixed protocol, classify the newer population, and develop an appropriate and systematic type. This algorithm achieves various supervised learning methods by considering a set of training and testing samples.

In this framework, the primary objective of the algorithm is in the foremost phase, computing along with the classification concept (determining either present or not) and building attributes for every performance. All the attributes are categorized as nodes which everyone will proceed in a decision like yes or no. A single yes/no condition would be acknowledged, and finally, there will be no other data that has to be divided again.

If this tree achieved an appropriate level in train data, it would not be acknowledged as the best classifier. The small tree will not be suitable for all types of train data. The better accuracy will model to an advanced decision tree in all time. Changsheng et al. (2019)

The main objective function:

$$E\left(s\right) = \sum_{i=1}^{c} - p_i \log_2 p_i \tag{9}$$

Here E is the entropy function, and p is the probability function.

Pseudocode

1. Select a better parameter of feature selection to segregate the attributes from the dataset.
2. Form the particular feature in the dataset as a decision node.

3. Split the entire dataset into lesser subsets (features).
4. Initiate the construction of the tree by doing again in a recursive manner for every child till the following aspect is satisfied (one of the conditions):
   a. All the objects apply to similar features.
   b. There should not be any surplus features.
   c. There should not be non-occurrence.

Normalization of the data is not mandatory to use the decision tree algorithm. This algorithm can be implemented without doing the data scaling. Imputation of missing variables is not required for this algorithm. It is not vital to code more and analyzes the data to preprocess. Also, the computational time will be less to preprocess the data. The theory beyond this algorithm is simple for coders and not difficult to learn as much as various algorithms. The arithmetic computation of this algorithm needs high memory space. Also, it takes a large time to execute the mathematical computation. The execution of this model is higher sensitive when there is a little modification in data. It finally produces an immense variation in the model of the tree. The complexity of time and space is high in this algorithm. The time requires to train the data in the decision tree algorithm is higher than other algorithms. This algorithm is not satisfactory for the prediction of continuous variables and handling regression problems.

Random Forest

One of the supervised learning algorithms is Random Forest. It is utilized for decision-making for both regression and classification problems. It is also said as ensemble leaner, which creates more number of classifier and the results of the classifier are accumulated. The random forest can create more number classification and regression trees (CART) in which training is given based on the sample of bootstrap of the unique training data and search is based on the random method that is selected based on the sub-division of the input variables that is used for defining the split among them. Classification and regression trees are binary Decision Trees built by the split of data in the node to the child node starting from the root node, which includes the whole sample node.

The working process of random forest is selecting samples, the decision is calculated based on tree and result is predicted, next the voting method is accomplished. Finally, the result is predicted based on the vote.

Pseudocode

Step 1: Read the dataset.
Step 2: Start with singe region.

Step 3: Set number of iteration, split.

Step 4: Test the dataset for accuracy.

Step 5: The average of voting combines prediction.

Step 6: Repeat from step 2 for maximum accuracy.

The random forest has minimum variance.Random forest is more flexible and gives more accuracy even when the dataset is not scaled and has missing values. It alsocombines the various decision trees for more accuracy.Random forest is more complex for execution and construction.Random forest consumes more time.Random forest requires more computational resources.

Multi-Layer Perceptron

A Multilayer perceptron (MLP) is a feed-forward artificial neural network. There are minimum nodes of 3 layers as input, hidden, and output layers. Other than the input node, every node is a neuron that utilizes a non-linearity activation function. MLP needs a supervised learning method (backpropagation) to train. Both the non-linear activation function and multiple layers categorize MLP from linear perceptron. It will categorize the data, which is separating in linear. Sultana et al., (2019)

The concept of MLP is mainly used equivocally, almost to any feedforward artificial neural network, also defined as the network combined of a multi-layerperceptron. These perceptrons are commonly known as vanilla neural networks in colloquial, especially when one hidden layer is held.

Activation Function

If multiple layer perceptron has activation function linearly in neurons, it means the linear function will sketch the inputs (weighted) to output in all neurons. Further linear algebra defines either layer could be modified to 2 layered input, output model. In Multilayer perceptron, few neurons arenonlinear. It was evolved to the frequency model of biological neurons, which is action potentials. There are 2 accepted activation functions in sigmoid. Mekha et al., (2019) They are,

$$y\left(v_i\right) = tanh\left(v_i\right) and y\left(v_i\right) = \left(1 + e^{-v_i}\right)^{-1} \tag{10}$$

Modern advancement in deep learning, Rectifier Linear Unit (ReLU) is high intermittently utilized as the potential method to overwhelm the problems in numerical relevant to sigmoid.

In this, the hyperbolic tangent sort from -1 to 1, also the remaining is the logistic function related to the shape but sort from 0 to 1. Now, y_i is the output of the *i*th neuron, and v_i is the input connections of the weighted sum. Here alter activation function is developed for both rectifier and soft plus activation functions. The most specific activation function comprisesthe radial basis function.

Learning

Learning arises in perceptron by adjusting the connection of the weights; subsequently, all data is being measured as mentioned in Naga Srinivasu P. et al. (2021),depending on the number of errors during the execution (output) to the desired result. It is an illustration of supervised learning that then achievesbackpropagation, the proposal of the algorithm of least meanssquare to the linear perceptron.

Here the degree of the output node error j in the nth data point by $e_j(n) = d_h(n) - y_j(n)$, where d is a target variable, and y is a perceptron value. The weights of the node are further modified, which depends on the corrections that increase the error in the result, which is given by

$$\in (n) = \frac{1}{2} \sum_j e_j^2 (n) \tag{11}$$

Now gradient descent is used to alter every weight is

$$\Delta w_{ji}(n) = -\eta \frac{\partial \in (n)}{\partial v_j (n)} y_i (n) \tag{12}$$

Where y_i is the output of the preceding neuron and η is the learning rate, has preferred to assure that the weights suddenly converge to feedback excluding oscillations.

The derivation must be computed based on activated local field v_j, which changes. Also, it is simple to validate for an output node. This derivation can be made simple to

$$\frac{\partial \in (n)}{\partial v_j (n)} y_i (n) = e_j (n) \varnothing' (v_j (n)) \tag{13}$$

Where $\varnothing'$ is the derivation of the activation function mentioned above, which did not change. The study is complicated for the adjustment of weights in hidden node, yet it can program that known derivation is

$$-\frac{\partial \in (n)}{\partial v_j (n)} = \varnothing' (v_j (n)) \sum_k -\frac{\partial \in (n)}{\partial v_k (n)} w_{kj}(n) \tag{14}$$

This is dependent on the variation in weights of *k*th nodes, which means the output layer. Soto modify the weights of the hidden layer, the weights of the output layer may vary according to the derivation of the activation function. Thus this algorithm performs backpropagation of the activation function.

Feedforward neural networks (FFNNs) are the prominent model of Artificial Neural Network that can recognize and approximately computemodels utilizing their advancement in correlating layered design. They are comprised of neurons set, which performs as processing component, scattered over a list of entirely connected heap layers. MLP is a peculiar class of FFNN. In Multilayer perceptron, neurons have arranged in 1 direction. Data transition happens among three layers: input layer, hidden layer, and output layer. It explains the Multilayer perceptron network with 1 hidden layer. Medisetty et al., (2018) The inter-connection between those layers should be outlined by various weights [-1 to 1]. Every node in MLP will achieve 2 functions: one is activation, and another is the summation. The summation function is summed by the inputs, weights, and bias products.

$$S_j = \sum_{i=1}^{n} w_{ij} I_i + \beta_j \tag{15}$$

Where n is the no. of inputs, I_i represents input i, β_j is bias, and w_{ij} is weight connection.

Next, an activation function has been stimulated using Eq. (15), various models of activation functions can be handled in Multilayer perceptron. Laghmati et al., (2019) The function has outlined in Eq. (16)

$$f_j (x) = \frac{1}{1 + e^{-S_j}} \tag{16}$$

Subsequently, the final result of neuron j can be acquired in Eq. (17)

$$y_i = f_j \left(\sum_{i=1}^{n} \omega_{ij} I_i + \beta_j \right) \tag{17}$$

The framework of Artificial Neural Network is modeled, the learning step is observed and fine-tuned, then the network weights are modified. Eltrass et al., (2018) Those weights are rationalized to compute the result and decrease the error.

This model is utilized as a metaphor for biological/medical neural networks. It computes competent 51 z, so that it can be parallelized simply.In this model, the training process can influence local minima. Adel (2018)

EVALUATION METRICS

Accuracy

Accuracy is calculated by the total sum of true positive and true negative by the sum of classification attributes of true and false values.

$$Accuracy = \frac{TP + TN}{TP + TN + FP + EN} \tag{18}$$

$$Sensitivity = \frac{TP}{TP + FN} \tag{19}$$

$$Specificity = \frac{TN}{TN + FP} \tag{20}$$

RESULTS AND DISCUSSION

Different Algorithms like Decision tree, Logistic Regression, Random Forest, and Multilayer perceptron have been implemented as given in the pseudo code section. Figure2 demonstrates that the accuracy of various machine learning algorithms is performed in the Breast Cancer Wisconsin (diagnostic) dataset. The accuracy is predicted using a confusion matrix. It is found that the accuracy of Multilayer perceptron of deep learning algorithm has higher accuracy of 97% than the accuracy of Random Forest of 95%, Logistic Regression of 91% and Decision Tree of 93% which is the lowest. The outcome is shown in figure 2.

Table 3. Accuracy of various algorithms

Algorithm	Accuracy (%)	Sensitivity (%)	Specificity (%)
Logistic Regression	91	90	91
Decision Tree	93	91	92
Random Forest	95	93	92
Multilayer Perceptron Neural Network	97	95	94

Figure 2. Comparison ofthe accuracy of various algorithms

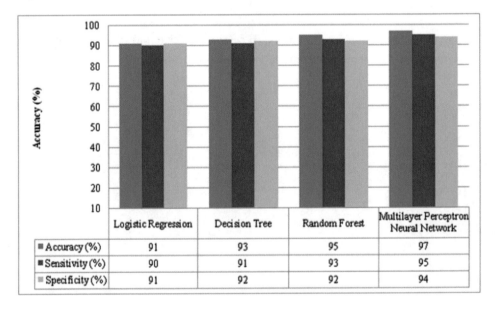

CONCLUSION

Breast Cancer tops the deadlierdiseases that cause more death rates in women worldwide. But this deadlier disease can be treated to cure if it was diagnosed in its earlier stages.Since manual diagnosis is quite time-consuming and inaccurate in most cases, the need of the hour is any innovation for analysis and predicting cancer that can save millions of lives.In this chapter, three machines and one Deep Learning algorithm for the prediction of disease classification were studied and investigated for the prediction of breast cancer. In this work, Logistic Regression, Random Forest, and Decision Tree are the threemachine learning models utilized to categorizedisease. Efficiency in applying Machine and deep Learning modelsisanalyzed based on performance metrics like accuracy, sensitivity, and specificity. The proposedMLP

(Multi-Layer Perceptron) model exhibits the highest performance with an accuracy of 97%. In the future, this chapter can be improved by implementing other different Deep and machinelearning algorithms and different optimization techniquesfor analysis and prediction of disease, which is severe cancer type.

REFERENCES

Adel, M., Kotb, A., Farag, O., Darweesh, M. S., & Mostafa, H. (2019). Breast Cancer Diagnosis Using Image Processing and Machine Learning for Elastography Images. *2019 8th International Conference on Modern Circuits and Systems Technologies (MOCAST),* 1-4. 10.1109/MOCAST.2019.8741846

Asria, H., Mousannifb, H., Al Moatassimec, H., & Noeld, T. (2016). Using Machine Learning Algorithms for Breast Cancer Risk Prediction and Diagnosis. *Procedia Computer Science, 83,* 1064–1069. doi:10.1016/j.procs.2016.04.224

Bayrak, E. A., Kırcı, P., & Ensari, T. (2019). Comparison of Machine Learning Methods for Breast Cancer Diagnosis. *2019 Scientific Meeting on Electrical-Electronics & Biomedical Engineering and Computer Science (EBBT),* 1-3. 10.1109/EBBT.2019.8741990

Deepalakshmi, P., Prudhvi Krishna, T., Siri Chandana, S., & Lavanya, K. (2021). Plant Leaf Disease Detection Using CNN Algorithm *International Journal of Information System Modeling and Design, 12*(1), 1–21. doi:10.4018/IJISMD.2021010101

Easttom, C., Thapa, S., & Lawson, J. (2020). A Comparative Study of Machine Learning Algorithms for Use in Breast Cancer Studies. *2020 10th Annual Computing and Communication Workshop and Conference (CCWC),* 412-416. 10.1109/CCWC47524.2020.9031266

Eltrass & Salama. (2018). Fully automated scheme for computer-aided detection and breast cancer diagnosis using digitised mammograms. *IET Image Processing, 14*(3), 495-505. . doi:10.1049/iet-ipr.2018.5953

Heidari, A. A., Faris, H., Aljarah, I., & Mirjalili, S. (2018). An Efficient Hybrid Multilayer Perceptron Neural Network with Grasshopper Optimization. *Soft Computing, 2018.* Advance online publication. doi:10.100700500-018-3424-2

Iqbal, H. T., Majeed, B., Khan, U., & Bin Altaf, M. A. (2019). An Infrared High classification Accuracy Hand-held Machine Learning based Breast-Cancer Detection System. *2019 IEEE Biomedical Circuits and Systems Conference (BioCAS),* 1-4. 10.1109/BIOCAS.2019.8918687

Kajala, A., & Jain, V. K. (2020). Diagnosis of Breast Cancer using Machine Learning Algorithms-A Review. *2020 International Conference on Emerging Trends in Communication, Control and Computing (ICONC3), Lakshmangarh, Sikar, India*, 1-5. 10.1109/ICONC345789.2020.9117320

Khuriwal, N., & Mishra, N. (2018). Breast cancer diagnosis using adaptive voting ensemble machine learning algorithm. *2018 IEEMA Engineer Infinite Conference (eTechNxT)*, 1-5. 10.1109/ETECHNXT.2018.8385355

Krishna & Rao. (2018). Prediction Of Breast Cancer Using Machine Learning Techniques. *International Journal of Management, Technology And Engineering, 8*(12).

Laghmati, S., Tmiri, A., & Cherradi, B. (2019). Machine Learning based System for Prediction of Breast Cancer Severity. *2019 International Conference on Wireless Networks and Mobile Communications (WINCOM)*, 1-5. 10.1109/WINCOM47513.2019.8942575

Mekha, P., & Teeyasuksaet, N. (2019). Deep Learning Algorithms for Predicting Breast Cancer Based on Tumor Cells. *2019 Joint International Conference on Digital Arts, Media and Technology with ECTI Northern Section Conference on Electrical, Electronics, Computer and Telecommunications Engineering (ECTI DAMT-NCON)*, 343-346. 10.1109/ECTI-NCON.2019.8692297

Mojrian, S. (2020). Hybrid Machine Learning Model of Extreme Learning Machine Radial basis function for Breast Cancer Detection and Diagnosis; a Multilayer Fuzzy Expert System. *2020 RIVF International Conference on Computing and Communication Technologies (RIVF)*, 1-7. 10.1109/RIVF48685.2020.9140744

Naga Srinivasu, P., & Balas, V. E. (2021). Performance Measurement of Various Hybridized Kernels for Noise Normalization and Enhancement in High-Resolution MR Images. In Bio-inspired Neurocomputing. Studies in Computational Intelligence (vol. 903). Springer. doi:10.1007/978-981-15-5495-7_1

Niţică, Ş., Czibula, G., & Tomescu, V. (2020). A comparative study on using unsupervised learning based data analysis techniques for breast cancer detection. *2020 IEEE 14th International Symposium on Applied Computational Intelligence and Informatics (SACI)*, 99-104. 10.1109/SACI49304.2020.9118783

Sharma & Nair. (2019). Efficient Breast Cancer Prediction Using Ensemble Machine Learning Models. *2019 4th International Conference on Recent Trends on Electronics, Information, Communication & Technology (RTEICT)*, 100-104. 10.1109/RTEICT46194.2019.9016968

Sivapriya, J., Aravind Kumar, V., Siddarth Sai, S., & Sriram, S. (2019). Breast Cancer Prediction using Machine Learning. *International Journal of Recent Technology and Engineering, 8*(4).

Sultana, J., Sadaf, K., Jilani, A. K., & Alabdan, R. (2019). Diagnosing Breast Cancer using Support Vector Machine and Multi-Classifiers. *2019 International Conference on Computational Intelligence and Knowledge Economy (ICCIKE)*, 449-451. 10.1109/ICCIKE47802.2019.9004356

Teixeira, F., Montenegro, J. L. Z., da Costa, C. A., & da Rosa Righi, R. (2019). An Analysis of Machine Learning Classifiers in Breast Cancer Diagnosis. *2019 XLV Latin American Computing Conference (CLEI)*, 1-10. 10.1109/CLEI47609.2019.235094

Thomas, T., Pradhan, N., & Dhaka, V. S. (2020). Comparative Analysis to Predict Breast Cancer using Machine Learning Algorithms: A Survey. *2020 International Conference on Inventive Computation Technologies (ICICT)*, 192-196. 10.1109/ICICT48043.2020.9112464

Wang, Y., Lei, B., Elazab, A., Tan, E.-L., Wang, W., Huang, F., Gong, X., & Wang, T. (2020). Breast Cancer Image Classification via Multi-Network Features and Dual-Network Orthogonal Low-Rank Learning. *IEEE Access: Practical Innovations, Open Solutions, 8*, 27779–27792. doi:10.1109/ACCESS.2020.2964276

Yarabarla, M. S., Ravi, L. K., & Sivasangari, A. (2019). Breast Cancer Prediction via Machine Learning. *2019 3rd International Conference on Trends in Electronics and Informatics (ICOEI)*, 121-124. 10.1109/ICOEI.2019.8862533

Zhu, C., Idemudia, C., & Feng, W. (2019). Improved logistic regression model for diabetes prediction by integrating PCA and K-means techniques. *Informatics in Medicine Unlocked, 17*, 100179. Advance online publication. doi:10.1016/j.imu.2019.100179

Chapter 10
A Model–Based Approach for Extracting Emotional Status From Immobilized Beings Using EEG Signals

Namana Murali Krishna
AVN Institute of Engineering and Technology, Hyderabad, India

G. Raja Vikram
Vignan Institute of Technology and Science, Hyderabad, India

Harikrishna Kamatham
AVN Institute of Engineering and Technology, Hyderabad, India

J. Sirisha Devi
Institute of Aeronautical Engineering, Hyderabad, India

ABSTRACT

Human-computer interaction is a potential area of interest since the birth of the computer era. The chapter highlights the usage of electroencephalogram (EEG wave) signals to initiate a conveying medium for immobilized persons, who are not able to express their feelings, by the use of human brain waves or signals. In order to recognize the human feelings or expressions with some emotion by an disable persons, a classifier based on a gamma distribution is utilized. The characteristic of the human brain waves are extracted with the usage of cepstral coefficients. The extracted characteristic is classified into various emotion states using generalized gamma distribution. In order to experiment the proposed model, six healthy persons or subjects are taken aged between from 20 and 28, and a 64 electrode channel EEG system is considered to gather the EEG brain signals under audio as well as visual stimuli. In this chapter, the authors focused the study on four basic human emotions: boredom, sad, happy, and neutral.

DOI: 10.4018/978-1-6684-3791-9.ch010

INTRODUCTION

Human Emotion identification shows a vital role in recognize the psychological attitude of the individuals. Huge of investigation is projected in this wing to identify the human emotions through the audio signal of Audio (Patel, 2021), (Suhaimi et al., 2020),(Chen, 2000),(Krishna, 2019) and classify these audio speech signal into non identical emotions there by paving the way to recognize the individual's behavior. Emotion recognition has its strong roots in Telephone Conversation, Business Process Outsourcing (BPO) where, the independent and discrete human emotion features are bring out through either spectral speech signal features or the temporal. However, in generally the techniques are maximum used for recognition of human emotion based on the elaborate from audio files, where these signals are artificial or generated through the acting sequence and these signals can be generated if the subject is healthy. In case of immobilized persons, the above acquisition of emotion signals is not feasible. In this research article we are extracted human emotions, it can be broadly excerpt using two different groups, categorical (discrete) descriptor as well as dimensional (continuous) descriptor. Human behavior like Emotion which are identified with the help of categorical descriptors build, the fundamental feelings or emotions like Angry, neutral, sad, happy, and boredom. However, the main limitation of the brain signal acquire from categorical descriptor which include, the large training data set is required for training purpose as well as analysis point of view, and it is limited to classification of a unique emotion from the Brain signals and the emotions are extract from the EEG signal comprises a mixtures the different emotions.

Moreover, the continuous descriptor evaluates the signals effectively in case of mobilized persons and to overcome the above disadvantage dimensional descriptor can be of more use. The term, dimension refers to the exact set of attributes, which form the basis of a particular emotion. A two-dimensional graph is used to depict the model, that contains the activation along the Y-axis and evaluation along the X-axis.

The Activation referred to intensity of the human emotions and evaluation of the human emotion is measured, the emotion is to be extract from the disable or immobilize people, Electroencephalography (EEG) is used, which is to be measures the electrical activity of the human brain. The brain electrical activity's is measured or obtained the input data with the help of EEG electrodes which are placing on the brain scalp.

Huge works have been placed in Literature (Pitsikalis, 2003), (Krishna, 2013), (Ververidis, 2006) based on the different physiological signals like heartbeat, skin conductivity, as well as EMG. Very little bit work projected through EEG data to analyze the human emotion state of physically disabled people like immobilized persons who does not express their feelings, using model-based techniques. Hence in this research article an attempt is prepared to identify the emotion state of mind

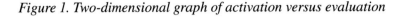

Figure 1. Two-dimensional graph of activation versus evaluation

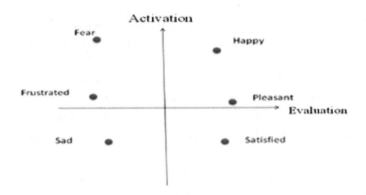

among head Diseased persons like Brain disabled. The parameters of initial vales is evaluates with the model of Generalized Gamma Distribution is updated through the Expectation–Maximization (EM algorithm), which is proposed by Mr. McLachlan and Krishnan in the year of 1997. This research article is organized as, in Section-2 of the paper, a brief introduction about emotion recognition is presented, in section -3, Generalized Gamma Distributions is introduced, section Four of the article presents the experimental results & the finally concludes the paper in section-5.

EMOTION RECOGNITION AND SYSTEM EXPERIMENTATION PROCESS

Emotions are inherent features of our daily life and all the non-verbal communications can be interpreted by means of emotions. In generally the human emotions cannot quantitatively determined, but can be estimated through identifying the expressions of face, few psycho physiological parameters like rate of heart beat and skin conductance changes abruptly, in a particular emotion state. The emotions generated are sensed by brain areas and to extract these signals, sophisticated equipments, which can extract these dynamic changes in the brain signals, are needed. To understand the relationship between the emotion generated and the physiological change that takes place, in the brain can be assessed by using Neurophysiology, and these modifications can be estimated from the system of central nervous (Park, 2003) (Nakasone, 2005) (Cai, 2009). To study the emotion state of mind, in a case of diseased person, EEG signals are used.

The Human emotions are initiated by the brain which are interpreted from the signals of EEG through the limbic system. These signals trigger the physiological

Table 1. Type of emotion and regions of the brain

Type of emotion	Regions of Brain
Fear	Bilateral Temporal activation
Sadness	Left Temporal areas
sadness, happiness and disgust	Right Prefrontal Cortex area

effects like heart rate, respiration rate and blood volume pressure, which was earlier, used to detect the emotion. But, the experiments demonstrated the reality that various other parts of brain also has vital role in provoking emotions specifically the motions viz. fear, disgust and surprise.In the Brain system we have several regions, which are contribute in assessing the emotions include, following regions.

As well as the above things, all human emotions portion the areas viz., temporal cortex cingulated gyrus and prefrontal cortex

Figure 2. Different emotional states of several regions in human brain

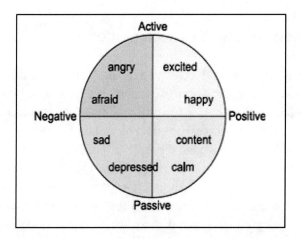

Equipment

In generally the system of EEG recording having 64 bit electrodes with the media of conductive, A to D converters (Analog to digital) filters with inbuilt amplifiers as well as maintain the recording device which is collecting the EEG signals and store the EEG data. With the support of electrode gel we maintain the connectivity between electrodes and scalp surface to sense the brain signals. In EEG system

Figure 3. Block diagram for the classification of human emotion based on EEG signal

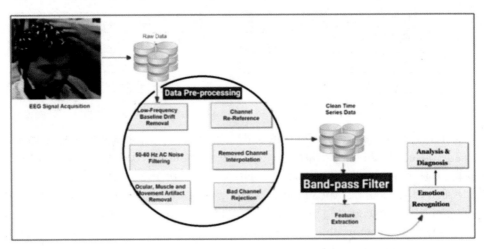

generally we consider microvolt signals and nanovolt through amplifier where we can recognize the accurate ranges.

EEG Measurement and Experimentation

The human brain signal in the EEG's data are measured in terms of five different rhythms as follows gamma (γ), mu (μ), alpha (∞), delta (δ), beta (β) and Theta (θ). Here the specified rhythms having different ranges of frequency and here each ranges of frequency denotes a specific effect of the mind. The range and the effect of the individual rhythms are placed in the table-2. The brain signals like EEG data is extracted from the physically diseased people using the EEG Nero Scan Equipment, after receiving the data, next activity is pre-processor, the EEG Signals to avoid the unwanted noise and which is extracted from the amplitude signals, normalized into various frequency ranges based on Rhythm, for the purpose of dimensionality minimizing.

These features like rytham are extracted trough Probability Density function as well as Generalized Gamma Distribution of each and individual rhythms are extracted, as well as for each of the emotion state that are shows the subject either person, we are the calculated the PDF value (Probability density functions) and estimate the Maximum likelihood value of each and every input signal, classified the various emotion states.

In order to acquire the data from EEG signals, firstly we will trained the subjects, if the subjected is mentally ready to experiments, then only place the EEG Cap of Nero Scan system on top of the scalp after explained the electrodes position. Here

Figure 4. Real-time display of the EEG data stream of different frequencies

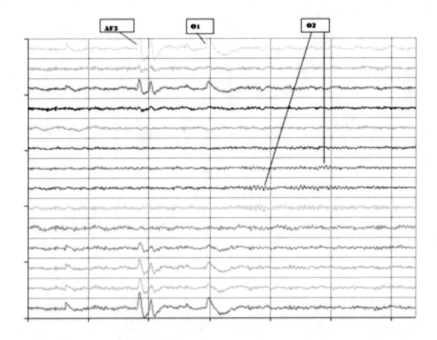

the duration of time factor should have a vital role in the elaborate and extract procedure; the procedure should be done in the procedure of trained technician of Nero scan machine.

In this research paper, we focused only four (4) different emotions from 10 different subjects. Through Nero scan EEG equipment, extracted EEG Brain signals to recognize the emotions, The reference electrode located in between F3, Fp and Fp2. The acquired Brain signals like EEG are processed through the distribution of generalized gamma. The Variance and mean of the EEG signals is initiate and PDF value (probability density function) of gamma distribution is calculated for each and every input EEG signal. This procedure facilitates in facilitate of noise as well as determine to which emotions the I/P (input) signals exactly belongs to.

Acquisition of EEG Signals using Nero Scan Machine -64 Bit "Sequence of Phases:"

- Phase 1. Initially train the Signal database
- Phase 2. From the train database, find the SIGMA & MU values
- Phase 3. For each and every emotional dataset, find out the PDF value (Probability Density Function)

Table 2. The range and the effect of the individual rhythms

Rhythm	Frequency	Range Location	Reason	Frequency bands
Delta (δ)	(0-4) Hz	Location of Frontal lobe	Deep sleep	
Theta (θ)	(4-7) Hz	Midline as well as temporal	meditation & Drowsiness	
Alpha (∞)	(8-13) Hz	Frontal, Occipital	closed eyes, Relaxing	
Mu (μ)	(8-12) Hz	Central location	Contra lateral Motor acts	
Beta (β)	(13-30) Hz	Frontal & central	thinking & Concentration	
Gamma (γ)	(30- 100+) Hz		Cognitive functions	

- Phase 4. Collect the brain signals means EEG wave and consider as test database
- Phase 5. For test database, estimate the SIGMA as well as MU

- Phase 6. Calculated the PDFs value of the testing data.
- Phase 7. Compare the train database versus EEG test data and finally identify which data of emotion state does the EEG (brain signals) data matches with the verified or existing EEG dataset.
- Phase 8. Display the state of emotion.

Figure 5. Electrodes position of EEG 64 channel

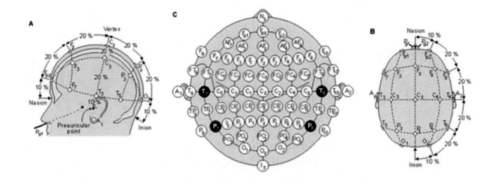

GENERALIZED GAMMA DISTRIBUTION: GENERALIZED GAMMA MIXTURE MODEL

To extract the accurate results of feature extraction based on EEG signals from human Brain, models of maximum posterior estimation are utilized (Krishna et al., 2017). In this research paper, we consider Generalize Gamma distribution for classification the human brain signals into different emotions. The classifier, it signifies the Variables like the sum of n-Exponential Distributed Random both parameters of the shape and scale, which are positive integer values only (Yang, 2010). Here the main parameters like Shape and Scale are defined using (Wei, 2009). The Generalized Gamma Mixture model is given by

$$f\left(x, k, c, a, b\right) = \frac{c\left(x - a\right)^{ck-1} e^{-\left(\frac{x-a}{b}\right)^{\sigma}}}{b^{ck} r\left(k\right)} \tag{1}$$

Here 'a' denotes the parameter of location, and parameter 'b' denotes the scale, k well as c both are the shape parameters respectively. Based on generalized gamma distribution, the parameters of Scale and shape, one can easily classifying the different emotions of EEG or brain signals

$$y = (x/\beta)\delta \tag{2}$$

a standard gamma distribution with parameter α is obtained

$$f(x, \alpha, \beta, \delta)dx = \frac{\ddot{a}}{\hat{a}^{\ddot{a}\acute{a}}\tilde{A}(\acute{a})} x\delta - 1e - (\frac{x}{\hat{a}})\delta \tag{3}$$

$$f(x) = \frac{1}{\tilde{A}(\acute{a})} y^{\alpha-1}e^{-y} - \tag{4}$$

Here we find out the random number which is related to y in density of Gamma, then only link this no to the generalized gamma by following the equation

$$x = \hat{a}y^{\frac{1}{\acute{a}}} \tag{5}$$

Expectation-Maximization Algorithm (EM Algo) for Estimation of the model parameters For good accurate emotion reorganization system, it is necessary to calculate the main parameters of the subject model efficiently. Through EM Algorithm, calculating or estimating the parameters which are maximizes the likely hood function of the models for sequence i, Let $xi=(x1, x2......xt)$, be the training vectors drawn from a brain signal and are differentiate by the value of PDF of the Generalized Gamma Distribution as given to above equation-1, the updated equation for the shape parameters are given by

$$c = \frac{1}{\dfrac{1}{r}\dfrac{\partial f}{\partial c} - k\log\dfrac{(x-a)}{b} + \dfrac{(x-a)^c}{b^c\log\left(\dfrac{x-a}{b}\right)}} \tag{6}$$

Figure 6. Analyzing when δ decreases or increases

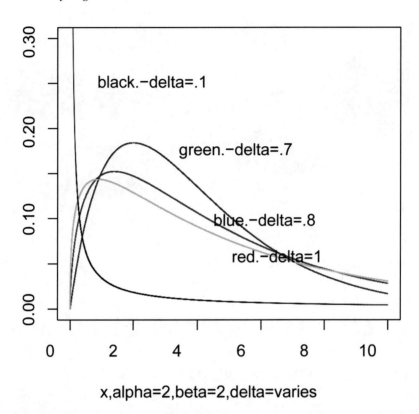

black.−delta=.1

green.−delta=.7

blue.−delta=.8

red.−delta=1

x,alpha=2,beta=2,delta=varies

$$\left(k\right)^{(I+1)} = 1 + \frac{\left[\int_0^\infty e^{-t}\left(\log e^t\right)t^{k-1}dt\right]}{\ddot{A}(k-1)\left[c\log\left(\frac{x-a}{b}\right)\frac{1}{r}\frac{\partial f}{\partial c}\right]} \tag{7}$$

The updated equation for the scale parameters is given by

$$b^{(l+1)} = \frac{ck}{\frac{c}{b^{c+1}}(x-a)^c - \frac{1}{f}\frac{\partial f}{\partial b}} \tag{8}$$

With the using of the equations (6) to (8) The updated derivation is derived to scale parameters and Generalized Gamma distribution is modelled:

0 2 4 6 8 10

Figure 7. Hardware setup for EEG signal acquisition

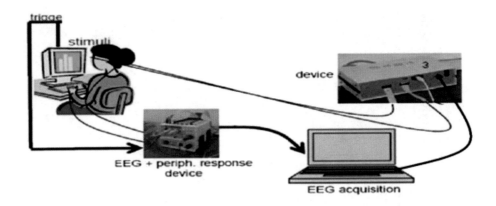

x,alpha=2,beta=2,delta=varies

Whenever the generalized gamma distribution ä either decreases. or else increases, it have two shape parameters like á as well as ä. Whenever ä is increasing, A plot with several graphs is increasing is shown in above figure.

METHODOLOGY FOR ACQUIRING EEG SIGNALS

Through Nero Scan equipment, acquiring the EEG/ brain signals. After collecting the Brain Signals calculate the frequency of each and every signal. For the experimentation point of view we consider 10-20 electrode system. Initially each subject/person is trained regarding the system as well as a test acquisition is organized; after acquainted the EEG Signals through the system, we noted the generated of actual readings as well as noted the frequencies generated also. For 10 -20 System the position of the electrodes F8, F7, F4, F2, FP2, Fp1, FpZ and F3 are considered. This electrodes position indicates or placed the frontal location of scalp and the human emotions can be well interpreted from these locations or particular potions. These frequencies were trained trough two different models, Generalized Gamma distribution. The Acquisition of EEG Signals using Nero Scan Machine -64 Bit- "Sequence of Phases which are specified in the above algorithm. For training and experimentation we considered more than 6 different subjects for training point of view and remaining half subjects for purpose of testing, for experimentation point of view we consider different emotions like neutral, sad, Happy and angry.

Figure 8. Participant wearing the EEG cap - 64 electrodes plugged

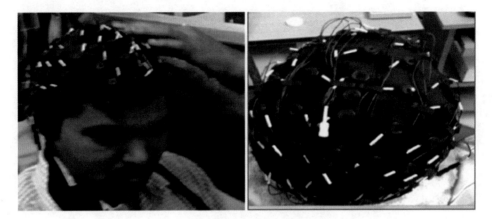

EMPIRICAL ANALYSIS AND EXPERIMENTAL RESULTS

The experimentation has been carried out on 5 different emotions of 6 healthy subjects and is conducted using MATLAB on Core i3 processor. The obtained signals have been utilized for experimentation and only some part of the dataset has been considered. The below figures show the signals and their corresponding emotion. The emotion classification accuracy is observed to about 80% and is as tabulated below. The emotions have been extracted from the subjects who were initially trained about the EEG data extraction pattern. The extracted signals have been preprocessed and the desired feature is extracted from the brain signals based on the rhythm. As there is a scope for noise present in the obtain EEG brain signal due to different reasons like movement of eye etc., the signals get distracted. Hence, minimize the noise present in the signals and obtain accurate classification, the brain signal data is further apply to proposed generalized gamma distribution. For classifying the the emotions, Alpha Features and Beta Features are considered. On self assessment section of experiments, it is found that five emotions (Boredom, Happy, Neutral, and Sad,) are extracted by subjects among six emotions. As the length of the initial extracted signals is more, only a part of the signal for about few seconds has been considered and the graphs below clearly show that the emotions identified are much accurate to the emotions identified as per the standards range of frequency of the wave.

The term, dimension refers to the exact set of attributes, which form the basis of a particular emotion. A two dimensional graph is used to depict the model, that considers the activation along the Y-axis and evaluation along the X-axis.

Figure 9. Features extracted frequency graphs with no of samples

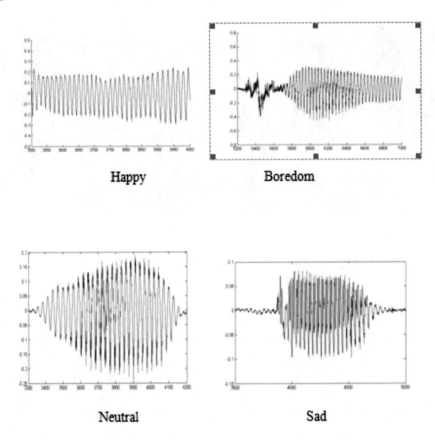

In our experimentation we consider four major emotional states for mobilized people like neutral, sad, angry and Happy. For suppose the EEG wave interpreted as happy, in case of not healthy or immobilized during the medical investigation

Table 3. comparisons between DTGMM and Generalized Gamma distribution based immobilized persons

Name of the classifier	Double Truncated Gaussian Mixture Model				Generalized Gamma distribution			
Data acquisition method	Happy	Sad	Angry	Neutral	Happy	Sad	Angry	Neutral
Acting sequences (Speech signal)	85	84	86	84	88	90	90	85
Electroencephalography (EEG)	88	85	90	80	90	86	92	82

Figure 10. Recognition rate of emotions of mobilized persons using generalized gamma distribution

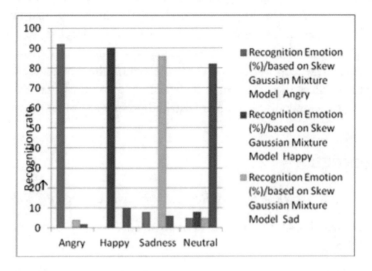

in a particular hospital, that implies/ shows that, the immobilized person simply responding to the particular medicine or drug, and result can be indicate via happy emotions state. Therefore to understand these EEG signals, it is lots of necessary to classify the brain signals(EEG) effectively.

CONCLUSION

Recognition of Emotions in case of immobilized persons.in our research the human emotions are classified into two different categories like, dimensional descriptor and another one is categorical descriptor. The reality of identification of human emotions we consider categorical descriptors, the basic emotions such as angry, happy, sad and neutral. Moreover, the continuous descriptor evaluates the signals effectively in case of mobilized persons and to overcome the above disadvantage dimensional descriptor can be of more use. The term, dimension refers to the exact set of attributes, which form the basis of a particular emotion. A two dimensional graph is used to depict the model, that considers the activation along the Y-axis and evaluation along the X-axis.

Finally we want just recall that, introduce a innovative approach for human emotion recognition based on Generalized Gamma Distribution using EEG dataset. As classification of human emotion recognition has vital in supporting to physically challenged persons, disease diagnosis like Alzheimer's patients, etc using the emotion recognition, the feedback of the usage of drug administered can be understand and thereby proper planning regarding the treatment can be done. EEG wave interpreted as happy, in case of not healthy or immobilized during the medical investigation in a particular hospital, that implies/ shows that, the immobilized person simply responding to the particular medicine or drug, and result can be indicate via happy emotions state. The scope of feature work is recognize the thought technology. We hope that the result of this research, it can be simply revive the Generalized Gamma Distribution, the Generalized Gamma Distribution in many other areas

REFERENCES

Cai. (2009). *The Research on Emotion Recognition from ECG Signal*. Academic Press.

Chen. (2000). *Emotional Expressions in Audiovisual Human Computer Interaction*. Academic Press.

Krishna. (2019). *An Efficient Mixture Model Approach in Brain-Machine Interface Systems for Extracting the Psychological Status of Mentally Impaired Persons Using EEG Signals*. IEEE Access.

Krishna, N. (2013). Inferring the Human Emotional State of Mind using Asymetric Distrubution. *International Journal of Advanced Computer Science and Applications*, 116–118.

Krishna, N. M., Devi, J. S., & Yarramalle, S. (2017). A Novel Approach for Effective Emotion Recognition Using Double Truncated Gaussian Mixture Model and EEG. *I.J. Intelligent Systems and Applications*, 6(6), 33–42. doi:10.5815/ijisa.2017.06.04

Nakasone, A. (2005). Emotion Recognition from Electromyography and Skin Conductance. *The Fifth International Workshop on Biosignal Interpretation*.

Park. (2003). *Emotion Recognition and Acoustic Analysis from Speech Signal*. Academic Press.

Patel, P. (2021). EEG-based human emotion recognition using entropy as a feature extraction measure. Springer.

Pitsikalis. (2003). Some Advances on Speech Analysis using Generalized Dimensions. *ITRW on Non-Linear Speech Processing (NOLISP 03)*.

Suhaimi, N. S., Mountstephens, J., & Teo, J. (2020). EEG-Based Emotion Recognition: A State-of-the-Art Review of Current Trends and Opportunities. *Computational Intelligence and Neuroscience*, *2020*, 1–19. doi:10.1155/2020/8875426 PMID:33014031

Ververidis. (2006). *Emotional speech recognition: Resources, features, and methods*. Academic Press.

Wei, L. (2009). Emotion-induced Higher Wavelet Entropy in the EEG with Depression during a Cognitive Task. *International Conference of the IEEE EMBS, 22*, 5018-5021.

Yang, S. (2010). ECG Pattern Recognition Based on Wavelet Transform and BP Neural Network. *Second International Symposium on Networking and Network Security*, 246-249.

Chapter 11
Basic Issues and Challenges on Explainable Artificial Intelligence (XAI) in Healthcare Systems

Oladipo Idowu Dauda
https://orcid.org/0000-0002-1472-2237
University of Ilorin, Ilorin, Nigeria

Joseph Bamidele Awotunde
https://orcid.org/0000-0002-1020-4432
University of Ilorin, Ilorin, Nigeria

Muyideen AbdulRaheem
University of Ilorin, Ilorin, Nigeria

Shakirat Aderonke Salihu
University of Ilorin, Ilorin, Nigeria

ABSTRACT

Artificial intelligence (AI) studies are progressing at a breakneck pace, with prospective programs in healthcare industries being established. In healthcare, there has been an extensive demonstration of the promise of AI through numerous applications like medical support systems and smart healthcare. Explainable artificial intelligence (XAI) development has been extremely beneficial in this direction. XAI models allow smart healthcare equipped with AI models so that the results generated by AI algorithms can be understood and trusted. Therefore, the goal of this chapter is to discuss the utility of XAI in systems used in healthcare. The issues, as well as difficulties related to the usage of XAI models in the healthcare system, were also discussed. The findings demonstrate some examples of XAI's effective medical practice implementation. The real-world application of XAI models in healthcare will significantly improve users' trust in AI algorithms in healthcare systems.

DOI: 10.4018/978-1-6684-3791-9.ch011

INTRODUCTION

The application of artificial intelligence (AI) in mission-critical systems such as healthcare, self-driving automobiles, as well as the military has a direct influence on human life (Awotunde, et al., 2021a; Awotunde, et al., 2021b). The "black box" aspect of AI, on the other hand, makes deployment in mission-critical applications challenging, posing ethical and legal problems and leading to a deficit of confidence (Das & Rad 2020; Abiodun et al., 2021). A subfield of AI, known as Explainable Artificial Intelligence (XAI), supports a collection of instruments, algorithms, and tactics for producing natural, and human-comprehensible interpretations having high quality, for AI results. Other than offering detailed overview of XAI ecosystem using in AI currently, this chapter delves into XAI in the healthcare system.

The current interest in XAI by the researchers give birth to provide the European General Data Protection Regulation (GDPR) the government (AI, 2019), to regulate the data generated from medical captured data. For example, gives insight to the crucial actualization of AI's trust (Weld & Bansal 2019; Lui & Lamb 2018; Hengstler, Enkel & Duelli 2016), bias (Chen *et al.,* 2019; Challen, *et al.,* 2019; DeCamp & Lindvall 2020), influence of argumentative examples on misleading classifier results (Guo *et al.,* 2019; Su, Vargas & Sakurai 2019), and ethnics (Cath et al., 2018; Etzioni & Etzioni 2017; Bostrom & Yudkowsky 2014; Dignum, 2018). gives insight on the importance of XAI generally. Curiosity, according to the authors in (Miller 2019), is one of the primary reasons why people seek reasons for certain actions. An additional cause may be to make gaining knowledge less difficult to repeat model creation and achieve better results.

Every explanation must be consistent across identical datasets and produce good or comparable interpretations as time goes on (Sokol & Flach 2020). Explanations must make the AI system demonstrative with the aim of promoting comprehension for human beings, confidence in decision-making, and supporting unbiased and just results. As a result, an explanation or interpretable solution for AI systems is required to assure AI decision-making transparency, trust, and fairness. A way of confirming an AI agent`s or algorithm's output decision is known as an explanation.

To describe a cancer detection model based on microscopic pictures, a map of input pixels that make a contribution to the output of the model might be employed. A voice recognition model might be defined by the means of the power spectrum information accessible at a certain moment, which had a bigger effect on the current choice of output. Furthermore, the trained model's variables or activations can be the basis for explanations, which may be conveyed using surrogates such as decision trees, gradients, or other approaches. An explanation of why an agent selected one choice over another might be presented in the context of supervised learning. The concepts of readily understandable and explainable AI, on the other hand, are typically

Figure 1. Explainable artificial intelligence for healthcare systems

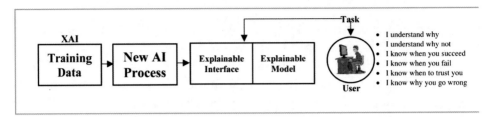

ambiguous and may be misleading (Rudin 2019), and they need incorporate some kind of reasoning (Doran, Schulz & Besold 2017).

Capabilities of artificial intelligence (AI) in healthcare have been extensively highlighted, having applicability in a variety of medical fields. As worldwide systems of healthcare strive to achieve the "quadruple objective," which involves improving patient experience, population health, cutting per capita healthcare expenditures (Berwick, Nolan, & Whittington 2008), and improving healthcare providers' work lives, this promise has been warmly accepted (Bodenheimer & Sinsky 2014). Figure 1 diplayed the general overview of XAI for healthcare systems.

When it comes to the deployment of artificial intelligence (AI) in healthcare systems, a growing number of researches have been conducted like interpreting chest radiographs (Hwang *et al.,* 2019) mammograms in detecting cancer (Geras *et al.,* 2017), tomography scans in analyzing computers (Benedek, *et al.,* 2021; Sh 2021), magnetic resonance images for the identification of brain tumors (Hua *et al.,* 2015; Kamnitsas *et al.,* 2016), position emission tomography for Alzheimer disease prediction (Ding *et al.,* 2019). However, there are currently few successful examples use of such procedures in clinical practice. This chapter discusses the measures that must be taken to tmove these potentially disruptive technologies from the lab to the clinic, as well as the major issues and limitations of explainable AI in healthcare. The goal of this chapter is to collect novel research articles that look at the approaches and technology infrastructures needed to boost AI trustworthiness for healthcare applications.

The Explainable Artificial Intelligence Framework in Healthcare Systems

The XAI framework is a general conceptual framework demonstrated in figure 2 where the explanators was use automatically has induced models for explainability, and these can be assessed using concepts and performance metrics. Researchers have acknowledged a varied set of notions and necessities that an explanation should meet in order to be easily understandable by end-users (Abiodun *et al.* 2022), In order to

Figure 2. The framework for explainable artificial intelligence with collaboration among methods for explanations and evaluation methods

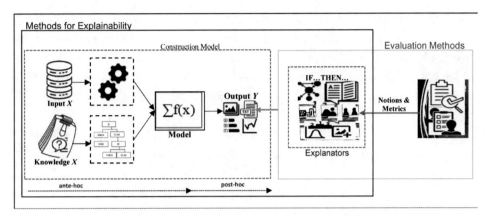

give appropriate relevant information to back up life choice processes, especially for laypeople. However, a detailed examination of these research revealed a lack of systematic arrangement of the different conceptions associated to the concept of explainability, as well as techniques to assessing the quality of explanations.

An overview of Explainable Artificial Intelligence Model using RETAIN

As show in Figure 2 the high-level of the model, where the central feature can be delegate for the prediction responsibility in the process of healthcare data generating from the captured data. This can be used to address the problems and difficulty with interpreting various AI-based models where in most cases the recurrent weights feed past data to the hidden layer like in CNN and RNN. Therefore, the RETAIN model consider both the visit-level and variable-level influence, the model use a linear embedding in the input of XAI, and this can be define as:

$$v_i = W_{cmb}x_i, \tag{1}$$

$v_i \in \mathbb{R}^m$ represented the embedding of the input XAI $x_i \in \mathbb{R}^r$, m is the size of the embedding dimension, $W_{cmb} \in \mathbb{R}^{m \times r}$ is the matrix to learn. One set of weights is used for visit-level focus, while the other is used for variable-level attention. The following equation is derived.

RETIAN Interpretation

The largest α_i is used to find the visits that contribute to prediction, which is a simple process. Finding influential variables, on the other hand, is a little more difficult because a visit is represented by a collection of medical variables, each of which has a different predictive value. Each variable's contribution is governed by v, β, and α, and interpreting α alone tells us which visits are important in prediction but not why.

A method to interpret the end-to-end behavior of RETAIN is used. We examine changes in the likelihood of each label y_i, 1, ..., y_i, s in relation to changes in the original input x_i, 1, ..., x_i, r, ..., x_i, 1, ..., x_i, r by maintaining and values fixed as the attention of doctors. The input variable with the biggest contribution will be the x_j, k that produces the largest change in y_i, d. In more technical terms, we're attempting to forecast the probability of the output vector y_i, $\in \left\{0, 1\right\}^s$, which may be represented as follows, given the sequence x_1, ..., x_i,

$$p\left(y_i | x_1, \ldots, x_i\right) = p\left(y_i | c_i\right) = softmax\left(W_{c_i} + b\right) \tag{2}$$

v_1, ..., v_i is the sum of the visit embedding and $\alpha's$ and $\beta's$ are the attentions weighted. Hence, Equation (2) can be expressed in the following way,

$$p\left(y_i | x_1, \ldots, x_i\right) = p\left(y_i | c_i\right) = softmax\left(W\left(\sum_{j=1}^{i}\alpha_j\beta_j \odot v_j\right) + b\right) \tag{3}$$

Eq (3) may be simplified as Eq 4, using the knowledge that the visit encoding vi is the sum of the columns of W_{cmb} weighted by each element of x_i.

$$p\left(y_i | x_1, \ldots, x_i\right) = softmax\left(W\left[\sum_{j=1}^{i}\alpha_j\beta_j \odot \sum_{k=1}^{r}x_{j, k}W_{cmb}[:, k]\right] + b\right) = softmax\left(\sum_{j=1}^{i}\sum_{k=1}^{r}x_{j, k}\alpha_jW\left(\beta_j \odot W_{cmb}[:, k]\right) + b\right) \tag{4}$$

The k_{-th} element of the input vector x_j is $x_{j, k}$. Eq (4) can be entirely reconstructed to the components at each input x_1, ..., x_i, allowing for the calculation of the contribution ω of the k_{-th} variable of the input x_j at time step $j < i$ allowing for the prediction of y_i as follows:

In the α_j and β_j, the index x_i of y_i is omitted. At time step I in the visit sequence $x_1, \ldots, x_T$. As a result, for $\alpha's \ and \ \beta's$, the index i is always assumed. Eq (5) also demonstrates that when utilizing a binary input value, the coefficient is the contribution. When utilizing a non-binary input value, however, we must multiply the coefficient and the input value $x_{j,\ k}$ to calculate the contribution correctly.

EXPLAINABLE ARTIFICAL INTELLIGENCE IN HEALTHCARE SYSTEMS

XAI is considered as a set of techniques and algorithms, assisting humans to interpret and trust machine learning algorithm outputs (Antoniadi *et al.*, 2021). "Explainable AI" is a term that refers to a model`s predicted effect and biases. It permits the assessment of the correctness, integrity, and transparency of a model, in addition to the result of AI-assisted decision-making. Organizations require XAI to create trust and confidence in the implementation process of AI models. Furthermore, the XAI aids organizations in implementing an accountable AI improvement strategy. Humans can have a tougher time decoding and retracing the computer's reasoning as AI advances.

The XAI has the ability to revolutionize virtually every aspect of medicine, -currently as well as in future. However, a lack of accountability in Machine learning (ML) and artificial intelligence (AI) has shown to be more problematic in quite a few sectors, including outside of health (Mathews 2019; Oladipo et al., 2022). This is especially true when users are required to comprehend the outcomes of AI systems. Explainable AI (XAI) provides a cause that lets users comprehend the reason a system produced a specific end result (Heinrichs & Eickhoff 2020; Awotunde et al., 2021c). In light of the conditions, the end result can also be comprehended. One place in which XAI is severely required is-a Clinical Decision Support Systems (CDSS). These systems, because of their inexplicability, help clinical practitioners making medical decisions, which may lead to worries about less or more outcomes from such model. Practitioners could be capable of making higher informed, and in a few instances, life-saving choices if the logic behind the recommendations is clarified. The necessity for XAI in CDSS and the healthcare commercial enterprise in general is exacerbated via the demand for ethical and fair decision-making (Bleher & Braun 2022), in addition to the truth that AI educated on historical data might reproduce historical acts and biases that should be identified.

Despite the growing demand for ethical AI, it is difficult for people to accept procedures that are generally not clearly interpretable, manageable, or predictable (Zhu, et al., 2018; Hall 2018). It is generally assumed that a focus on efficiency will lead to more transparent systems. This is correct because there is a trade-off between a model's performance and transparency (Awotunde et al., 2021a; Awotunde et al., 2021b; Rudin 2019). However, a better understanding of the process can eliminate the shortcomings. Interpretability is a key design factor that can improve the implementation capabilities of machine learning models for three reasons.

- By recognizing and correcting biases in the training data set, interpretability improves the objectivity of decision making.
- Interpretability improves robustness by identifying potential adversarial violations that could change the prediction.
- Interpretability can be used to ensure that only relevant variables are used to derive conclusions, i.e., that a model's inferences are based on true causality.

The system's interpretation must supply information approximately about the model's operations and predictions, an illustration of the model's discriminating rules, or information about what can disrupt the model in order to be considered realistic (Hall 2018).

The ability of explainable AI to help human beings in understanding and clarifying machine learning (ML) algorithms, deep learning, and neural networks is vital due to its significance in helping an organization to have a thorough understanding of the AI decision-making procedures, in addition to model monitoring and accountability, and to avoid trusting AI blindly, as neural networks and deep learning are a few of the most challenging for human beings to grasp.

For decades, the medical sector has deployed AI in the form of Clinical Decision Support Systems (DSSs) to aid physicians in diagnosing and categorizing patients. The effectiveness of machine learning models is restricted by the computer's inherent incapability to elucidate its behaviors and judgements to human beings, even though they are reliable. Although there is an increasing amount of research on machine learning algorithms that are transparent and easily understood, majority of the research focuses on technical users. A newly released article gives a comprehensive summary of explainable artificial intelligence research (Pierce 2019).

In (Samanta, Avleen, Rohit & Kary 2020), the author proposed an XAI for decision-support systems for humans in the clinical field. The study looked at the feasibility of XAI techniques for decision support in clinical image evaluation contexts. Increase the comprehension of Convolutional Neural Network (CNN) assessments by using three distinct explainable approaches on the same medical imaging data set was the goal of this study. To increase health practitioners' confidence in black box predictions, there were visible explanations of in-vivo gastral pictures recorded by video capsule endoscopy. (VCE).

They used the LIME and SHAP interpretable machine learning techniques, as well as the CIU alternative explanation technique, which is based on Contextual Value and Utility (CIU). Human judgment was used to evaluate the explanations provided. They showed the use of a neural network, namely a CNN, in medicine. Using explanations supplied by LIME, SHAP, and CIU as the basis, they conducted three user studies. Through a web-based survey, users without a background in medicine carried out a set of tests, providing information about their experiences and insights of the explanations. Accordingly, three possibly explainable approaches that may be used to a variety of medical data sets with future developments in implementation and give good decision-support for medical specialists were proposed.

The report XAI for Neuroscience, Behavioral Neurostimulation discusses several practical applications of XAI and machine learning in clinical and basic neuroscience, including new understandings of vital principles of brain function, brain disorder detection of higher accuracy, and more knowledgeable protocols for intervention. Authors in (Fellous et al., 2019) published a study on XAI for Neuroscience, Behavioral Neurostimulation, which details many practical applications of XAI and machine learning in fundamental and clinical research. They discussed XAI's possible benefits in the area of neurostimulation for fundamental clinical research and satisfying applications, as along with major concerns and hurdles to the XAI approach's viability.

Andreas (2020) gave emphasis to the necessity for XAI in the medicine in order to aid physicians to make explicable, clear, and comprehensible decisions. They projected that being able to clarify the choices of machine learning will increase the likelihood of it being used in medicine. Holzinger et al., (2017) used XAI in another research to emphasize the necessity of making simple and unambiguous judgments in the context of a digital pathology application. Sahiner et al., (2019) presented a summary of the history and existing state of DL study in imaging and radiation treatment of medicine, explore problems and solutions, and deduce with imminent prospects. Amann et al., (2020) conducted an analysis of the usage of XAI in clinical settings and find that the inclusion of explainability is a necessary precondition for minimizing objections to ethical standards. It may help maintain patients at the center of care by empowering them to make educated and autonomous health choices with the aid of medical professionals. A novel explanation approach, Local Interpretable Model-agnostic Explanations (LIME), established by (Ribeiro, Singh & Guestrin 2016) was proposed as a mechanism for reliably and interpretably explaining the classifier's predictions. The versatility of the model is evidenced by the fact that it contains explanations of text and graphics for a variety of models. It aided both experts and non-expert users in making model assessments by quantifying their confidence and providing insight into untrustworthy models' projections. Additionally, they examine the influence of explainability on confidence in systems of Computer Vision and AI in 2020, by increasing the comprehension and reliability of Computer Vision selections on medical diagnostic data based on deep learning. Additionally, they compared the recognition methodologies of two deep learning models utilising XAI: Multi-Layer Perceptron and CNN.

When AI is integrated with medical equipment and smart wearable technologies such as Fitbits, it can foresee the development of health problems in users using the data collected and analysed. While the integration of advanced AI and intelligent devices has a broad variety of potential applications in smart healthcare, there is a concern about the opaque operation of AI models' judgements, which has resulted in a lack of responsibility and confidence in the choices made. XAI is a branch of study that focuses on developing ways for explaining AI-based predictions (Lundberg & Lee 2017). XAI is seen as a way that AI-based systems may use to assess and diagnose health data, as well as a possible method for creating accountability. Transparency, tracking of result, and enhancement of model are all critical in the healthcare sector (Holzinger et al., (2017).

Smart healthcare is the use of technology such as cloud computing, the Internet of Things, and artificial intelligence to produce a more efficient, effective, and tailored healthcare system (Awotunde et al., 2021b; Lundberg & Lee 2017). Individuals may monitor their health in real time using healthcare applications on their smartphones or wearable devices, giving them control over their health (Wang, Yang, Abdul & Lim 2019). User-level health data may be shared with specialists for further diagnosis, and AI can be utilised for health screening, early illness detection, and treatment plan selection. In healthcare, the ethical concern over AI transparency, along with a lack of confidence in AI systems' black-box operation, mandates explainable AI models. XAI methods are a kind of artificial intelligence technology that is used to explain AI models and their predictions (Awotunde et al., 2021b; (Wang et al., 2019).

Numerous solutions in the area of XAI have been presented throughout the years, many of which have been applied to the healthcare sector. Certain AI models in the area of XAI, such as decision sets, are self-explanatory by their very nature, which academics have exploited and employed to explain illness prediction (asthma, diabetes, lung cancer). They are self-explanatory in that they were created by mapping an instance of data to an outcome based on certain criteria and are derived from a patient's health record (Ajagbe, Awotunde, Oladipupo & Oye 2022). For instance, prediction models will be developed to forecast lung cancer based on a condition: IF the individual is a smoker with a history of respiratory illness, then lung cancer will be anticipated. The disadvantage of self-explanatory AI models is that they impose a limit on the number of AI models that may be used to increase accuracy (Awotunde, Folorunso, Ajagbe, Garg & Ajamu 2022). There has been a surge in interest in XAI techniques capable of explaining any AI model in order to address the explainability of a broader variety of AI models. Model-agnostic XAI techniques are those that are not reliant on the AI model being presented. Local Interpretable Model-Agnostic Explanation (LIME) was developed by researchers as one of the most extensively used model-agnostic approaches for explaining predictions by quantifying the contribution of all components involved in prediction generation (Hofman et al., 2021). The researchers used LIME to explain how Recurrent Neural Networks (RNNs) anticipate heart failure, and their explanations assisted them in identifying the most common health problems related with a bigger threat of heart failure, as well as renal failure, anaemia, and diabetes. Numerous more model-agnostic XAI techniques, such as Anchors and Shapley values, have been developed and used in the healthcare domain. A framework for integrating human reasoning expertise into the creation of XAI techniques was proposed, with the objective of improving explanations via the incorporation of the user's reasoning goals (Jacovi, Marasović, Miller & Goldberg 2021; Colonna 2021) The paradigm developed here may be used to particular domains, such as smart healthcare, to produce human-friendly insights into the functioning of AI-based systems that employ XAI methods at different stages to assist clinicians in making clinical decisions. There are certain challenges associated with deploying XAI techniques. End users, who may be physicians with medical expertise or laypeople, should value the explanations provided by XAI techniques (Amparore Perotti & Bajardi 2021). It is feasible to design effective user interfaces for showing explanations. Model-independent XAI techniques have a number of problems, including higher processing costs and assumption-based operation, which are presently under investigation (Pauline-Graf et al., 2021).

Numerous publications provide measurable criteria for evaluating the explainability characteristics (such as clarity, comprehensiveness, proportionality, completeness, and accuracy) of various explanatory forms. They noted that some characteristics (clarification, comprehensiveness, and completeness), as well as the class of outstanding illustrative arguments, remain unquantifiable (Zhou, Gandomi Chen & Holzinger 2021). Further research by (Enas, Arunkumar & Gustavo 2021) identifies challenges and proposes solutions for a more trustworthy XIA judgment system, include but are not restricted to:

- AI technologies for precision medicine that can be explained
- Medical devices that use explainable AI and the IoMT-based system
- AI that can be explained for targeted medicine delivery
- An AI that can be explained for medical picture segmentation
- Effective Knowledge retention and development in health-care technology that can be explained
- Context-aware systems in healthcare and related applications
- Context-aware systems in healthcare and related applications
- AI-assisted healthcare decision-making

- AI-assisted surgery that can be explained
- ML-models and health informatics case studies with explainable AI

A clinical decision-making system (CDSS) is a type of health information technology that offers medical physicians, patients, staff, or different types of human beings having understanding and information that is specific to a particular person and is filtered or supplied intelligently at the right time to improve well-being and treatment (Awotunde, Adeniyi, Ajagbe & González-Briones 2022). CDS is a set of tools designed to help clinicians make better decisions in the clinic. Computerized alerts and reminders to caregivers and patients; medical guidelines; order sets that are condition-specific; data reports and summaries of focused patient; templates of documentation; diagnostic support, and referential information that are related and relevant are just a few of the tools available. "Clinical decision support systems combine health observations with health information to impact clinicians' health choices for enhanced health care", this is a working description developed by Robert Hayward of the Centre for Health Evidence. CDSSs are a hot topic in the artificial intelligence of the medical field (Joshi 2020).

A group of techniques along with the strategies that allow the results and output of machine learning algorithms to be understood and trusted by humans is known as Explainable artificial intelligence (XAI) (Mahbooba Timilsina Sahal & Serrano 2021). "Explainable AI", a phrase referring to the projected impact and probable biases of an AI model. XAI assists the evaluation of model transparency, fairness, accuracy, and results used in AI-assisted decision making. XAI is critical for the trust and confidence of an organization when bringing AI models into production (Dhanorkar *et al.*, 2021). Explainability of AI also aids in the development of AI in a responsible manner (Curia 2021).

Humans will find it more challenging to comprehend and follow how computer came to conclusions as AI continues to advance. The whole computing procedure is converted into a "black box" that is difficult to interpret. Black box models are generated using this data. The creators of the algorithm, the engineers and data scientists are clueless about what is going on inside them or how the AI algorithm achieve certain results. Artificial Intelligence (AI) Model, additionally referred to as black box, is any artificial intelligence system whose inputs and activities are concealed from the user or any other interested parties. A black box, in the broadest sense, is an impenetrable system (Matuchansky 2019; Rafia *et al.*, 2021).

This process is difficult for data scientists, programmers, and users to analyze since it is inherently independent. These models of a black box are built straight from data by an algorithm in machine learning, which means that human beings, including those who create them, have no idea the process involved in combining variables to make predictions (Newman & Furbank 2021; Angelov *et al.*, 2021).

A "black box" predictive model can be such a complex function of variables that people cannot figure out how the variables are related to each other to get the final prediction even when given a list of input variables. Interpretable models, that are precisely similar to the black box models but can be greater ethically, are distinct in that they are limited in order to provide improved comprehension of how predictions are formed (Barredo *et al.*, 2020).

In some instances, in which a handful of arguments are incuded in a brief reasonable statement, or when using a linear model in which the arguments are weighted and combined, it may be made abundantly clear how variables are associated to generate the ending forecast. Decomposable models are sometimes used to create interpretable models, or other limitations are imposed on the model to provide a new level of understanding (Rohitha 2019). A bulk of machine learning models, on the other hand, aren't built with interpretability in mind; instead, they're built to be predictors that are accurate on a predefined dataset which might or might not reflect the way the model would be used in reality.

ISSUES AND CHALLENGES OF EXPLAINABLE ARTIFICIAL INTELLIGENCE

Insufficient description for participants (e.g., physicians, patients, researchers, and the general public) concerning therapeutic and diagnostic solutions as well as treatments is one of the most critical difficulties in today's public and clinical health decision-making systems. Explainable Artificial Intelligence (XAI) suffers a number of flaws with lack of transparency and interpretability being the most serious. One of them is the trade-off between achieving algorithm transparency's simplicity while also having an impact on the high-performance nature of sophisticated yet opaque models (when one increases the transparency aspect, privacy and the security of sensitive data come into question). Another issue is selecting what information is appropriate for the user, which will necessitate different levels of knowledge (Braun & Clarke 2021).

Another trade-off in XAI is between correctness and interpretability, or between the simplicity of the information provided by the system's core knowledge and the comprehensiveness of this description (Ibarguren *et al.*, 2022). Intelligibility does not have to be at the same level whether the observer is a subject matter expert, a policy maker, or a user with no prior understanding of machine learning. One of the reasons why it is difficult for XAI to establish objective standards for what constitutes a good explanation is because of this (van der Waa, Nieuwburg, Cremers & Neerincx 2021). It's possible that an algorithm is confidential, in which case revealing it would be a security risk. Algorithms are well-understood, but they are

Figure 3. Summary of XAI challenges discussed in this overview and its impact on the principles for responsible AI

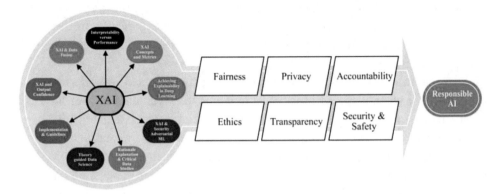

also extremely complicated. It makes conclusions based on legitimate data that are not reasonable, biased, or out of line (Szczepański, Choraś Pawlicki & Pawlicka 2021). Figure 3 displayed the summary of XAI challenges with its impact on the principles for Responsible AI.

Transparency is one attribute that can help with interpretability. Creating explainability approaches, on the other hand, is a difficult task. Explainable AI models have the disadvantage of limiting the use of other AI models that can be used to improve accuracy. Users who are physicians with medical experience or regular people will benefit from the explanations generated by the XAI technologies. It is also feasible to create proper user interfaces for displaying explanations efficiently.

Other concerns and issues in the areas of explainable AI include:

Bias

The AI system has a tendency to develop a skewed perspective of the world based on the shortcomings of the data sets, framework, or target value - possibly an impartial representation of such a subjective reality. For example, as regards to supervised learning, where a teacher is involved in the learning process, the teacher's bias will influence the AI system's decision (Yang, Ye & Xia 2022; Adadi & Berrada 2020).

Data Learning

The time it takes to learn and produce a good output is typically long, which might impede improvement or enhancement in some domains, particularly in Health Care Decision Systems.

Fairness

There is no way to tell whether or not an AI system's decisions are reasonable. Fairness is context-dependent, having different viewpoints based on the data supplied to machine learning techniques (Finocchiaro *et al.*, 2021; Taylor & Taylor 2021).

Hardware Dependence

Explainable Artificial Intelligence cannot function without some type of hardware, and this can impact some of its decisions (Senoner, Netland & Feuerriegel 2021; Jiménez-Luna, Skalic, Weskamp & Schneider 2021).

Complexity

While the goal of XAI is to help humans understand and accept the results of machine learning algorithms, it is still difficult and requires an expert in the subject to train the algorithm, particularly in the case of supervised learning, before desirable results can be obtained. Algorithms are sometimes simple to understand but quite difficult to implement. As a consequence, a layman's understanding is absurd, and that's an area where XAI techniques could be useful. Because XAI can create alternate, easier-to-understand algorithms (Puiutta & Veith 2020; Gilpin et al., 2018).

Inadequate Data

The amount of data required to train the AI may be insufficient for it to learn and make decisions that humans can understand. This might lead to underfitting of the model utilized, which can have a negative impact on future decisions based on new data.

Injustice

According to Phillips et al., (2020), humans may grasp how a machine algorithm works and the results it produces, but it remains unclear how the system is reliable using a legal or moral code.

Protection

Can clients have faith in the AI system's reliability without knowing how it comes to its conclusions? This is linked to the fundamental problem of generalization in statistical learning theory, which is how tightly can we bind errors on unseen data (Zubatiuk & Isayev 2021)

Computing Power

XAI demands the computational power of a supercomputer as they require a continuous increasing number of cores and GPUs to perform efficiently, and supercomputers remain not cheap (Vilone & Longo 2021).

Implementation Strategies

The lack of a well-defined implementation strategy is one of artificial intelligence's most significant issues. In order to be successful with AI, a strategic approach must be devised. This includes identifying areas for improvement, setting clear targets, and providing a continual process improvement feedback loop (Currie & Hawk 2021).

Abstractions

To make things easier to understand, abstractions are used. The foundation for articulating large-scale goals in small increments is elevated structures. It has always been difficult to automate the finding of concepts, and today's frontier of XAI research is understanding the discovery and sharing of abstractions in learning and explanation (Yang, Folke & Shafto 2021). Hence, the use of XAI in healthcare systems will helps the medical experts in understanding the results obtains from the AI-based models.

FUTURE DIRECTIONS

Combining deep learning technology with ontological approaches is one way to bridge the gap between artificial inference and human comprehension (Holzinger, Kieseberg, Weippl & Tjoa 2018). Deep Tensor (Maruhashi et al., 2018), a deep neural network designed for datasets with relevant graph-like properties, is an excellent current example, and it is advantageous for us that the disciplines of biology, chemistry, medicine, and drug creation, among others, provide many such datasets. Graphs can be used to encode the interactions between diverse things (mutations, genes, medications, diseases, and so on).

Consider a Deep Tensor network that learns to identify biological interaction pathways that lead to a specific disease. We would now be able to automatically identify and explain the inference elements that had a substantial impact on the classification findings. These criteria can also be used to filter a knowledge graph made up of publicly available medical research corpora (large ontologies) (Holzinger 2014). Furthermore, the resulting interaction pathways are bound by the domain's logical restrictions (in this example: Biology). As a result, the categorization is displayed as an annotated interaction path, with annotations on each edge referring to specific medical texts that give supporting evidence, which can then be explained by a human expert (Paulheim 2017).

As a result, effective mapping of results from high-dimensional spaces into lower-dimensional spaces is required in order to make them not only perceivable and manipulable by humans, but the increasing issue is that the best-performing approaches are the least transparent. Our greatest procedures are not retraceable, making them incomprehensible, making it impossible to explain why a decision was made. However, contemporary privacy trends necessitate transparent "glass box" alternatives.

CONCLUSION AND SUGGESTION FOR FURTHER STUDIES

The establishment of frameworks and models to aid in the understanding and interpretation of AI system decisions is a focus of XAI research. XAI methods can be used to describe and track AI-based autonomous system results. As previously stated, incorporating XAI approaches poses several difficulties. The choice of ways for providing explanations in a way that is both informative and efficient, and hence therapeutically effective, is still a fundamental issue. In order to include successful interpretability into the CDSS, there seems to be great amount of work that needs to be achieved. To better understand how explainability can be employed in this essential environment, research concentrating on each and every stages of CDSS evolution is needed. So as to better understand how comprehensibility can be employed in this essential environment, research concentrate on any and all stages of CDSS evolution are needed. Medical decision support has been provided using models of deep learning like CNN, LSTM, auto-encoder, fully convolutional models, deep belief networks, as well as system model suggestions such as decomposition modeling techniques, graph-based modeling techniques, predictor variables, pattern classification, information graph-based, neutral, and post hoc. The use of such novel methods to medical data can assist clinicians in making more accurate and faster diagnoses. According to the findings from this chapter, subjective assessments might provide useful information about functionality, there is really a general absence of established and trustworthy evaluation metrics.

REFERENCES

Abdulhay, E., Arunkumar, N., & Ramirez, G. (n.d.). *Explainable Artificial Intelligence for Medical Applications*. Hindawi. Retrieved September 20, 2021, from https://www.hindawi.com/journals/jhe/si/658251/

Abiodun, K. M., Awotunde, J. B., Aremu, D. R., & Adeniyi, E. A. (2022). Explainable AI for Fighting COVID-19 Pandemic: Opportunities, Challenges, and Future Prospects. In *Computational Intelligence for COVID-19 and Future Pandemics* (pp. 315–332). Springer. doi:10.1007/978-981-16-3783-4_15

Adadi, A., & Berrada, M. (2020). Explainable AI for healthcare: from black box to interpretable models. In *Embedded Systems and Artificial Intelligence* (pp. 327–337). Springer.

Ai, H. (2019). High-level expert group on artificial intelligence. *Ethics Guidelines for Trustworthy AI.*

Ajagbe, S. A., Awotunde, J. B., Oladipupo, M. A., & Oye, O. E. (2022). Prediction and Forecasting of Coronavirus Cases Using Artificial Intelligence Algorithm. In *Machine Learning for Critical Internet of Medical Things* (pp. 31–54). Springer.

Amann, J., Blasimme, A., Vayena, E., Frey, D., & Madai, V. I. (2020). Explainability for artificial intelligence in healthcare: A multidisciplinary perspective. *BMC Medical Informatics and Decision Making, 20*(1), 1–9.

Amparore, E., Perotti, A., & Bajardi, P. (2021). To trust or not to trust an explanation: Using LEAF to evaluate local linear XAI methods. *PeerJ. Computer Science, 7*, e479.

Andreas, J. (2020). Explainable machine learning for scientific insights and discoveries. *IEEE, 3*(8), 42.

Angelov, P. P., Soares, E. A., Jiang, R., Arnold, N. I., & Atkinson, P. M. (2021). Explainable artificial intelligence: An analytical review. *Wiley Interdisciplinary Reviews. Data Mining and Knowledge Discovery, 11*(5), e1424.

Antoniadi, A. M., Du, Y., Guendouz, Y., Wei, L., Mazo, C., Becker, B. A., & Mooney, C. (2021). Current Challenges and Future Opportunities for XAI in Machine Learning-Based Clinical Decision Support Systems: A Systematic Review. *Applied Sciences (Basel, Switzerland), 11*(11), 5088. https://doi.org/10.3390/app11115088

Awotunde, J. B., Adeniyi, A. E., Ajagbe, S. A., & González-Briones, A. (2022). Natural computing and unsupervised learning methods in smart healthcare data-centric operations. In *Cognitive and Soft Computing Techniques for the Analysis of Healthcare Data* (pp. 165–190). Academic Press.

Awotunde, J. B., Ajagbe, S. A., Oladipupo, M. A., Awokola, J. A., Afolabi, O. S., Mathew, T. O., & Oguns, Y. J. (2021, October). An Improved Machine Learnings Diagnosis Technique for COVID-19 Pandemic Using Chest X-ray Images. *Communications in Computer and Information Science, 2021, 1455 CCIS*, 319–330.

Awotunde, J. B., Folorunso, S. O., Ajagbe, S. A., Garg, J., & Ajamu, G. J. (2022). AiIoMT: IoMT-Based System-Enabled Artificial Intelligence for Enhanced Smart Healthcare Systems. *Machine Learning for Critical Internet of Medical Things*, 229-254.

Awotunde, J. B., Folorunso, S. O., Jimoh, R. G., Adeniyi, E. A., Abiodun, K. M., & Ajamu, G. J. (2021a). Application of artificial intelligence for COVID-19 epidemic: An exploratory study, opportunities, challenges, and future prospects. Studies in Systems. *Decision and Control, 2021*(358), 47–61. doi:10.1007/978-3-030-69744-0_4

Awotunde, J. B., Ogundokun, R. O., Jimoh, R. G., Misra, S., & Aro, T. O. (2021b). Machine learning algorithm for cryptocurrencies price prediction. *Studies in Computational Intelligence, 2021*(972), 421–447. doi:10.1007/978-3-030-72236-4_17

Barredo, A. A. (2020). Explainable Artificial Intelligence (XAI): Concepts, taxonomies, opportunities and challenges toward responsible AI. *Information Fusion, 58*, 82–115. https://doi.org/10.1016/j.inffus.2019.12.012

Benedek, Z., Todor-Boér, S., Kocsis, L., Bauer, O., Suciu, N., & Coroş, M. F. (2021). Psoas muscle index defined by computer tomography predicts the presence of postoperative complications in colorectal cancer surgery. *Medicina, 57*(5), 472.

Berwick, D. M., Nolan, T. W., & Whittington, J. (2008). The triple aim: Care, health, and cost. *Health Affairs, 27*(3), 759–769.

Bleher, H., & Braun, M. (2022). Diffused responsibility: attributions of responsibility in the use of AI-driven clinical decision support systems. *AI and Ethics*, 1-15.

Bodenheimer, T., & Sinsky, C. (2014). From triple to quadruple aim: Care of the patient requires care of the provider. *Annals of Family Medicine, 12*(6), 573–576.

Bostrom, N., & Yudkowsky, E. (2014). The ethics of artificial intelligence. The Cambridge handbook of artificial intelligence, 1, 316-334.

Braun, V., & Clarke, V. (2021). Can I use TA? Should I use TA? Should I not use TA? Comparing reflexive thematic analysis and other pattern-based qualitative analytic approaches. *Counselling & Psychotherapy Research, 21*(1), 37–47.

Cath, C., Wachter, S., Mittelstadt, B., Taddeo, M., & Floridi, L. (2018). Artificial intelligence and the 'good society': The US, EU, and UK approach. *Science and Engineering Ethics*, *24*(2), 505–528.

Challen, R., Denny, J., Pitt, M., Gompels, L., Edwards, T., & Tsaneva-Atanasova, K. (2019). Artificial intelligence, bias and clinical safety. *BMJ Quality & Safety*, *28*(3), 231–237.

Chen, L., Cruz, A., Ramsey, S., Dickson, C. J., Duca, J. S., Hornak, V., ... Kurtzman, T. (2019). Hidden bias in the DUD-E dataset leads to misleading performance of deep learning in structure-based virtual screening. *PLoS One*, *14*(8), e0220113.

Colonna, L. (2021). *Artificial Intelligence in the Internet of Health Things: Is the Solution to AI Privacy More AI? SSRN Electronic Journal*. doi:10.2139srn.3838571

Curia, F. (2021). Features and explainable methods for cytokines analysis of Dry Eye Disease in HIV infected patients. *Healthcare Analytics*, *1*, 100001.

Currie, G., & Hawk, K. E. (2021, March). Ethical and legal challenges of artificial intelligence in nuclear medicine. *Seminars in Nuclear Medicine*, *51*(2), 120–125.

Das, A., & Rad, P. (2020). *Opportunities and challenges in explainable artificial intelligence (xai): A survey*. arXiv preprint arXiv:2006.11371.

DeCamp, M., & Lindvall, C. (2020). Latent bias and the implementation of artificial intelligence in medicine. *Journal of the American Medical Informatics Association*, *27*(12), 2020–2023.

Dhanorkar, S., Wolf, C. T., Qian, K., Xu, A., Popa, L., & Li, Y. (2021, June). Who needs to know what, when?: Broadening the Explainable AI (XAI) Design Space by Looking at Explanations Across the AI Lifecycle. In *Designing Interactive Systems Conference 2021* (pp. 1591-1602). Academic Press.

Dignum, V. (2018). Ethics in artificial intelligence: Introduction to the special issue. *Ethics and Information Technology*, *20*(1), 1–3.

Ding, Y., Sohn, J. H., Kawczynski, M. G., Trivedi, H., Harnish, R., Jenkins, N. W., ... Franc, B. L. (2019). A deep learning model to predict a diagnosis of Alzheimer disease by using 18F-FDG PET of the brain. *Radiology*, *290*(2), 456–464.

Doran, D., Schulz, S., & Besold, T. R. (2017). *What does explainable AI really mean? A new conceptualization of perspectives*. arXiv preprint arXiv:1710.00794.

Etzioni, A., & Etzioni, O. (2017). Incorporating ethics into artificial intelligence. *The Journal of Ethics*, *21*(4), 403–418.

Fellous, J. M., Sapiro, G., Rossi, A., Mayberg, H., & Ferrante, M. (2019). Explainable Artificial Intelligence for Neuroscience, *Behavioral Neurostimulation. Frontiers in Neuroscience, 1*(1). Advance online publication. doi:10.3389/fnins.2019.01346

Finocchiaro, J., Maio, R., Monachou, F., Patro, G. K., Raghavan, M., Stoica, A. A., & Tsirtsis, S. (2021, March). Bridging machine learning and mechanism design towards algorithmic fairness. In *Proceedings of the 2021 ACM Conference on Fairness, Accountability, and Transparency* (pp. 489-503). ACM.

Geras, K. J., Wolfson, S., Shen, Y., Wu, N., Kim, S., Kim, E., . . . Cho, K. (2017). *High-resolution breast cancer screening with multi-view deep convolutional neural networks.* arXiv preprint arXiv:1703.07047.

Gilpin, L. H., Bau, D., Yuan, B. Z., Bajwa, A., Specter, M., & Kagal, L. (2018, October). Explaining explanations: An overview of interpretability of machine learning. In *2018 IEEE 5th International Conference on data science and advanced analytics (DSAA)* (pp. 80-89). IEEE.

Goodman, B., & Flaxman, S. (2017). European Union regulations on algorithmic decision-making and a "right to explanation". *AI Magazine, 38*(3), 50–57.

Guo, Q., Li, Z., An, B., Hui, P., Huang, J., Zhang, L., & Zhao, M. (2019, May). Securing the deep fraud detector in large-scale e-commerce platform via adversarial machine learning approach. In *The World Wide Web Conference* (pp. 616-626). Academic Press.

Hall, P. (2018). *On the art and science of machine learning explanations.* arXiv preprint arXiv:1810.02909.

Heinrichs, B., & Eickhoff, S. B. (2020). Your evidence? Machine learning algorithms for medical diagnosis and prediction. *Human Brain Mapping, 41*(6), 1435–1444.

Hengstler, M., Enkel, E., & Duelli, S. (2016). Applied artificial intelligence and trust—The case of autonomous vehicles and medical assistance devices. *Technological Forecasting and Social Change, 105*, 105–120. doi:10.1016/j.techfore.2015.12.014

Hofman, J. M., Watts, D. J., Athey, S., Garip, F., Griffiths, T. L., Kleinberg, J., ... Yarkoni, T. (2021). Integrating explanation and prediction in computational social science. *Nature, 595*(7866), 181–188.

Holzinger, A. (2014). *Biomedical informatics: discovering knowledge in big data.* Springer.

Holzinger, A., Biemann, C., Pattichis, C. S., & Kell, D. B. (2017). *What do we need to build explainable AI systems for the medical domain?* arXiv preprint arXiv:1712.09923.

Holzinger, A., Kieseberg, P., Weippl, E., & Tjoa, A. M. (2018, August). Current advances, trends and challenges of machine learning and knowledge extraction: from machine learning to explainable AI. In *International Cross-Domain Conference for Machine Learning and Knowledge Extraction* (pp. 1-8). Springer.

Hua, K. L., Hsu, C. H., Hidayati, S. C., Cheng, W. H., & Chen, Y. J. (2015). Computer-aided classification of lung nodules on computed tomography images via deep learning technique. *OncoTargets and Therapy*, 8.

Hwang, E. J., Park, S., Jin, K. N., Im Kim, J., Choi, S. Y., Lee, J. H., ... Park, C. M. (2019). Development and validation of a deep learning–based automated detection algorithm for major thoracic diseases on chest radiographs. *JAMA Network Open*, 2(3), e191095–e191095.

Ibarguren, I., Pérez, J. M., Muguerza, J., Arbelaitz, O., & Yera, A. (2022). PCTBagging: From inner ensembles to ensembles. A trade-off between discriminating capacity and interpretability. *Information Sciences*, *583*, 219–238.

Inam, R., Terra, A., Mujumdar, A., Fersman, E., & Feljan, A. V. (2021, April). *Explainable AI: How humans can trust Artificial Intelligence*. Ericsson White Paper. https://www.ericsson.com/en/reports-and-papers/white-papers/explainable-ai--how-humans-can-trust-ai

Jacovi, A., Marasović, A., Miller, T., & Goldberg, Y. (2021, March). Formalizing trust in artificial intelligence: Prerequisites, causes and goals of human trust in AI. In *Proceedings of the 2021 ACM conference on fairness, accountability, and transparency* (pp. 624-635). ACM.

Jiménez-Luna, J., Skalic, M., Weskamp, N., & Schneider, G. (2021). Coloring molecules with explainable artificial intelligence for preclinical relevance assessment. *Journal of Chemical Information and Modeling*, *61*(3), 1083–1094.

Joshi, N. (2020). *5 Artificial intelligence implementation challenges in healthcare* [Blog]. Retrieved from https://www.bbntimes.com/technology/5-artificial-intelligence-implementation-challenges-in-healthcare

Kamnitsas, K., Ferrante, E., Parisot, S., Ledig, C., Nori, A. V., Criminisi, A., ... Glocker, B. (2016, October). DeepMedic for brain tumor segmentation. In *International workshop on Brainlesion: Glioma, multiple sclerosis, stroke and traumatic brain injuries* (pp. 138-149). Springer.

Lui, A., & Lamb, G. W. (2018). Artificial intelligence and augmented intelligence collaboration: Regaining trust and confidence in the financial sector. *Information & Communications Technology Law*, *27*(3), 267–283. doi:10.1080/13600834.201 8.1488659

Lundberg, S. M., & Lee, S. I. (2017). A unified approach to interpreting model predictions. *Advances in Neural Information Processing Systems*, *30*, 4765–4774.

Mahbooba, B., Timilsina, M., Sahal, R., & Serrano, M. (2021). Explainable artificial intelligence (xai) to enhance trust management in intrusion detection systems using decision tree model. *Complexity*.

Maruhashi, K., Todoriki, M., Ohwa, T., Goto, K., Hasegawa, Y., Inakoshi, H., & Anai, H. (2018, April). Learning multi-way relations via tensor decomposition with neural networks. *Proceedings of the AAAI Conference on Artificial Intelligence*, *32*(1).

Mathews, S. M. (2019, July). Explainable artificial intelligence applications in NLP, biomedical, and malware classification: a literature review. In *Intelligent computing-proceedings of the computing conference* (pp. 1269–1292). Springer.

Matuchansky, C. (2019). Deep medicine, artificial intelligence, and the practicing clinician. *Lancet*, *394*(10200), 736.

Miller, T. (2019). Explanation in artificial intelligence: Insights from the social sciences. *Artificial Intelligence*, *267*, 1–38.

Newman, S. J., & Furbank, R. T. (2021). Explainable machine learning models of major crop traits from satellite-monitored continent-wide field trial data. *Nature Plants*, *7*(10), 1354–1363.

Oladipo, I. D., AbdulRaheem, M., Awotunde, J. B., Bhoi, A. K., Adeniyi, E. A., & Abiodun, M. K. (2022). Machine Learning and Deep Learning Algorithms for Smart Cities: A Start-of-the-Art Review. *IoT and IoE Driven Smart Cities*, 143-162.

Paulheim, H. (2017). Knowledge graph refinement: A survey of approaches and evaluation methods. *Semantic Web*, *8*(3), 489–508.

Pauline-Graf, D., Mandel, S. E., Allen, H. W., & Devnew, L. E. (2021). Assumption Validation Process for the Assessment of Technology-Enhanced Learning. *Contemporary Educational Technology*, *13*(4).

Phillips, P. J., Hahn, C. A., Fontana, P. C., Broniatowski, D. A., & Przybocki, M. A. (2020). Four principles of explainable artificial intelligence. Academic Press.

Pierce, R. (2019). *AI in Healthcare: Solutions, Challenges, and Dilemmas in Medical Decision-Making. SSRN Electronic Journal.* doi:10.2139srn.3806767

Puiutta, E., & Veith, E. (2020, August). Explainable reinforcement learning: A survey. In *International cross-domain conference for machine learning and knowledge extraction* (pp. 77-95). Springer.

Ribeiro, M. T., Singh, S., & Guestrin, C. (2016). why should I trust you?: Explaining the predictions of any classifier. *Proceedings of the 22nd ACM SIGKDD International Conference on Knowledge Discovery and Data Mining*, 1135–1144. https://github.com/marcotcr/lime

Rohitha, E. P. (2019, December 13). *Explainability of AI: The challenges and possible workarounds.* https://medium.com/@rohithaelsa/explainability-of-ai-the-challenges-and-possible-workarounds-14d8389d2515

Rudin, C. (2019). Stop explaining black box machine learning models for high stakes decisions and use interpretable models instead. *Nature Machine Intelligence*, *1*(5), 206–215.

Sahiner, B., Pezeshk, A., Hadjiiski, L. M., Wang, X., Drukker, K., & Cha, K. H. (2019). Deep learning in medical imaging and radiation therapy. *Medical Physics*, *6*(1), 36.

Samanta, K., Avleen, M., Rohit, S., & Kary, F. (2020). Explainable Artificial Intelligence for Human Decision-Support System in Medical Domain. *Medical Physics*, *46*(1), 336.

Senoner, J., Netland, T., & Feuerriegel, S. (2021). Using explainable artificial intelligence to improve process quality: Evidence from semiconductor manufacturing. *Management Science*.

Sh, K. F. (2021). Advantages of Magnetic Resonance Computer Tomography in the Diagnosis of Thyroid Cancer. *Pindus Journal of Culture, Literature, and ELT*, *9*, 80–84.

Sokol, K., & Flach, P. (2020, January). Explainability fact sheets: a framework for systematic assessment of explainable approaches. In *Proceedings of the 2020 Conference on Fairness, Accountability, and Transparency* (pp. 56-67). Academic Press.

Su, J., Vargas, D. V., & Sakurai, K. (2019). One pixel attack for fooling deep neural networks. *IEEE Transactions on Evolutionary Computation*, *23*(5), 828–841.

Szczepański, M., Choraś, M., Pawlicki, M., & Pawlicka, A. (2021, June). The methods and approaches of explainable artificial intelligence. In *International Conference on Computational Science* (pp. 3-17). Springer.

Taylor, J. E. T., & Taylor, G. W. (2021). Artificial cognition: How experimental psychology can help generate explainable artificial intelligence. *Psychonomic Bulletin & Review*, *28*(2), 454–475.

van der Waa, J., Nieuwburg, E., Cremers, A., & Neerincx, M. (2021). Evaluating XAI: A comparison of rule-based and example-based explanations. *Artificial Intelligence*, *291*, 103404.

Vilone, G., & Longo, L. (2021). Notions of explainability and evaluation approaches for explainable artificial intelligence. *Information Fusion*, *76*, 89–106.

Wang, D., Yang, Q., Abdul, A., & Lim, B. Y. (2019, May). Designing theory-driven user-centric explainable AI. *Proceedings of the 2019 CHI conference on human factors in computing systems*, 1-15.

Weld, D. S., & Bansal, G. (2019). The challenge of crafting intelligible intelligence. *Communications of the ACM*, *62*(6), 70–79. doi:10.1145/3282486

Yang, G., Ye, Q., & Xia, J. (2022). Unbox the black-box for the medical explainable ai via multi-modal and multi-centre data fusion: A mini-review, two showcases and beyond. *Information Fusion*, *77*, 29–52.

Yang, S. C. H., Folke, T., & Shafto, P. (2021). Abstraction, validation, and generalization for explainable artificial intelligence. *Applied AI Letters*, *2*(4), e37.

Zhou, J., Gandomi, A. H., Chen, F., & Holzinger, A. (2021). Evaluating the Quality of Machine Learning Explanations: A Survey on Methods and Metrics. *Electronics (Basel)*, *10*(5), 593. https://doi.org/10.3390/electronics10050593

Zhu, J., Liapis, A., Risi, S., Bidarra, R., & Youngblood, G. M. (2018, August). Explainable AI for designers: A human-centered perspective on mixed-initiative co-creation. In *2018 IEEE Conference on Computational Intelligence and Games (CIG)* (pp. 1-8). IEEE.

Zubatiuk, T., & Isayev, O. (2021). Development of multimodal machine learning potentials: Toward a physics-aware artificial intelligence. *Accounts of Chemical Research*, *54*(7), 1575–1585.

Chapter 12
Principles and Methods of Explainable Artificial Intelligence in Healthcare:
Framework for Classifying Alzheimer's Disease Using Machine Learning

Manimekalai K.
Sri G. V. G. Visalakshi College for Women, India

Abirami D.
Sri G. V. G. Visalakshi College for Women, India

ABSTRACT

Alzheimer's disease (AD) is a degenerative brain illness that primarily affects elderly adults. This sickness takes away people's capacity to think, read, and do many other things. Clinical trials investigating medications to treat this disease have a high failure rate, due to the difficulty in identifying the patients affected by this disease early on. It affects around 45 million people worldwide. Machine learning, a branch of artificial intelligence, incorporates a range of probabilistic methods. Several approaches showed potential prediction accuracies; however, they were tested using distinct pathologically untested data sets making a fair comparison difficult. Alzheimer's disease (AD) is a degenerative brain disease that mostly affects the elderly. Pre-processing, feature selection, and classification are just a few of the various factors that go into making the framework. This proposed approach directs researchers in the right direction for early Alzheimer's disease detection and can distinguish AD from other disorders.

DOI: 10.4018/978-1-6684-3791-9.ch012

INTRODUCTION

Alzheimer's Disease is caused by brain cells, where it starts at the age of sixty, which was named by Dr. Alosis Alzheimer in the year 1906. The exact reason for the disease is not known. People affected by this disease have trouble doing their day-to-day activities like driving, cooking, remembering things, and thinking clearly. The loss of cognitive function is called dementia. It is common among old age.

Data is interpreted and analysed using machine learning. It can also classify patterns and model data. It enables judgments to be made that would otherwise be impossible to make using routine procedures while saving time and effort. ML methods have been widely utilised in mining, retrieval and a variety of other applications, most notably in the identification and categorization of brain illnesses using Cathode Ray Tube (CRT) images and x-rays. AD researchers have just lately attempted to apply ML to AD prediction. As a result, there is a limitation of knowledge in AD prediction and ML. Today's imaging technologies and high-throughput diagnostics, on the other hand, have left us overwhelmed by a great number (even hundreds) of cellular, clinical, and molecular parameters. Standard measurements and human instinct don't always work in today's environment.

LITERATURE REVIEW

Neuropsychological examinations contain the Mini Mental State Examination(MMSE), Beth Israel Deaconess Medical Center (BIDMC), Cognitive Assessment (COG), Blessed Orientation Memory and Concentration test(BOMC), Montreal Cognitive Assessment(MoCA) and General Practitioner Assessment of Cognition (GP CoG). Though MMSE is popular, it has a drawback. The MMSE has the disadvantage of being unresponsive to the primary indicator, which emphasizes the importance of having a diagnostic test that may be used on participants of any gender, including religion, culture, or intellectual level. The Alzheimer's Association's changes are generally studied group studied people of various ages in several developing countries to address this issue. (Sosa et al., 2009) stated that the CSI for Dementia battery was established by these researchers, and normative scores for different age groups were established.

The research concentrates on leveraging knowledge discovery from data to diagnose Alzheimer's disease. The subject will be asked a predetermined series of questions in this battery. Each response will be assessed. According to (Sosa et al., 2009) the subjects will be classed as AD patients or not based on their score. An important step is data analysis and decision-making. The Psychologist's knowledge is necessary for investigation and decision-making. Human error is unavoidable. o solve this, DM must be used to discover knowledge based on (Jiawei Han, Micheline Kamber, 2012).

Data Mining (DM) is used to diagnose disease in this study. DM has been utilized by several researchers to diagnose various diseases. (Soni et al., 2011) analyzed datasets of heart disease patients using supervised techniques. In the identification of breast cancer (Hu, 2011), (Fallahi & Jafari, 2011) and (Zheng et al., 2014) employed a DM approach. Artificial neural networks were employed (Mahjabeen Mirza Beg, 2012) to diagnose breast cancer. In their study (Luo & Cheng, 2010) discuss the use of decision trees and SVM in diagnosing breast cancer.

(Breetha & Kavinila, 2013) studied hierarchical clustering in cancer identification and classification. (Rahman & Afroz, 2013) examined different classification approaches on diabetic patient data sets utilizing WEKA, Matlab, and Tanagra technologies. (Joshi et al., 2011) examined DM to predict cardiac disease. (S. R. Bhagya Shree, 2014) assessed different classification techniques in identifying AD. Based on their observation, the techniques utilized were outperforming.

(Ferreira et al., 2012) identified neonatal jaundice using decision trees and neural networks. (Abhishek et al., 2012) compared two categories of NN. WEKA is employed as an analytical tool. To identify the disease, researchers have utilized a variety of classification systems, some of which are as follows (Sriram et al., 2013) compared the outcomes of classification algorithms for diagnosing Parkinson's disease. (Patil & Sherekar, 2013) examined Naive Bayes classification in their study. Several researchers discussed pre-processing feature selection and classification. Various techniques were demonstrated and compared to various algorithms. The following table contains a list of these.

DM requires the use of a software program for data analysis. Other tools are available, including WEKA, See5, Wiz Why, and others. WEKA has been used as a tool by the vast majority of scholars. (Othman & Yau, 2007) and (Singhal & Jena, 2013) discussed several classification methodologies to identify breast cancer using WEKA. According to(Andreeva et al., 2012), WEKA forecasts the bulk of the data.

METHODOLOGY

Weka includes modules for data classification and disease prediction accuracy. Weka has been used in the medical profession to diagnose and analyze datasets related to Alzheimer's disease. Weka algorithms can accurately construct predictive models by extracting meaningful information from Alzheimer's datasets using WEKA. This research discusses DM strategies for properly predicting the survivability of ADby classification of several algorithms. Figure 1 depicts the WEKA GUI Chooser

Table 1. Techniques used and comparison to various algorithms

Author	Methods used or compared	Result
(Fong et al., 2020)	Faster R CNN, SSD and YOLOv3	Accuracy was obtained.
(Bharathi & Arunachalam, 2021)	Arithmetic mean, median, Gaussian, bilateral and Fast Fourier Transform (FFT)	The outliers removed.
(Natarajan & Sathiamoorthy, 2018)	Equalization of histograms, thresholding, are used.	Noise reduced.
(Khatami et al., 2017).	Wavelet transform (WT), Kolmogorov Smirnov (KS) test	Enhanced the execution of DBNs.
(Gupta & Roy, 2019)	Medav Filter	Filter has great noise removal characteristics.
(Alashwal et al., 2020)	Random forest classifier	Provided evidence for protective factors against the development of AD.
(Trambaiolli et al., 2017)	Several Filters used.	Accuracy improved.
(Divya & Shantha Selva Kumari, 2021)	Support vector machine (SVM)	Produced better results.
(Sarwinda & Arymurthy, 2013)	Kernel PCA	Method achieved accuracy of 100%
(Shi et al., 2020)	Multi-modality feature selection method	Well demonstrated
(Li et al., 2017)	MKSCDDL Algorithm used.	A useful tool for illness detection in its early stages.
(Zhu et al., 2014)	Joint regression and classification (JRC)	Diagnosed AD or MCI effectively.
(Q. Li et al., 2017)	Multimodal discriminative dictionary learning	Efficient machine learning method.
(Liu et al., 2012)	Ensemble method	Method showed promising performance
(Duda et al., 2016)	Voxel-wise features	Low performance.
(Singh & Aswani, 2018)	KNN classifier	Dispensed with the noise.
(Amitab et al., 2018)	hybrid drive noise filter	Expelled noise from the influenced pixel.
(Albright, 2019)	All-Pairs	Effective in predicting the progression of AD.
(Klosowski & Frahm, 2017)	Filter fitting	Condition noise was killed without providing obscure, spreading, or repairing ancient oddities.
(Gunja et al., 2017)	Trans-spiral coronary angiography (TRA)	Diminished radiation measurements
(Bhadouria et al., 2017)	Algorithm	PSNR was compared with other filtering strategies.
(Anitha et al., 2017)	Versatile worldwide limit	Recognized the anomalies

Figure 1. WEKA GUI Chooser's Point of View

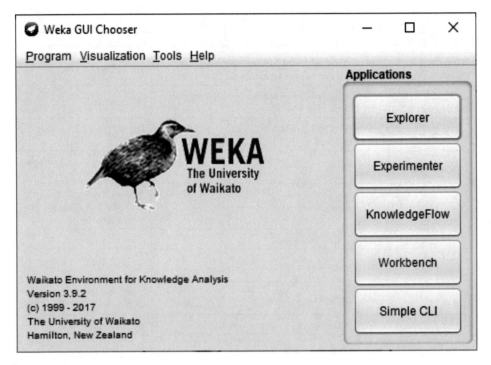

tool. It includes four applications: Explorer, Experimenter, Knowledge Flow, and Simple CLI.

Figure 2 shows a description of the Alzheimer's dataset. The dataset contains 3873 instances and 83 characteristics. For analysis, various algorithms were used using the WEKA DM tool.

DM TECHNIQUES

DM is a highly specialized discipline in computer science. The implicit extraction of previously unidentified and possibly relevant information from historical data sources has been termed DM. It uses MLand statistical techniques to discover and communicate knowledge understandably. To uncover knowledge patterns, several methods have been created. The Weka interface used in this paper is Explorer.

It preprocesses the data and analyses the classification accuracy result using the Decision Table, ZeroR, OneR, JRIP, Naïve Bayes, and proposed algorithms. Figure 3 depicts the Explorer interface with Alzheimer's dataset, opened using a CSV file and its graphical display.

Figure 2. The datasets are saved in the Comma Separated Value (CSV) format

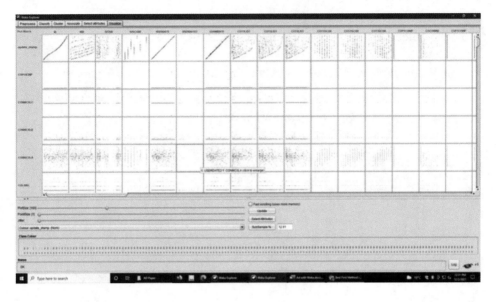

Figure 3. View of CSV ADDataset File open in Explorer interface

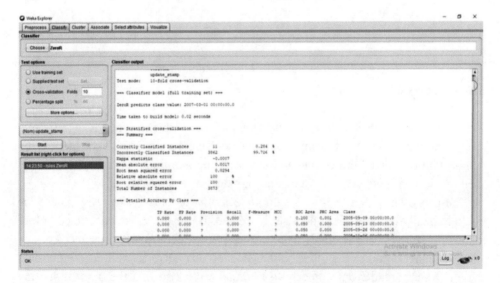

Proposed Model

There are three steps in the suggested model.

- Pre-Processing
- Feature Selection
- Classification

The Framework for Classifying AD Using ML is depicted in Figure 4.

Figure 4. Framework for Classifying AD using ML

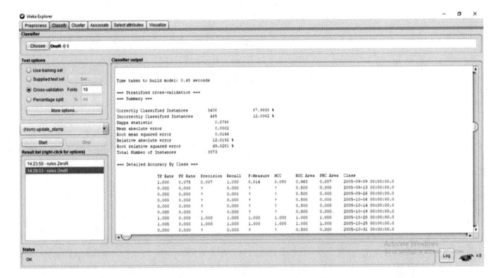

Pre-processing

The first stage is to gather information on the subjects. Data is frequently insufficient, noisy, and inconsistent in the physical universe. Detecting missing data, identifying abnormalities, correcting errors, and lowering the amount of data to be analyzed will result in large payoffs for decision-making.

Pre-processing is the initial step in effectively classifying AD data. The pathologically demonstrated data set is treated to prevent class imbalance before being transformed to a readable data format. When the number of instances of one class is nearly equal to the other class, ML methods perform well. The input data type is transformed from numeric to nominal values so that the algorithms that employ that data type as input can be used.

Excel sheets are commonly used to present data. The common format of WEKA is ARFF. It shifted to the CSV file and then altered to an ARFF format.

Model Evaluation

WEKA comes with two learning performance evaluations. The data set can be assessed using the following criteria:

1. Training set: A data set is split into training and test data by the classifier. In this situation, each model's outcome can be preserved and viewed.
2. Cross-validation: WEKA generates five models and ten models for Fivefold and Tenfold cross validation, respectively.

The List of ML Algorithms tab displays a list of ML algorithms. In general, these methods run a classification process numerous times. The algorithm parameters and the weight of the input data can be changed to improve the classifier's accuracy. The classification method, ZeroR, OneR, JRIP, Naïve Bayes, and proposed algorithms are used on pre-processed data, and the results are saved. Only the qualities that contribute to the findings are selected for the same preprocessed data, and the rest attributes are deleted. The same categorization algorithm is used for this data, and the same results are obtained. The outcomes are tabulated. This is how the results of various neuropsychological tests are prepared. The explorer, the WEKA tool's knowledge flow, and the Java API investigate the prepared dataset. Explorer is a data exploration tool. The explorer can be used to preprocess data, specify result-oriented attributes, and display results. Experimenter is a program that allows to create and running of statistical tests.

Knowledge flow, like Explorer, employs a drag & drop interface. The user can drag and drop boxes representing learning algorithms and data sources on the knowledge flow interface to establish the required configuration.

Naive Bayes algorithm is a supervised learning method for classification tasks. As a result, the Naive Bayes Classifier is another name for it. To forecast a target variable, Naive Bayes uses attributes like other supervised learning algorithms. The fundamental difference is that Naive Bayes assumes that features are unrelated and there is no correlation between them. However, this is not the case in reality. The name of this method comes from the erroneous notion that attributes are unrelated.

A Naive Bayesian is a classifier that analyzes probabilities.

It is based on the total probability theorem and Bayes theory. The chance that a document d with vector x conforms to hypotheses h is provided by Equation (1) to (3).

$$\text{The } P\left(h1 \mid dx\right) = \frac{P\left(xi|h1\right)P\left(h1\right)}{P\left(xi|h1\right)P\left(h1\right) + P\left(xi|h2\right)P\left(h2\right)} \tag{1}$$

$$P\left(h1|xi\right) = \frac{P\left(xi|h1\right)P\left(h1\right)}{P\left(x1\right)} \tag{2}$$

$$P\left(h1|xi\right) = \sum_{j=1}^{n} P\left(xi|hj\right)P\left(hj\right) \tag{3}$$

accuracy of a classifier is defined as the proportion of test set tuples successfully identified by the classifier on a given set. The proportion returned is truly related to the query is defined as precision. It is defined in Equation (4).

$$Precision = \frac{\left|\{relavant\} \cap \{retrieved\}\right|}{\{retrieved\}} \tag{4}$$

The recall is the fraction of retrieved cases among all relevant cases. It is the % of documents returned that were relevant to the query. It is explained in the Equation (5).

$$Recall = \frac{\left|\{relavant\} \cap \{retrieved\}\right|}{\{retrieved\}} \tag{5}$$

A useful way to describe information or knowledge is to utilize a rule-based classification strategy. A rule-based classifier employs IF-THEN rules to categorize the data.

IF Condition THEN Conclusion

According to (Sheshadri et al., 2015) A rule R's coverage and accuracy may be measured.

Let Ncovers stands the number of tuples covered by R

|D| stands the number of tuples in D, given a tuple, X, from a class labeled data collection D, then R's precision and coverage are defined as

$$Accuracy = \frac{N_{covers}}{|D|} \tag{6}$$

$$Coverage = \frac{N_{covers}}{N_{correct}} \qquad (7)$$

RESULTS AND DISCUSSION

WEKA is used to import the CSV file. There are 3873 instances and 83 characteristics, as can be seen. The data is divided into five-folds and tenfold cross-validation. In that case, the ultimate fold will only yield good outcomes.

Feature Selection

Best First Search (BFS)

A graph search strategy is called BFS. Based on an evaluation function f(n), it will select a node for expansion Because the assessment gauges the distance to the goal, the node with the lowest evaluation is traditionally chosen for the explanation. A priority queue, a data structure that keeps the fringe in ascending order of f values, can be used to perform the best first search within a general search framework. The depth-first and BFS methods are combined in this search algorithm. The BFS algorithm is sometimes denoted as a greedy algorithm since it tackles the most desirable path as soon as its heuristic weight becomes the most desirable.

Algorithm

Step 1: Add the root or starting node to the queue.

Step 2: When the queue is empty, stop and return.

Step 3: When the first node in the queue is our target node, we will halt and move to success.

Step 4: If not, eliminate the first item in the queue. Calculate the projected goal distance for each child by expanding it. Arrange the individuals in the queue in increasing order.

Step 5: Return back to step 3.

Step 6: End.

The best-first approach is employed in this investigation. As an Attribute Evaluator, CfsSubset Evaluator is employed.

Attribute Evaluator: CfsSubset Evaluator

Search Method: BestFirst

Figure 5. Best first search using the full training set

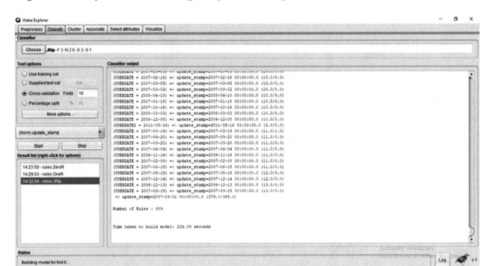

Figure 5,6,7 denotes Best First Search using the full training set, best first search using five-fold Cross-Validation, and Best First Search using 10 Fold Cross-Validation.

Search Method: Greedy Stepwise

In the Greedy Algorithm, the collection of resources is recursively partitioned based on the resource's maximal, firsthand availability at each execution stage. There are two steps when employing the greedy strategy to solve a problem.

- We are examining the things on the list.
- Optimization.

Algorithm

Step 1:   Go through the data, starting with Index 0 as the starting point.

Step 2:   Check the remaining activities when more activities can be done by the time the considered activity is concluded.

Step 3:   If no more activities remain, the current remaining activity is deemed the next activity to be reviewed. Repeat Steps 1 and 2 for the new activity under consideration. If there are no more activities available, continue to step 4.

Step 4:   Return the union of the indices that were taken into account. These are the activity indicators that will be used to attain the maximum throughput achievable.

Figure 8 shows the Search Method using Greedy Algorithm.

Figure 6. Best first search using 5-Fold Cross-Validation

	A	B	C	D	E	F	G	H	I	J	K	L	M	N	O
1	ID	RID	SITEID	VISCODE	USERDATE	USERDA	EXAMDATE	COT1LIST	COT2LIST	COT3LIST	COT1SCOI	COT2SCOI	COT3SCOI	COP1CON	COCOMN
2	4	2	107 bl		09.09.2005		08.09.2005	1:2:7:8:9	1:3:4:5:7:9	3:5:6:7:8:9	5	7	7	-4	1:2:3:4:5
3	6	5	107 bl		09.09.2005		07.09.2005	1:2:3:7:9	1:3:5:7:8:9	2:3:4:5:7:9	5	7	7	-4	
4	8	3	107 bl		13.09.2005		12.09.2005		7:09:10	1:7:9:10	5:7:8:9:10	3	4	5	-4	1:2:3:4
5	10	8	107 bl		26.09.2005		19.09.2005	1:2:4:5:7:8	1:2:3:4:5:6	1:2:3:4:5:6	8	10	9	-4	1:2:3:4:5
6	12	7	10 bl		06.10.2005		06.10.2005		-4	7:8:9:10	4:8:9:10	0	4	4	-4	1:2:3:4
7	14	16	107 bl		14.10.2005		13.10.2005	1:2:3:9:10	2:3:4:5:6:9	1:2:3:5:9:1	5	6	6	-4	1:2:3:4:5
8	16	15	4 bl		19.10.2005		18.10.2005	1:2:3:4:5:6	1:2:3:4:7:8	2:3:4:5:7:8	8	8	8	-4	1:2:3:4:5
9	18	30	11 bl		20.10.2005		20.10.2005	1:4:7:9:10	1:2:3:10	2:09:10	5	4	3	-4	1:2:3:4:5
10	20	22	107 bl		20.10.2005		19.10.2005	2:3:6:7:8:1	1:5:6:7:8:1	1:3:4:5:7:9	6	6	7	-4	1:2:3:4:5
11	22	31	11 bl		25.10.2005		24.10.2005	1:2:3:4:5:7	1:2:3:4:5:6	1:2:3:4:5:6	8	10	10	-4	1:2:3:4:5
12	24	21	107 bl		25.10.2005		24.10.2005	1:2:3:5:8:9	1:2:3:4:5:7	1:2:3:4:5:6	6	9	10	-4	1:2:3:4:5
13	26	29	32 bl		31.10.2005		31.10.2005		-4	3:06	5:09:10	0	2	3	-4	1:2:3:5
14	28	14	10 bl		07.11.2005		04.11.2005	1:4:5:6:7:9	1:2:3:4:5:7	2:3:4:5:7:8	7	8	8	-4	1:2:3:4:5
15	30	4	10 bl		08.11.2005		08.11.2005	4:5:6:10	2:4:7:8:10	1:3:4:5:6:7	4	5	8	-4	1:2:3:4:5
16	32	35	4 bl		08.11.2005		08.11.2005	1:5:6:7:8:9	1:2:3:4:5:6	2:3:4:5:6:8	6	8	7	-4	1:2:3:4:5
17	34	23	107 bl		09.11.2005		08.11.2005	1:2:3:6:8	1:2:3:4:5:6	1:2:3:5:6:7	5	8	8	-4	1:2:3:4:5
18	36	10	107 bl		11.11.2005		10.11.2005		7:09:10	1:5:7:9:10	1:3:4:6:9:1	3	5	6	-4	1:2:3:4:5
19	38	42	11 bl		14.11.2005		10.11.2005	1:3:9:10	3:5:6:7:9:1	3:6:8:9:10	4	6	5	-4	1:2:3:4:5
20	40	41	2 bl		15.11.2005		15.11.2005		10	9:10	5:6:8:9:10	1	2	5	-4	1:2:3:4:5
21	42	19	32 bl		23.11.2005		23.11.2005	1:2:3:4:5:6	1:2:3:4:5:6	1:2:3:4:5:6	10	10	10	-4	1:2:3:4:5

Figure 7. Best first search using 10-Fold Cross-Validation

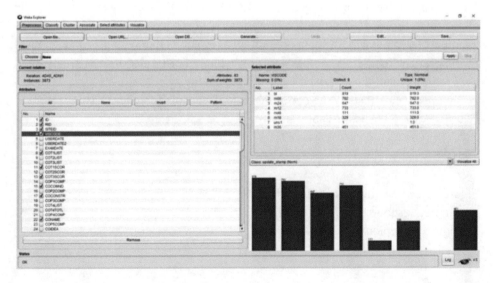

Figure 8. Search method using Greedy Algorithm

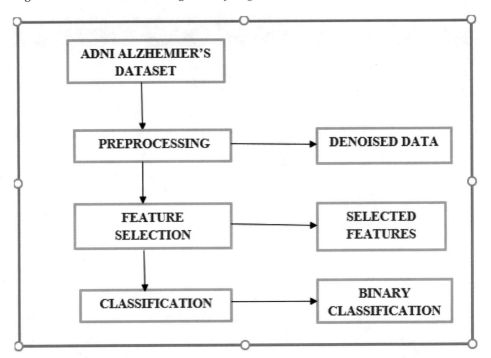

Classification

Decision Table

The decision table algorithm is found under Rules in the classifiers of Weka. The most straightforward technique of representing ML output is to use the same format as the input. To summarise the data, it employs a decision table with the same features as the primary dataset. A simple decision table majority classifier is created and used to implement the classifier rules decision table.

Figures 9 and 10 show the classifier using Decision Table and Visualization of Classifier using Decision Table.

ZeroR

Figure 11 depicts the ZeroR algorithm.
Figure 12 shows the OneR algorithm.
Figure 13 depicts the JipR algorithm.

Figure 9. Classifier using decision table

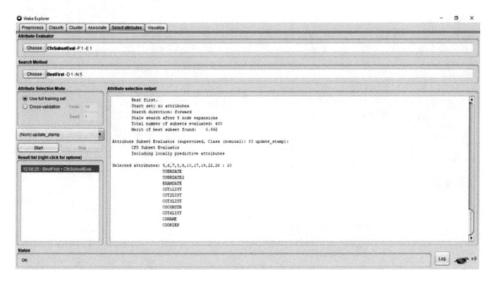

RESULTS AND DISCUSSION

Metrics of Performance

The proposed technique combination's performance for AD data is assessed using the widely used quantitative measurement Mean Squared Error (MSE).

Figure 10. Visualization of classifier using decision table

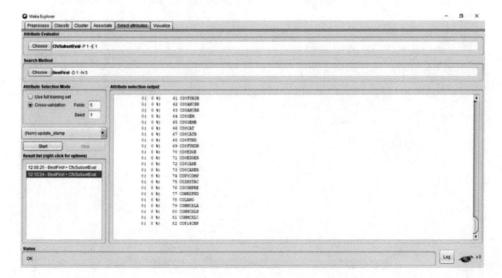

Figure 11. ZeroR

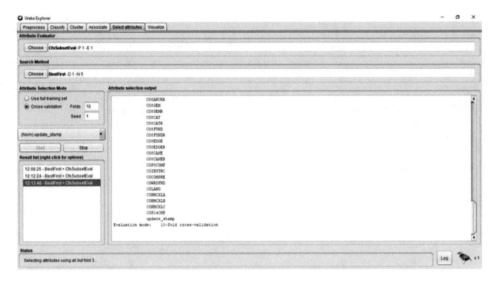

The performance of the proposed approach combination for AD data is evaluated using the commonly used quantitative measurement Mean squared error (MSE).

Table 2 depicts the comparison of Classification algorithms based on Metrics.

Figure 12. OneR

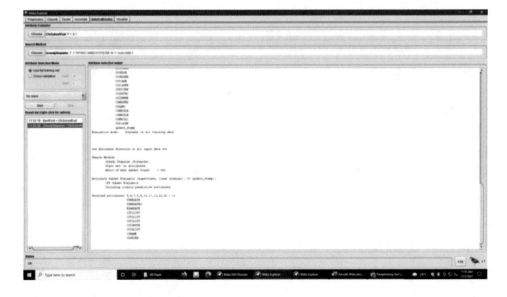

Figure 13. JipR

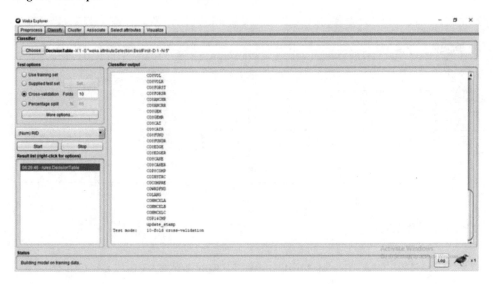

MSE

The difference between the denoised data and the original data is the Mean Square Error, abbreviated as MSE. The MSE for AD data is calculated using the equation (8) and RMSE is calculated using the equation (9).

$$MSE = \frac{1}{M} \sum_{j=1}^{M} \left(y(j) - \overline{y(j)} \right)^2 \tag{8}$$

Where, $y(j)$:Original data, $y(j)$: Denoised data

RMSE

RMSE = Sqrt (MSE) (9)

The classification Algorithms ZeroR, OneR, JRIP, Decision Table, Naïve Bayes, and proposed algorithms are given in Table 1. MSE, RMSE, and Kappa statistics were tabulated when it took to create the model. Compared to the table above, the proposed model established a model in the shortest amount of time, 0.01 Seconds, and the Mean Absolute Error is 0.0015.

Table 2. Comparison of classification algorithms based on metrics

Algorithms	Time taken	MSE	RMSE	Kappa Statistics
Decision Table	3.87 Seconds	0.0052	0.0023	0.5432
Zero R	0.02 Seconds	0.0017	0.0294	-0.0007
One R	0.45 Seconds	0.0002	0.0144	0.8798
JRip	2.09 Seconds	0.0017	0.0294	-0.0007
Naïve Bayes	0.02 Seconds	0.2367	0.0378	0.6542
Proposed algorithm	**0.01 Seconds**	0.0015	0.0204	-0.0005

CONCLUSION

This research is based on comparing and evaluating recent work in AD prognosis and prediction utilizing ML algorithms. Recent ML trends, including the types of data used and the performance of ML algorithms in forecasting AD in its early stages, have been explicitly reported. ML enhances prediction accuracy, especially when compared to classical statistical tools, self-evident. The proposed approach is based on a single modality to avoid the additional expense of calculating and merging different modalities. The pathologically established data will improve accuracy and validity, and a balanced class will aid classifiers in producing accurate findings. This model can assist physicians in enhancing their prediction performance while also addressing the constraints identified in prior research. One framework was produced in this study. Features have been chosen. It has categorized itself as a result of this.

REFERENCES

Abhishek. (2012). Proposing Efficient Neural Network Training Model for Kidney Stone Diagnosis. *International Journal of Computer Science and Information Technologies, 3*(11), 3900–3904.

Alashwal, H., Abdalla, A., El Halaby, M., & Moustafa, A. A. (2020). Feature selection for the classification of Alzheimer's disease data. *ACM International Conference Proceeding Series*, 41–45. 10.1145/3378936.3378982

Albright, J. (2019). Forecasting the progression of Alzheimer's disease using neural networks and a novel preprocessing algorithm. *Alzheimer's & Dementia (New York, N. Y.), 5*(1), 483–491. doi:10.1016/j.trci.2019.07.001 PMID:31650004

Amitab, K., Medhi, K., Kandar, D., & Paul, B. S. (2018). Impulse noise reduction in digital images using fuzzy logic and artificial neural network. *Proceedings of the International Conference on Computing and Communication Systems*, 155–165. 10.1007/978-981-10-6890-4_14

Andreeva, P., Dimitrova, M., & Radeva, P. (2012). *Data mining learning models and algorithms*. Academic Press.

Anitha, J., Dinesh Peter, J., & Immanuel Alex Pandian, S. (2017). A dual stage adaptive thresholding (DuSAT) for automatic mass detection in mammograms. *Computer Methods and Programs in Biomedicine*, *138*, 93–104. doi:10.1016/j. cmpb.2016.10.026 PMID:27886719

Bhadouria, V. S., Tanase, A., Schmid, M., Hannig, F., Teich, J., & Ghoshal, D. (2017). A Novel Image Impulse Noise Removal Algorithm Optimized for Hardware Accelerators. *Journal of Signal Processing Systems for Signal, Image, and Video Technology*, *89*(2), 225–242. doi:10.100711265-016-1187-5

Bhagya Shree, S. R., H. S. S. (2014). An initial investigation in the Diagnosis of AD using various Classification Techniques. *IEEE International Conference on Computational Intelligence and Computing Research*, 1–5. 10.1109/ ICCIC.2014.7238300

Bharathi, A., & Arunachalam, A. S. (2021). *Pre-Processing on Alzheimer MRI images*. Academic Press.

Breetha, S., & Kavinila, R. (2013). *Hierarchical Clustering For Cancer Discovery Using Range Check And Delta Check*. Academic Press.

Divya, R., & Shantha Selva Kumari, R. (2021). Genetic algorithm with logistic regression feature selection for Alzheimer's disease classification. *Neural Computing & Applications*, *33*(14), 8435–8444. doi:10.100700521-020-05596-x

Duda, R. O., Hart, P. E., Stork, D. G., & Wiley, J. (2016). *Pattern Classification All materials in these slides were taken from Pattern Classification* (2nd ed.). Academic Press.

Fallahi, A., & Jafari, S. (2011). An Expert System for Detection of Breast Cancer Using Data Preprocessing and Bayesian Network. *International Journal of Advanced Science and Technology*, *34*, 65–70.

Ferreira, D., Oliveira, A., & Freitas, A. (2012). Applying data mining techniques to improve diagnosis in neonatal jaundice. *BMC Medical Informatics and Decision Making*, *12*(1), 143. doi:10.1186/1472-6947-12-143 PMID:23216895

Fong, J. X., Shapiai, M. I., Tiew, Y. Y., Batool, U., & Fauzi, H. (2020). Bypassing MRI Pre-processing in Alzheimer's Disease Diagnosis using Deep Learning Detection Network. *2020 16th IEEE International Colloquium on Signal Processing & Its Applications (CSPA)*, 219–224.

Gunja, A., Pandey, Y., Xie, H., Wolska, B. M., Shroff, A. R., Ardati, A. K., & Vidovich, M. I. (2017). Image noise reduction technology reduces radiation in a radial-first cardiac catheterization laboratory. *Cardiovascular Revascularization Medicine; Including Molecular Interventions*, *18*(3), 197–201. doi:10.1016/j. carrev.2016.12.017 PMID:28089778

Gupta, S., & Roy, S. (2019). Medav filter—filter for removal of image noise with the combination of median and average filters. In *Recent Trends in Signal and Image Processing* (pp. 11–19). Springer. doi:10.1007/978-981-10-8863-6_2

Han & Kamber. (2012). *Data Mining: Concepts and Techniques*. Academic Press.

Hu, R. (2011). Medical Data Mining Based on Decision Tree Algorithm. *Medical Data Mining Based on Decision Tree Algorithm.*, *4*(5), 14–19. doi:10.5539/cis.v4n5p14

Joshi, S., Szweda, P., Szweda, P., Bichara, D., & Iggidr, A. (2011). *Expert Systems with Applications*. https://www.tandfonline.com/doi/full/10.1080/23737867.2016. 1211495%0A

Khatami, A., Khosravi, A., Nguyen, T., Lim, C. P., & Nahavandi, S. (2017). Medical image analysis using wavelet transform and deep belief networks. *Expert Systems with Applications*, *86*, 190–198. doi:10.1016/j.eswa.2017.05.073

Klosowski, J., & Frahm, J. (2017). Image denoising for real-time MRI. *Magnetic Resonance in Medicine*, *77*(3), 1340–1352. doi:10.1002/mrm.26205 PMID:27079944

Li, J., Cheng, K., Wang, S., Morstatter, F., Trevino, R. P., Tang, J., & Liu, H. (2017). Feature selection: A data perspective. *ACM Computing Surveys*, *50*(6), 1–45. doi:10.1145/3136625

Li, Q., Wu, X., Xu, L., Chen, K., Yao, L., & Li, R. (2017). Multi-modal discriminative dictionary learning for Alzheimer's disease and mild cognitive impairment. *Computer Methods and Programs in Biomedicine*, *150*, 1–8. doi:10.1016/j.cmpb.2017.07.003 PMID:28859825

Liu, M., Zhang, D., Shen, D., & Initiative, A. D. N. (2012). Ensemble sparse classification of Alzheimer's disease. *NeuroImage*, *60*(2), 1106–1116. doi:10.1016/j. neuroimage.2012.01.055 PMID:22270352

Luo, S., & Cheng, B. (2010). *Diagnosing Breast Masses in Digital Mammography Using Feature Selection and Ensemble Methods.* doi:10.1007/s10916-010-9518-8

Mahjabeen Mirza Beg, M. J. (2012). An Analysis of the Methods Employed for Breast Cancer Diagnosis. *International Journal of Research in Computer Science*, 2(3), 25–29. doi:10.7815/ijorcs.23.2012.025

Natarajan, M., & Sathiamoorthy, S. (2018). *A Novel Pre-Processing Approach for the Denoising of Alzheimer Disease Image Dataset.* Academic Press.

Othman, M. F. Bin, & Yau, T. M. S. (2007). Comparison of different classification techniques using WEKA for breast cancer. *3rd Kuala Lumpur International Conference on Biomedical Engineering 2006*, 520–523. 10.1007/978-3-540-68017-8_131

Patil, T. R., & Sherekar, S. S. (2013). *Performance Analysis of Naive Bayes and J48 Classification Algorithm for Data Classification.* Academic Press.

Rahman, R. M., & Afroz, F. (2013). *Comparison of Various Classification Techniques Using Different Data Mining Tools for Diabetes Diagnosis.* Academic Press.

Sarwinda, D., & Arymurthy, A. M. (2013). Feature selection using kernel PCA for Alzheimer's disease detection with 3D MR Images of brain. *2013 International Conference on Advanced Computer Science and Information Systems (ICACSIS)*, 329–333. 10.1109/ICACSIS.2013.6761597

Sheshadri, H. S., Shree, S. R. B., & Krishna, M. (2015). Diagnosis of Alzheimer's disease employing neuropsychological and classification techniques. *2015 5th International Conference on IT Convergence and Security (ICITCS)*, 1–6.

Shi, Y., Zu, C., Hong, M., Zhou, L., Wang, L., Wu, X., & Zhou, J. (2020). ASMFS: Adaptive-Similarity-based Multi-modality Feature Selection for Classification of Alzheimer's Disease. *Computer Vision and Pattern Recognition*, 1–27.

Singh, V., & Aswani, D. (2018). Face detection in hybrid color space using HBF-KNN. *Proceedings of International Conference on Recent Advancement on Computer and Communication*, 489–498. 10.1007/978-981-10-8198-9_52

Singhal, S., & Jena, M. (2013). A Study on WEKA Tool for Data Preprocessing. *Classification and Clustering.*, 6, 250–253.

Soni, J., Ansari, U., Sharma, D., & Soni, S. (2011). Predictive data mining for medical diagnosis: An overview of heart disease prediction. *International Journal of Computers and Applications*, 17(8), 43–48. doi:10.5120/2237-2860

Sosa, A. L., Albanese, E., Prince, M., Acosta, D., Ferri, C. P., Guerra, M., Huang, Y., Jacob, K. S., de Rodriguez, J. L., Salas, A., Yang, F., Gaona, C., Joteeshwaran, A., Rodriguez, G., de la Torre, G. R., Williams, J. D., & Stewart, R. (2009). Population normative data for the 10/66 Dementia Research Group cognitive test battery from Latin America, India and China: A cross-sectional survey. *BMC Neurology*, *9*(1), 48. doi:10.1186/1471-2377-9-48 PMID:19709405

Sriram, T. V. S., Rao, M. V., Narayana, G. S., Kaladhar, D., & Vital, T. P. R. (2013). Intelligent Parkinson disease prediction using machine learning algorithms. *Int. J. Eng. Innov. Technol*, *3*, 212–215.

Trambaiolli, L. R., Spolaôr, N., Lorena, A. C., Anghinah, R., & Sato, J. R. (2017). Feature selection before EEG classification supports the diagnosis of Alzheimer's disease. *Clinical Neurophysiology*, *128*(10), 2058–2067. doi:10.1016/j. clinph.2017.06.251 PMID:28866471

Zheng, B., Yoon, S. W., & Lam, S. S. (2014). Breast cancer diagnosis based on feature extraction using a hybrid of K-means and support vector machine algorithms. *Expert Systems with Applications*, *41*(4, Part 1), 1476–1482. doi:10.1016/j.eswa.2013.08.044

Zhu, X., Suk, H.-I., & Shen, D. (2014). A novel matrix-similarity based loss function for joint regression and classification in Alzheimer's Disease diagnosis. *NeuroImage*, *100*, 91–105. doi:10.1016/j.neuroimage.2014.05.078 PMID:24911377

Compilation of References

Abadi, M., Barham, P., Chen, J., Chen, Z., Davis, A., Dean, J., & Isard, M. (2016). *Tensorflow: A system for large-scale machine learning.* Paper presented at the 12th USENIX symposium on operating systems design and implementation (OSDI 16).

Abdollahi, A., & Rahbaralam, M. (2020). Effect of temperature on the transmission of COVID-19: A machine learning case study in Spain. MedRxiv. Doi:10.1101/2020.05.01.20087759

Abdulhay, E., Arunkumar, N., & Ramirez, G. (n.d.). *Explainable Artificial Intelligence for Medical Applications.* Hindawi. Retrieved September 20, 2021, from https://www.hindawi.com/journals/jhe/si/658251/

Abhishek. (2012). Proposing Efficient Neural Network Training Model for Kidney Stone Diagnosis. *International Journal of Computer Science and Information Technologies, 3*(11), 3900–3904.

Abiodun, K. M., Awotunde, J. B., Aremu, D. R., & Adeniyi, E. A. (2022). Explainable AI for Fighting COVID-19 Pandemic: Opportunities, Challenges, and Future Prospects. In *Computational Intelligence for COVID-19 and Future Pandemics* (pp. 315–332). Springer. doi:10.1007/978-981-16-3783-4_15

Abolhassani, M., Ehsani, S., Esfandiari, H., Hajiaghayi, M., Kleinberg, R., & Lucier, B. (2017, June). Beating 1-1/e for ordered prophets. In *Proceedings of the 49th Annual ACM SIGACT Symposium on Theory of Computing* (pp. 61-71). ACM.

Action plan for the prevention and control of noncommunicable diseases in the WHO European region 2016–2025. (2017, August 15). https://www.euro.who.int/en/health-topics/noncommunicable-diseases/pages/policy/publications/action-plan-for-the-prevention-and-control-of-noncommunicable-diseases-in-the-who-european-region-20162025

Adadi, A., & Berrada, M. (2018). undefined. *IEEE Access: Practical Innovations, Open Solutions, 6,* 52138–52160. doi:10.1109/ACCESS.2018.2870052

Adadi, A., & Berrada, M. (2020). Explainable AI for healthcare: from black box to interpretable models. In *Embedded Systems and Artificial Intelligence* (pp. 327–337). Springer. doi:10.1007/978-981-15-0947-6_31

Adel, M., Kotb, A., Farag, O., Darweesh, M. S., & Mostafa, H. (2019). Breast Cancer Diagnosis Using Image Processing and Machine Learning for Elastography Images. *2019 8th International Conference on Modern Circuits and Systems Technologies (MOCAST)*, 1-4. 10.1109/MOCAST.2019.8741846

Administrator. (2017, September 11). *Noncommunicable diseases*. WHO. https://www.emro.who.int/annual-report/2016/noncommunicable-diseases.html

Agrawal, S., Ding, Y., Saberi, A., & Ye, Y. (2012). Price of correlations in stochastic optimization. *Operations Research*, *60*(1), 150–162.

Agrebi, S., & Larbi, A. (2020). Use of artificial intelligence in infectious diseases. In *Artificial intelligence in precision health* (pp. 415–438). Academic Press. doi:10.1016/B978-0-12-817133-2.00018-5

Ahad, M. A. R., Antar, A. D., & Shahid, O. (2019). *Vision-based Action Understanding for Assistive Healthcare: A Short Review*. Paper presented at the CVPR Workshops.

Ai, H. (2019). High-level expert group on artificial intelligence. *Ethics Guidelines for Trustworthy AI*.

Ajagbe, S. A., Awotunde, J. B., Oladipupo, M. A., & Oye, O. E. (2022). Prediction and Forecasting of Coronavirus Cases Using Artificial Intelligence Algorithm. In *Machine Learning for Critical Internet of Medical Things* (pp. 31–54). Springer.

Akbulut, A., Ertugrul, E., & Topcu, V. (2018). Fetal health status prediction based on maternal clinical history using machine learning techniques. *Computer Methods and Programs in Biomedicine*, *163*, 87–100. doi:10.1016/j.cmpb.2018.06.010 PMID:30119860

Alaei, S. (2014). Bayesian combinatorial auctions: Expanding single buyer mechanisms to many buyers. *SIAM Journal on Computing*, *43*(2), 930–972.

Alaei, S., Hajiaghayi, M., & Liaghat, V. (2012, June). Online prophet-inequality matching with applications to ad allocation. In *Proceedings of the 13th ACM Conference on Electronic Commerce* (pp. 18-35). ACM.

Alashwal, H., Abdalla, A., El Halaby, M., & Moustafa, A. A. (2020). Feature selection for the classification of Alzheimer's disease data. *ACM International Conference Proceeding Series*, 41–45. 10.1145/3378936.3378982

Albahri, A. S., Al-Obaidi, J. R., Zaidan, A. A., Albahri, O. S., Hamid, R. A., Zaidan, B. B., Alamoodi, A. H., & Hashim, M. (2020). Multi-biological laboratory examination framework for the prioritization of patients with COVID-19 based on integrated AHP and group VIKOR methods. *International Journal of Information Technology & Decision Making*, *19*(05), 1247–1269. doi:10.1142/S0219622020500285

Albahri, O. S., Al-Obaidi, J. R., Zaidan, A. A., Albahri, A. S., Zaidan, B. B., Salih, M. M., Qays, A., Dawood, K. A., Mohammed, R. T., Abdulkareem, K. H., Aleesa, A. M., Alamoodi, A. H., Chyad, M. A., & Zulkifli, C. Z. (2020). Helping doctors hasten COVID-19 treatment: Towards a rescue framework for the transfusion of best convalescent plasma to the most critical patients based on biological requirements via ml and novel MCDM methods. *Computer Methods and Programs in Biomedicine*, *196*, 105617. doi:10.1016/j.cmpb.2020.105617 PMID:32593060

Albright, J. (2019). Forecasting the progression of Alzheimer's disease using neural networks and a novel preprocessing algorithm. *Alzheimer's & Dementia (New York, N. Y.)*, *5*(1), 483–491. doi:10.1016/j.trci.2019.07.001 PMID:31650004

Aliberti, A., Pupillo, I., Terna, S., Macii, E., Di Cataldo, S., Patti, E., & Acquaviva, A. (2019). A multi-patient data-driven approach to blood glucose prediction. *IEEE Access: Practical Innovations, Open Solutions*, *7*, 69311–69325.

Ali, F., El-Sappagh, S., Islam, S. R., Kwak, D., Ali, A., Imran, M., & Kwak, K. (2020). A smart healthcare monitoring system for heart disease prediction based on ensemble deep learning and feature fusion. *Information Fusion*, *63*, 208–222. doi:10.1016/j.inffus.2020.06.008

Aliyeva, T., Rzayeva, U., & Azizova, R. (2021). SEIRD Model for Control of COVID-19: Case of Azerbaijan. *SHS Web of Conference, Volume 92. The 20th International Scientific Conference Globalization and its Socio-Economic Consequences 2020*.

Allibhai, E. (2018). *Building a Deep Learning Model using Keras*. Towards Data Science.

Al-Najjar, H., & Al-Rousan, N. (2020). A classifier prediction model to predict the status of Coronavirus COVID-19 patients in South Korea. *European Review for Medical and Pharmacological Sciences*. Advance online publication. doi:10.26355/eurrev_202003_20709 PMID:32271458

Amann, J., Blasimme, A., Vayena, E., Frey, D., & Madai, V. I. (2020). Explainability for artificial intelligence in healthcare: A multidisciplinary perspective. *BMC Medical Informatics and Decision Making*, *20*(1), 1–9.

Ameena, R. R., & Ashadevi, B. (2020). Predictive analysis of diabetic women patients using R. In *Systems Simulation and Modeling for Cloud Computing and Big Data Applications* (pp. 99–113). Academic Press.

Amitab, K., Medhi, K., Kandar, D., & Paul, B. S. (2018). Impulse noise reduction in digital images using fuzzy logic and artificial neural network. *Proceedings of the International Conference on Computing and Communication Systems*, 155–165. 10.1007/978-981-10-6890-4_14

Amma, N. B. (2012, February). Cardiovascular disease prediction system using genetic algorithm and neural network. In *2012 International Conference on Computing, Communication and Applications* (pp. 1-5). IEEE. 10.1109/ICCCA.2012.6179185

Amparore, E., Perotti, A., & Bajardi, P. (2021). To trust or not to trust an explanation: Using LEAF to evaluate local linear XAI methods. *PeerJ. Computer Science*, *7*, e479.

Anastassopoulou, C., Russo, L., Tsakris, A., & Siettos, C. (2020). Data-based analysis, modelling and forecasting of the COVID-19 outbreak. *PLoS One*, *15*(3), e0230405.

An, C., Lim, H., Kim, D. W., Chang, J. H., Choi, Y. J., & Kim, S. W. (2020). Machine learning prediction for mortality of patients diagnosed with COVID-19: A nationwide Korean cohort study. *Scientific Reports*, *10*(1), 1–11. doi:10.103841598-020-75767-2 PMID:33127965

Andreas, J. (2020). Explainable machine learning for scientific insights and discoveries. *IEEE*, *3*(8), 42.

Andreeva, P., Dimitrova, M., & Radeva, P. (2012). *Data mining learning models and algorithms*. Academic Press.

Angelov, P. P., Soares, E. A., Jiang, R., Arnold, N. I., & Atkinson, P. M. (2021). Explainable artificial intelligence: An analytical review. *Wiley Interdisciplinary Reviews. Data Mining and Knowledge Discovery*, *11*(5), e1424.

Anitha, J., Dinesh Peter, J., & Immanuel Alex Pandian, S. (2017). A dual stage adaptive thresholding (DuSAT) for automatic mass detection in mammograms. *Computer Methods and Programs in Biomedicine*, *138*, 93–104. doi:10.1016/j.cmpb.2016.10.026 PMID:27886719

Antoniadi, A. M., Du, Y., Guendouz, Y., Wei, L., Mazo, C., Becker, B. A., & Mooney, C. (2021). Current Challenges and Future Opportunities for XAI in Machine Learning-Based Clinical Decision Support Systems: A Systematic Review. *Applied Sciences (Basel, Switzerland)*, *11*(11), 5088. https://doi.org/10.3390/app11115088

Arora, K., & Bist, A. S. (2020). Artificial intelligence based drug discovery techniques for covid-19 detection. *Aptisi Transactions on Technopreneurship*, *2*(2), 120–126. doi:10.34306/att.v2i2.88

Arunachalam, S. (2020). Cardiovascular disease prediction model using machine learning algorithms. *International Journal for Research in Applied Science and Engineering Technology*, *8*(6), 1006–1019. doi:10.22214/ijraset.2020.6164

Ashiquzzaman, A., Kawsar Tushar, A., Islam, R., Shon, D., Im, K., Park, J., Lim, D., & Kim, J. (2017). *Reduction of Overfitting in Diabetes Prediction Using Deep Learning Neural Network*. Computer Vision and Pattern Recognition.

Asria, H., Mousannifb, H., Al Moatassimec, H., & Noeld, T. (2016). Using Machine Learning Algorithms for Breast Cancer Risk Prediction and Diagnosis. *Procedia Computer Science*, *83*, 1064–1069. doi:10.1016/j.procs.2016.04.224

Aung, M. S., Kaltwang, S., Romera-Paredes, B., Martinez, B., Singh, A., Cella, M., & Shafizadeh, M. (2015). The automatic detection of chronic pain-related expression: Requirements, challenges, and the multimodal EmoPain dataset. *IEEE Transactions on Affective Computing*, *7*(4), 435–451. doi:10.1109/TAFFC.2015.2462830 PMID:30906508

Awotunde, J. B., Ajagbe, S. A., Oladipupo, M. A., Awokola, J. A., Afolabi, O. S., Mathew, T. O., & Oguns, Y. J. (2021, October). An Improved Machine Learnings Diagnosis Technique for COVID-19 Pandemic Using Chest X-ray Images. *Communications in Computer and Information Science, 2021, 1455 CCIS*, 319–330.

Awotunde, J. B., Folorunso, S. O., Ajagbe, S. A., Garg, J., & Ajamu, G. J. (2022). AiIoMT: IoMT-Based System-Enabled Artificial Intelligence for Enhanced Smart Healthcare Systems. *Machine Learning for Critical Internet of Medical Things*, 229-254.

Awotunde, J. B., Folorunso, S. O., Bhoi, A. K., Adebayo, P. O., & Ijaz, M. F. (2021). Disease diagnosis system for IoT-based wearable body sensors with machine learning algorithm. *Hybrid Artificial Intelligence and IoT in Healthcare*, 201-222. doi:10.1007/978-981-16-2972-3_10

Awotunde, J. B., Adeniyi, A. E., Ajagbe, S. A., & González-Briones, A. (2022). Natural computing and unsupervised learning methods in smart healthcare data-centric operations. In *Cognitive and Soft Computing Techniques for the Analysis of Healthcare Data* (pp. 165–190). Academic Press.

Awotunde, J. B., Folorunso, S. O., Jimoh, R. G., Adeniyi, E. A., Abiodun, K. M., & Ajamu, G. J. (2021a). Application of artificial intelligence for COVID-19 epidemic: An exploratory study, opportunities, challenges, and future prospects. Studies in Systems. *Decision and Control, 2021*(358), 47–61. doi:10.1007/978-3-030-69744-0_4

Awotunde, J. B., Ogundokun, R. O., Jimoh, R. G., Misra, S., & Aro, T. O. (2021b). Machine learning algorithm for cryptocurrencies price prediction. *Studies in Computational Intelligence, 2021*(972), 421–447. doi:10.1007/978-3-030-72236-4_17

Ayman, M., & Dhage, S. N. (2018). Diabetes Disease Prediction Using Machine Learning on Big Data of Healthcare. *2018 Fourth International Conference on Computing Communication Control and Automation (ICCUBEA)*, 1-6. 10.1109/ICCUBEA.2018.8697439

Azar, Y., Chiplunkar, A., & Kaplan, H. (2018, June). Prophet secretary: Surpassing the 1-1/e barrier. In *Proceedings of the 2018 ACM Conference on Economics and Computation* (pp. 303-318). ACM.

Babaioff, M., Immorlica, N., Lucier, B., & Weinberg, S. M. (2020). A simple and approximately optimal mechanism for an additive buyer. *Journal of the Association for Computing Machinery, 67*(4), 1–40.

Bae, T. W., Kwon, K. K., & Kim, K. H. (2020). Mass Infection Analysis of COVID-19 Using the SEIRD Model in Daegu-Gyeongbuk of Korea from April to May 2020. *Journal of Korean Medical Science, 3*(34), e317. doi:10.3346/jkms.2020.35.e317

Bai, X., Fang, C., Zhou, Y., Bai, S., Liu, Z., Xia, L., . . . Chen, W. (2020). Predicting COVID-19 malignant progression with AI techniques. doi:10.1101/2020.03.20.20037325

Barbat, M. M., Wesche, C., Werhli, A. V., & Mata, M. M. (2019). An adaptive machine learning approach to improve automatic iceberg detection from SAR images. *ISPRS Journal of Photogrammetry and Remote Sensing, 156*, 247–259. doi:10.1016/j.isprsjprs.2019.08.015

Barredo, A. A. (2020). Explainable Artificial Intelligence (XAI): Concepts, taxonomies, opportunities and challenges toward responsible AI. *Information Fusion*, *58*, 82–115. https://doi.org/10.1016/j.inffus.2019.12.012

Bastani, O. (2017). *Interpreting Blackbox models via model extraction*. arxiv.org/abs/1705.08504.

Bateni, M., Dehghani, S., Hajiaghayi, M., & Seddighin, S. (2015). Revenue maximization for selling multiple correlated items. In *Algorithms-ESA 2015* (pp. 95–105). Springer.

Bayrak, E. A., Kırcı, P., & Ensari, T. (2019). Comparison of Machine Learning Methods for Breast Cancer Diagnosis. *2019 Scientific Meeting on Electrical-Electronics & Biomedical Engineering and Computer Science (EBBT)*, 1-3. 10.1109/EBBT.2019.8741990

Beck, B. R., Shin, B., Choi, Y., Park, S., & Kang, K. (2020). Predicting commercially available antiviral drugs that may act on the novel coronavirus (SARS-CoV-2) through a drug-target interaction deep learning model. *Computational and Structural Biotechnology Journal*, *18*, 784–790. doi:10.1016/j.csbj.2020.03.025 PMID:32280433

Benedek, Z., Todor-Boér, S., Kocsis, L., Bauer, O., Suciu, N., & Coroş, M. F. (2021). Psoas muscle index defined by computer tomography predicts the presence of postoperative complications in colorectal cancer surgery. *Medicina*, *57*(5), 472.

Berwick, D. M., Nolan, T. W., & Whittington, J. (2008). The triple aim: Care, health, and cost. *Health Affairs*, *27*(3), 759–769.

Beulah, J. R., Cyril, C. P. D., Geetha, S., Irene, D. S., & Nadu, T. (2021). Towards Improved Detection of Intrusions with Constraint-Based Clustering (CBC). *International Journal of Computer Networks and Applications*, *8*(1), 28–43. doi:10.22247/ijcna/2021/207980

Bhadouria, V. S., Tanase, A., Schmid, M., Hannig, F., Teich, J., & Ghoshal, D. (2017). A Novel Image Impulse Noise Removal Algorithm Optimized for Hardware Accelerators. *Journal of Signal Processing Systems for Signal, Image, and Video Technology*, *89*(2), 225–242. doi:10.100711265-016-1187-5

Bhagya Shree, S. R., H. S. S. (2014). An initial investigation in the Diagnosis of AD using various Classification Techniques. *IEEE International Conference on Computational Intelligence and Computing Research*, 1–5. 10.1109/ICCIC.2014.7238300

Bharathi, A., & Arunachalam, A. S. (2021). *Pre-Processing on Alzheimer MRI images*. Academic Press.

Bhateja, V., Tiwari, H., & Srivastava, A. (2015). A non-local means filtering algorithm for restoration of Rician distributed MRI. *Emerging ICT for Bridging the Future-Proceedings of the 49th Annual Convention of the Computer Society of India CSI*. 10.1007/978-3-319-13731-5_1

Bildirici, M., Guler Bayazit, N., & Ucan, Y. (2020). Analyzing crude oil prices under the impact of covid-19 by using lstargarchlstm. *Energies*, *13*(11), 2980. doi:10.3390/en13112980

Compilation of References

Birlasoft. (n.d.). *Demystifying explainable artificial intelligence: Benefits, use cases, and Models.* Retrieved October 23, 2021, from https://www.birlasoft.com/articles/demystifying-explainable-artificial-intelligence

Bleher, H., & Braun, M. (2022). Diffused responsibility: attributions of responsibility in the use of AI-driven clinical decision support systems. *AI and Ethics*, 1-15.

Bodenheimer, T., & Sinsky, C. (2014). From triple to quadruple aim: Care of the patient requires care of the provider. *Annals of Family Medicine*, *12*(6), 573–576.

Bostrom, N., & Yudkowsky, E. (2014). The ethics of artificial intelligence. The Cambridge handbook of artificial intelligence, 1, 316-334.

Bradac, D., Gupta, A., Singla, S., & Zuzic, G. (2019). *Robust algorithms for the secretary problem.* arXiv preprint arXiv:1911.07352.

Braun, V., & Clarke, V. (2021). Can I use TA? Should I use TA? Should I not use TA? Comparing reflexive thematic analysis and other pattern-based qualitative analytic approaches. *Counselling & Psychotherapy Research*, *21*(1), 37–47.

Breetha, S., & Kavinila, R. (2013). *Hierarchical Clustering For Cancer Discovery Using Range Check And Delta Check.* Academic Press.

Browning, L., Colling, R., Rakha, E., Rajpoot, N., Rittscher, J., James, J. A., Salto-Tellez, M., Snead, D. R. J., & Verrill, C. (2021). Digital pathology and artificial intelligence will be key to supporting clinical and academic cellular pathology through COVID-19 and future crises: The PathLAKE consortium perspective. *Journal of Clinical Pathology*, *74*(7), 443–447. doi:10.1136/jclinpath-2020-206854 PMID:32620678

Brownlee, J. (2017). *A Gentle Introduction to Long Shor-Term Memory Networks by the experts.* Machine Learning Mastery.

Cai. (2009). *The Research on Emotion Recognition from ECG Signal.* Academic Press.

Carpenter, K. A., Cohen, D. S., Jarrell, J. T., & Huang, X. (2018). Deep learning and Virtual drug screening. *Future Medicinal Chemistry*, *10*(21), 2557–2567. doi:10.4155/fmc-2018-0314 PMID:30288997

Carvalho, D. V., Pereira, E. M., & Cardoso, J. S. (2019). Machine learning Interpretability: A survey on methods and metrics. *Electronics (Basel)*, *8*(8), 832. doi:10.3390/electronics8080832

Castro, J., Gamez, D., & Tejada, J. (2009). Polynomial calculation of the shapley value based on sampling. *Computers & Operations Research*, *36*(5), 1726–1730. doi:10.1016/j.cor.2008.04.004

Cath, C., Wachter, S., Mittelstadt, B., Taddeo, M., & Floridi, L. (2018). Artificial intelligence and the 'good society': The US, EU, and UK approach. *Science and Engineering Ethics*, *24*(2), 505–528.

Challen, R., Denny, J., Pitt, M., Gompels, L., Edwards, T., & Tsaneva-Atanasova, K. (2019). Artificial intelligence, bias and clinical safety. *BMJ Quality & Safety*, *28*(3), 231–237.

Chandra, G., Gupta, R., & Agarwal, N. (2020). *Role of artificial intelligence in transforming the justice delivery system in covid-19 pandemic.* . doi:10.1038/nrd.2016.104

Chan, J. F. W., Yao, Y., Yeung, M. L., Deng, W., Bao, L., Jia, L., Li, F., Xiao, C., Gao, H., Yu, P., Cai, J.-P., Chu, H., Zhou, J., Chen, H., Qin, C., & Yuen, K. Y. (2015). Treatment with lopinavir/ritonavir or interferon-β1b improves outcome of MERS-CoV infection in a nonhuman primate model of common marmoset. *The Journal of Infectious Diseases*, *212*(12), 1904–1913. doi:10.1093/infdis/jiv392 PMID:26198719

Chan, J. F., Chan, K. H., Kao, R. Y., To, K. K., Zheng, B. J., Li, C. P., Li, P. T. W., Dai, J., Mok, F. K. Y., Chen, H., Hayden, F. G., & Yuen, K. Y. (2013). Broad-spectrum antivirals for the emerging Middle East respiratory syndrome coronavirus. *The Journal of Infection*, *67*(6), 606–616. doi:10.1016/j.jinf.2013.09.029 PMID:24096239

Charikar, M., Steinhardt, J., & Valiant, G. (2017, June). Learning from untrusted data. In *Proceedings of the 49th Annual ACM SIGACT Symposium on Theory of Computing* (pp. 47-60). ACM.

Chatterjee, S., Sarkar, A., Karmakar, M., Chatterjee, S., & Paul, R. (2020). SEIRD model to study the asymptomatic growth during COVID-19 pandemic in India. *Indian Journal of Physics*. . doi:10.1007/s12648-020-01928-8

Chaudhry, R. (2020). Coronavirus disease (2019) (COVID-19): Forecast of an emerging urgency in Pakistan. *Cureus*, *12*(5).

Chavhan, G. B., Babyn, P. S., Thomas, B., Shroff, M. M., & Haacke, E. (2009). *Principles, techniques, and applications of T2*-based MR imaging and its special applications*. Academic Press.

Chawla, S., Hartline, J. D., Malec, D. L., & Sivan, B. (2010, June). Multi-parameter mechanism design and sequential posted pricing. In *Proceedings of the forty-second ACM symposium on Theory of computing* (pp. 311-320). ACM.

Chawla, S., Malec, D., & Sivan, B. (2015). The power of randomness in bayesian optimal mechanism design. *Games and Economic Behavior*, *91*, 297–317.

Chen, C., Jafari, R., & Kehtarnavaz, N. (2015). *UTD-MHAD: A multimodal dataset for human action recognition utilizing a depth camera and a wearable inertial sensor*. Paper presented at the 2015 IEEE International conference on image processing (ICIP). 10.1109/ICIP.2015.7350781

Chen, H., Lundberg, S., & Lee, S. (2020). Explaining models by propagating Shapley values of local components. *Explainable AI in Healthcare and Medicine*, 261-270. doi:10.1007/978-3-030-53352-6_24

Chen, Y., Ouyang, L., Bao, F. S., Li, Q., Han, L., Zhu, B., . . . Chen, S. (2020). *An interpretable machine learning framework for accurate severe vs non-severe covid-19 clinical type classification*. doi:10.1101/2020.05.18.20105841

Chen, Y., Xie, Y., Zhou, Z., Shi, F., Christodoulou, A. G., & Li, D. (2018). *Brain MRI super resolution using 3D deep densely connected neural networks*. Paper presented at the 2018 IEEE 15th International Symposium on Biomedical Imaging (ISBI 2018). 10.1109/ISBI.2018.8363679

Chen, Y., Yang, W., & Zhang, B. (2020). *Using mobility for electrical load forecasting during the covid-19 pandemic*. arXiv preprint arXiv:2006.08826.

Chen. (2000). *Emotional Expressions in Audiovisual Human Computer Interaction*. Academic Press.

Cheng, V.C., Lau, S.K., Woo, P.C., & Yuen, K.Y. (2007). Severe acute respiratory syndrome coronavirus as an agent of emerging and reemerging infection. *Clinical Microbiology Reviews*, *20*(4), 660–694.

Chen, L., Cruz, A., Ramsey, S., Dickson, C. J., Duca, J. S., Hornak, V., ... Kurtzman, T. (2019). Hidden bias in the DUD-E dataset leads to misleading performance of deep learning in structure-based virtual screening. *PLoS One*, *14*(8), e0220113.

Chen, S., Kuhn, M., Prettner, K., & Bloom, D. E. (2018). The macroeconomic burden of noncommunicable diseases in the United States: Estimates and projections. *PLoS One*, *13*(11), e0206702. doi:10.1371/journal.pone.0206702 PMID:30383802

Chenthamarakshan, V., Das, P., Hoffman, S., Strobelt, H., Padhi, I., Lim, K. W., ... Mojsilovic, A. (2020). Cogmol: Target-specific and selective drug design for covid-19 using deep generative models. *Advances in Neural Information Processing Systems*, *33*, 4320–4332.

Chen, Z. (2020). Applications of Artificial Intelligence in drug development using real-world data. *Drug Discovery Today*. Advance online publication. doi:10.1016/j.drudis.2020.12.013 PMID:33358699

Chockanathan, U., DSouza, A. M., Abidin, A. Z., Schifitto, G., & Wismüller, A. (2019). Automated diagnosis of HIV-associated neurocognitive disorders using large-scale Granger causality analysis of resting-state functional MRI. *Computers in Biology and Medicine*, *106*, 24–30. doi:10.1016/j.compbiomed.2019.01.006 PMID:30665138

Choi, S., Lee, J., Kang, M. G., Min, H., Chang, Y. S., & Yoon, S. (2017). Large-scale machine learning of media outlets for understanding public reactions to nation-wide viral infection outbreaks. *Methods (San Diego, Calif.)*, *129*, 50–59. doi:10.1016/j.ymeth.2017.07.027 PMID:28813689

Chollet, F. (2015). *Keras*. https://keras.io

Choudhary, A. (2018). *Generate quick and accurate time series forecasts using Facebook's Prophet (with Python & R codes)*. Analytics Vidya.

Clancey, W. J., & Shortliffe, E. H. (1984). Readings in medical artificial intelligence: The first decade. Addison-Wesley Longman Publishing Co., Inc.

Coley, W., Green, W. H., & Jensen, K. F. (2018). Machine Learning in computer-aided synthesis planning. *Accounts of Chemical Research*, *51*(5), 1281–1289. doi:10.1021/acs.accounts.8b00087 PMID:29715002

Colonna, L. (2021). *Artificial Intelligence in the Internet of Health Things: Is the Solution to AI Privacy More AI? SSRN Electronic Journal.* doi:10.2139srn.3838571

Colubri, A., Hartley, M. A., Siakor, M., Wolfman, V., Felix, A., Sesay, T., Shaffer, J. G., Garry, R. F., Grant, D. S., Levine, A. C., & Sabeti, P. C. (2019). Machine-learning prognostic models from the 2014–16 Ebola outbreak: Data-harmonization challenges, validation strategies, and mHealth applications. *EClinicalMedicine, 11,* 54–64. doi:10.1016/j.eclinm.2019.06.003 PMID:31312805

Correa, J., Foncea, P., Hoeksma, R., Oosterwijk, T., & Vredeveld, T. (2017, June). Posted price mechanisms for a random stream of customers. In *Proceedings of the 2017 ACM Conference on Economics and Computation* (pp. 169-186). ACM.

Correa, J., Saona, R., & Ziliotto, B. (2021). Prophet secretary through blind strategies. *Mathematical Programming, 190*(1), 483–521.

Curia, F. (2021). Features and explainable methods for cytokines analysis of Dry Eye Disease in HIV infected patients. *Healthcare Analytics, 1,* 100001.

Currie, G., & Hawk, K. E. (2021, March). Ethical and legal challenges of artificial intelligence in nuclear medicine. *Seminars in Nuclear Medicine, 51*(2), 120–125.

Daghistani, T., & Alshammari, R. (2020). Comparison of statistical logistic regression and randomforest machine learning techniques in predicting diabetes. *Journal of Advances in Information Technology, 11*(2).

Darapaneni, N., Jain, P., Khattar, R., Chawla, M., Vaish, R., & Paduri, A. R. (2020, December). Analysis and Prediction of COVID-19 Pandemic in India. In *2020 2nd International Conference on Advances in Computing, Communication Control and Networking (ICACCCN)* (pp. 291-296). IEEE.

Das, A. (2006). *Opportunities and challenges in explainable artificial intelligence (XAI): A survey.* IEEE. https://arxiv.org/abs/2006.11371

Das, A., & Rad, P. (2020). *Opportunities and challenges in explainable artificial intelligence (xai): A survey.* arXiv preprint arXiv:2006.11371.

Das, A., Mishra, S., Hassanien, A. E., Salam, A., & Darwish, A. (2020). Artificial intelligence approach to predict the covid-19 patient's recovery. *EasyChair Preprint, 3223.* Advance online publication. doi:10.1007/978-3-030-63307-3_8

Davagdorj, K., Bae, J., Pham, V., Theera-Umpon, N., & Ryu, K. (2021). Explainable Artificial Intelligence Based Framework for Non-Communicable Diseases Prediction. *IEEE Access: Practical Innovations, Open Solutions, 9,* 123672–123688. doi:10.1109/ACCESS.2021.3110336

Davagdorj, K., Lee, J. S., Park, K. H., Huy, P. V., & Ryu, K. H. (2020). Synthetic oversampling based decision support framework to solve class imbalance problem in smoking cessation program. *International Journal of Applied Science and Engineering, 17,* 223–235. doi:10.6703/IJASE.202009_17(3).223

Davagdorj, K., Lee, J. S., Pham, V. H., & Ryu, K. H. (2020). A comparative analysis of machine learning methods for class imbalance in a smoking cessation intervention. *Applied Sciences (Basel, Switzerland), 10*(9), 3307. doi:10.3390/app10093307

Davagdorj, K., Pham, V. H., Theera-Umpon, N., & Ryu, K. H. (2020). Xgboost-based framework for smoking-induced noncommunicable disease prediction. *International Journal of Environmental Research and Public Health, 17*(18), 6513. doi:10.3390/ijerph17186513 PMID:32906777

Davagdorj, K., Yu, S. H., Kim, S. Y., Huy, P. V., Park, J. H., & Ryu, K. H. (2019). Prediction of 6 months smoking cessation program among women in Korea. *International Journal of Machine Learning and Computing, 9*(1), 83–90. doi:10.18178/ijmlc.2019.9.1.769

de Moraes Batista, A. F., Miraglia, J. L., Donato, T. H. R., & Chiavegatto Filho, A. D. P. (2020). COVID-19 diagnosis prediction in emergency care patients: a machine learning approach. MedRxiv. doi:10.1101/2020.04.04.20052092

DeCamp, M., & Lindvall, C. (2020). Latent bias and the implementation of artificial intelligence in medicine. *Journal of the American Medical Informatics Association, 27*(12), 2020–2023.

Deepalakshmi, P., Prudhvi Krishna, T., Siri Chandana, S., & Lavanya, K. (2021). Plant Leaf Disease Detection Using CNN Algorithm *International Journal of Information System Modeling and Design, 12*(1), 1–21. doi:10.4018/IJISMD.2021010101

Deore. (2019). The Stages of Drug Discovery and Development Process. *Asian Journal of Pharmaceutical Research and Development.*

Dey, S. (2018). Predicting adverse drug reactions through interpretable deep learning framework. *International Conference on Intelligent Biology and Medicine (ICIBM): Bioinformatics.* 10.118612859-018-2544-0

Dey, S. K., Hossain, A., & Rahman, M. M. (2018). Implementation of a Web Application to Predict Diabetes Disease: An Approach Using Machine Learning Algorithm. *21st International Conference of Computer and Information Technology (ICCIT)*, 1-5. 10.1109/ICCITECHN.2018.8631968

Dhanorkar, S., Wolf, C. T., Qian, K., Xu, A., Popa, L., & Li, Y. (2021, June). Who needs to know what, when?: Broadening the Explainable AI (XAI) Design Space by Looking at Explanations Across the AI Lifecycle. In *Designing Interactive Systems Conference 2021* (pp. 1591-1602). Academic Press.

Diakonikolas, I. (2018). *Algorithmic high-dimensional robust statistics.* http://www. iliasdiakonikolas. org/simons-tutorial-robust. html

Diakonikolas, I., Kamath, G., Kane, D. M., Li, J., Moitra, A., & Stewart, A. (2018). Robustly learning a gaussian: Getting optimal error, efficiently. In *Proceedings of the Twenty-Ninth Annual ACM-SIAM Symposium on Discrete Algorithms* (pp. 2683-2702). Society for Industrial and Applied Mathematics.

Diakonikolas, I., Kamath, G., Kane, D., Li, J., Moitra, A., & Stewart, A. (2019). Robust estimators in high-dimensions without the computational intractability. *SIAM Journal on Computing*, *48*(2), 742–864.

Dignum, V. (2018). Ethics in artificial intelligence: Introduction to the special issue. *Ethics and Information Technology*, *20*(1), 1–3.

DiMasi, J. A., & Faden, L. B. (2011). Competitiveness in follow-on drug R&D: A race or imitation? *Nature Reviews. Drug Discovery*, *10*(1), 23–27. doi:10.1038/nrd3296 PMID:21151030

Dinesh, K. G., Arumugaraj, K., Santhosh, K. D., & Mareeswari, V. (2018, March). Prediction of cardiovascular disease using machine learning algorithms. In *2018 International Conference on Current Trends towards Converging Technologies (ICCTCT)* (pp. 1-7). IEEE. 10.1109/ICCTCT.2018.8550857

Ding, Y., Sohn, J. H., Kawczynski, M. G., Trivedi, H., Harnish, R., Jenkins, N. W., ... Franc, B. L. (2019). A deep learning model to predict a diagnosis of Alzheimer disease by using 18F-FDG PET of the brain. *Radiology*, *290*(2), 456–464.

Dinh, A., Miertschin, S., Young, A., & Mohanty, S. D. (2019). A data-driven approach to predicting diabetes and cardiovascular disease with machine learning. *BMC Medical Informatics and Decision Making*, *19*(1), 1–15. doi:10.118612911-019-0918-5 PMID:31694707

Divya, R., & Shantha Selva Kumari, R. (2021). Genetic algorithm with logistic regression feature selection for Alzheimer's disease classification. *Neural Computing & Applications*, *33*(14), 8435–8444. doi:10.100700521-020-05596-x

Dong, C., Loy, C. C., He, K., & Tang, X. (2014). *Learning a deep convolutional network for image super-resolution.* Paper presented at the European conference on computer vision. 10.1007/978-3-319-10593-2_13

Donge. (2021). *Neural Networks and LSTM Networks. Built in expert contributor network.* Academic Press.

Doran, D., Schulz, S., & Besold, T. R. (2017). *What does explainable AI really mean? A new conceptualization of perspectives.* arXiv preprint arXiv:1710.00794.

Dou, Q., Wei, S., Yang, X., Wu, W., Liu, K. (2018). *Medical image super-resolution via minimum error regression model selection using random forest.* Academic Press.

Dourado Jr, C. M., da Silva, S. P. P., da Nobrega, R. V. M., Barros, A. C. D. S., Reboucas Filho, P. P., & de Albuquerque, V. H. C. (2019). Deep learning IoT system for online stroke detection in skull computed tomography images. *Computer Networks*, *152*, 25–39. doi:10.1016/j.comnet.2019.01.019

Du, J., Wang, L., Liu, Y., Zhou, Z., He, Z., & Jia, Y. (2020). *Brain MRI Super-Resolution Using 3D Dilated Convolutional Encoder–Decoder Network.* Academic Press.

Duda, R. O., Hart, P. E., Stork, D. G., & Wiley, J. (2016). *Pattern Classification All materials in these slides were taken from Pattern Classification* (2nd ed.). Academic Press.

Dutting, P., Feldman, M., Kesselheim, T., & Lucier, B. (2020). Prophet inequalities made easy: Stochastic optimization by pricing nonstochastic inputs. *SIAM Journal on Computing*, *49*(3), 540–582.

Dütting, P., & Kesselheim, T. (2019, June). Posted pricing and prophet inequalities with inaccurate priors. In *Proceedings of the 2019 ACM Conference on Economics and Computation* (pp. 111-129). ACM.

Duval, A. (2019). Explainable artificial intelligence (XAI). MA4K9 Scholarly Report, Mathematics Institute, The University of Warwick.

Easttom, C., Thapa, S., & Lawson, J. (2020). A Comparative Study of Machine Learning Algorithms for Use in Breast Cancer Studies. *2020 10th Annual Computing and Communication Workshop and Conference (CCWC)*, 412-416. 10.1109/CCWC47524.2020.9031266

Eck, N. J. V., & Waltman, L. (2014). Visualizing bibliometric networks. In *Measuring scholarly impact* (pp. 285–320). Springer.

Ehsani, S., Hajiaghayi, M., Kesselheim, T., & Singla, S. (2018). Prophet secretary for combinatorial auctions and matroids. In *Proceedings of the twenty-ninth annual acm-siam symposium on discrete algorithms* (pp. 700-714). Society for Industrial and Applied Mathematics.

Ekins, S., Freundlich, J. S., & Coffee, M. (2014). A common feature pharmacophore for FDA-approved drugs inhibiting the Ebola virus. *F1000 Research*, *3*, 277. Advance online publication. doi:10.12688/f1000research.5741.1 PMID:25653841

Ekins, S., Mottin, M., Ramos, P. R., Sousa, B. K., Neves, B. J., Foil, D. H., Zorn, K. M., Braga, R. C., Coffee, M., Southan, C., Puhl, A. C., & Andrade, C. H. (2020). Déjà vu: Stimulating open drug discovery for SARS-CoV-2. *Drug Discovery Today*, *25*(5), 928–941. doi:10.1016/j.drudis.2020.03.019 PMID:32320852

Ellis, C., Masood, S. Z., Tappen, M. F., LaViola, J. J. Jr, & Sukthankar, R. (2013). Exploring the trade-off between accuracy and observational latency in action recognition. *International Journal of Computer Vision*, *101*(3), 420–436. doi:10.100711263-012-0550-7

El-Sappagh, S., Alonso, J. M., Islam, S. M. R., Sultan, A. M., & Kwak, K. S. (2021). A multilayer multimodal detection and prediction model based on explainable artificial intelligence for Alzheimer's disease. *Scientific Reports*, *11*(1), 2660. Advance online publication. doi:10.103841598-021-82098-3 PMID:33514817

El-Sappagh, S., Saleh, H., Sahal, R., Abuhmed, T., Islam, S. R., Ali, F., & Amer, E. (2021). Alzheimer's disease progression detection model based on an early fusion of cost-effective multimodal data. *Future Generation Computer Systems*, *115*, 680–699. doi:10.1016/j.future.2020.10.005

Elshawi, R., Al-Mallah, M. H., & Sakr, S. (2019). On the interpretability of machine learning-based model for predicting hypertension. *BMC Medical Informatics and Decision Making*, *19*(1), 146. Advance online publication. doi:10.118612911-019-0874-0 PMID:31357998

ElShawi, R., Sherif, Y., Al-Mallah, M., & Sakr, S. (2021). Interpretability in healthcare: A comparative study of local machine learning interpretability techniques. *Computational Intelligence*, *37*(4), 1633–1650. doi:10.1111/coin.12410

Eltrass & Salama. (2018). Fully automated scheme for computer-aided detection and breast cancer diagnosis using digitised mammograms. *IET Image Processing*, *14*(3), 495-505. . doi:10.1049/iet-ipr.2018.5953

Escobar, J. D., Guillén, N. E. O., Reyes, S. V., Mosqueda, A. G., Kober, V., Rodriguez, R. R., & Rizk, J. E. L. (2021). Deep-learning based detection of COVID-19 using lung ultrasound imagery. *PLOS global. Public Health*, *16*(8), e0255886. Advance online publication. doi:10.1371/journal.pone.0255886

Esfandiari, H., Korula, N., & Mirrokni, V. (2018). Allocation with traffic spikes: Mixing adversarial and stochastic models. *ACM Transactions on Economics and Computation*, *6*(3-4), 1–23.

Etzioni, A., & Etzioni, O. (2017). Incorporating ethics into artificial intelligence. *The Journal of Ethics*, *21*(4), 403–418.

Ezra, T., Feldman, M., & Nehama, I. (2018). *Prophets and secretaries with overbooking.* arXiv preprint arXiv:1805.05094.

Ezra, T., Feldman, M., Gravin, N., & Tang, Z. G. (2020, July). Online stochastic max-weight matching: Prophet inequality for vertex and edge arrival models. In *Proceedings of the 21st ACM Conference on Economics and Computation* (pp. 769-787). ACM.

Fallahi, A., & Jafari, S. (2011). An Expert System for Detection of Breast Cancer Using Data Preprocessing and Bayesian Network. *International Journal of Advanced Science and Technology*, *34*, 65–70.

Faruque, M., Asaduzzaman, & Sarker, I. (2019). Performance Analysis of Machine Learning Techniques to Predict Diabetes Mellitus. In *2019 International Conference on Electrical, Computer and Communication Engineering (ECCE)*. IEEE Xplore.

Fatima, S. S., Wooldridge, M., & Jennings, N. R. (2008). A linear approximation method for the shapley value. *Artificial Intelligence, 172*(14), 1673 – 1699. doi:10.1016/j.artint.2008.05.003

Feldman, M., Gravin, N., & Lucier, B. (2014, December). Combinatorial auctions via posted prices. In *Proceedings of the twenty-sixth annual ACM-SIAM symposium on Discrete algorithms* (pp. 123-135). Society for Industrial and Applied Mathematics.

Feldman, M., Svensson, O., & Zenklusen, R. (2016). Online contention resolution schemes. In *Proceedings of the twenty-seventh annual ACM-SIAM symposium on Discrete algorithms* (pp. 1014-1033). Society for Industrial and Applied Mathematics.

Fellous, J. M., Sapiro, G., Rossi, A., Mayberg, H., & Ferrante, M. (2019). Explainable Artificial Intelligence for Neuroscience, *Behavioral Neurostimulation. Frontiers in Neuroscience*, *1*(1). Advance online publication. doi:10.3389/fnins.2019.01346

Feng, C., Wang, L., Chen, X., Zhai, Y., Zhu, F., Chen, H., . . . Li, T. (2021). A Novel Triage Tool of Artificial Intelligence-Assisted Diagnosis Aid System for Suspected COVID-19 Pneumonia in Fever Clinics. MedRxiv, 2020-03. doi:10.1101/2020.03.19.20039099

Ferreira, D., Oliveira, A., & Freitas, A. (2012). Applying data mining techniques to improve diagnosis in neonatal jaundice. *BMC Medical Informatics and Decision Making*, *12*(1), 143. doi:10.1186/1472-6947-12-143 PMID:23216895

Finocchiaro, J., Maio, R., Monachou, F., Patro, G. K., Raghavan, M., Stoica, A. A., & Tsirtsis, S. (2021, March). Bridging machine learning and mechanism design towards algorithmic fairness. In *Proceedings of the 2021 ACM Conference on Fairness, Accountability, and Transparency* (pp. 489-503). ACM.

Foley, J. D., & Van Dam, A. (1982). Fundamentals of interactive computer graphics. Addison-Wesley Longman Publishing Co., Inc.

Fong, J. X., Shapiai, M. I., Tiew, Y. Y., Batool, U., & Fauzi, H. (2020). Bypassing MRI Pre-processing in Alzheimer's Disease Diagnosis using Deep Learning Detection Network. *2020 16th IEEE International Colloquium on Signal Processing & Its Applications (CSPA)*, 219–224.

Fong, R. C., & Vedaldi, A. (2017). Interpretable explanations of black boxes by meaningful perturbation. *IEEE International Conference on Computer Vision (ICCV)*, 3449–3457.

Gao, F., You, J., Wang, J., Sun, J., Yang, E., & Zhou, H. (2017). A novel target detection method for SAR images based on shadow proposal and saliency analysis. *Neurocomputing*, *267*, 220–231. doi:10.1016/j.neucom.2017.06.004

Gautret, P., Lagier, J. C., Parola, P., Meddeb, L., Mailhe, M., Doudier, B., ... Raoult, D. (2020). Hydroxychloroquine and azithromycin as a treatment of COVID-19: Results of an open-label non-randomized clinical trial. *International Journal of Antimicrobial Agents*, *56*(1), 105949. doi:10.1016/j.ijantimicag.2020.105949 PMID:32205204

GBD 2015 Risk F Collaborators. (2016). Global, regional, and national comparative risk assessment of 79 behavioural, environmental and occupational, and metabolic risks or clusters of risks, 1990-2015: a systematic analysis for the Global Burden of Disease Study 2015. *Lancet, 388*(10053), 1659–1724. . doi:10.1016/S0140-6736(16)31679-8

Geetha, S., Deepalakshmi, P., & Pande, S. (2019, December). Managing Crop for Indian Farming Using IOT. In *2019 IEEE International Conference on Clean Energy and Energy Efficient Electronics Circuit for Sustainable Development (INCCES)* (pp. 1-5). IEEE. 10.1109/INCCES47820.2019.9167699

Geetha, S., Nanda, P., Joshua Samuel Raj, R., & Prince, T. (2021). Early Recognition of Herb Sickness Using SVM. In *Intelligence in Big Data Technologies—Beyond the Hype* (pp. 543–550). Springer. doi:10.1007/978-981-15-5285-4_54

Gemmar, P. (2020). An interpretable mortality prediction model for COVID-19 patients–alternative approach. MedRxiv. doi:10.1101/2020.06.14.20130732

Geras, K. J., Wolfson, S., Shen, Y., Wu, N., Kim, S., Kim, E., . . . Cho, K. (2017). *High-resolution breast cancer screening with multi-view deep convolutional neural networks.* arXiv preprint arXiv:1703.07047.

Ge, Y., Tian, T., Huang, S., Wan, F., Li, J., Li, S., Wang, X., Yang, H., Hong, L., Wu, N., Yuan, E., Luo, Y., Cheng, L., Hu, C., Lei, Y., Shu, H., Feng, X., Jiang, Z., Wu, Y., ... Zeng, J. (2021). An integrative drug repositioning framework discovered a potential therapeutic agent targeting COVID-19. *Signal Transduction and Targeted Therapy*, *6*(1), 1–16. doi:10.103841392-021-00568-6 PMID:33895786

Ghosh, P., Azam, S., Jonkman, M., Karim, A., Shamrat, F. J. M., Ignatious, E., Shultana, S., Beeravolu, A. R., & De Boer, F. (2021). Efficient prediction of cardiovascular disease using machine learning algorithms with relief and LASSO feature selection techniques. *IEEE Access: Practical Innovations, Open Solutions*, *9*, 19304–19326. doi:10.1109/ACCESS.2021.3053759

Gilpin, L. H., Bau, D., Yuan, B. Z., Bajwa, A., Specter, M., & Kagal, L. (2018, October). Explaining explanations: An overview of interpretability of machine learning. In *2018 IEEE 5th International Conference on data science and advanced analytics (DSAA)* (pp. 80-89). IEEE.

Gilvary. (2019). The Missing Pieces of Artificial Intelligence in Medicine. *Rise of Machines in Medicine*. doi: 10.1016/j.tips.2019.06.001

Gns, H. S., Saraswathy, G. R., Murahari, M., & Krishnamurthy, M. (2019). An update on Drug Repurposing: Re-written saga of the drug's fate. *Biomedicine and Pharmacotherapy*, *110*, 700–716. doi:10.1016/j.biopha.2018.11.127 PMID:30553197

Godio, A., Pace, F., & Vergnano, A. (2020). SEIR Modeling of the Italian Epidemic of SARS-CoV-2 Using Computational Swarm Intelligence. *International Journal of Environmental Research and Public Health*, *2020*(17), 3535. doi:10.3390/ijerph17103535 PMID:32443640

Gohel, P., Singh, P., & Mohanty, M. (2017). *Explainable AI: Current status and future directions.* IEEE Access Preprint.

Goh, G. K. M., Dunker, A. K., Foster, J. A., & Uversky, V. N. (2020). A novel strategy for the development of vaccines for SARS-CoV-2 (COVID-19) and other viruses using AI and viral shell disorder. *Journal of Proteome Research*, *19*(11), 4355–4363. doi:10.1021/acs.jproteome.0c00672 PMID:33006287

Goodman, B., & Flaxman, S. (2017). European Union regulations on algorithmic decision-making and a "right to explanation". *AI Magazine*, *38*(3), 50–57.

Greenspan, H. (2009). *Super-resolution in medical imaging.* Academic Press.

Guang, Y. (2021). Unbox the black-box for the medical Explainable AI via Multi-modal and Multi-center Data Fusion: a mini-review, two showcases and beyond. *Information Fusion*. doi: 1016/j.inffus.2021.07.016

Guida, J. P. (2020). Chloroquine, Hydroxychloroquine and Covid-19: A systematic review of literature. *InterAmerican Journal of Medicine and Health*, *3*, 1–10. doi:10.31005/iajmh.v3i0.79

Compilation of References

Guleria, P., Ahmed, S., Alhumam, A., & Srinivasu, P. N. (2022, January). Empirical Study on Classifiers for Earlier Prediction of COVID-19 Infection Cure and Death Rate in the Indian States. In Healthcare (Vol. 10, No. 1, p. 85). Multidisciplinary Digital Publishing Institute.

Guleria, P., Ahmed, S., Alhumam, A., & Srinivasu, P. N. (2022). Empirical Study on Classifiers for Earlier Prediction of COVID-19 Infection Cure and Death Rate in the Indian States. *Health Care, 10*(1), 85. https://doi.org/10.3390/healthcare10010085

Gunja, A., Pandey, Y., Xie, H., Wolska, B. M., Shroff, A. R., Ardati, A. K., & Vidovich, M. I. (2017). Image noise reduction technology reduces radiation in a radial-first cardiac catheterization laboratory. *Cardiovascular Revascularization Medicine; Including Molecular Interventions, 18*(3), 197–201. doi:10.1016/j.carrev.2016.12.017 PMID:28089778

Gunning, D., & Aha, D. (2019). DARPA's Explainable Artificial Intelligence (XAI) Program. *AI Magazine, 40*(2), 44–58. doi:10.1609/aimag.v40i2.2850

Guo, Q., Li, Z., An, B., Hui, P., Huang, J., Zhang, L., & Zhao, M. (2019, May). Securing the deep fraud detector in large-scale e-commerce platform via adversarial machine learning approach. In *The World Wide Web Conference* (pp. 616-626). Academic Press.

Gupta,, A., Gupta, S., & Katarya, R. (2021). InstaCovNet-19: A deep learning classification model for the detection of COVID-19 patients using Chest X-ray. *Applied Soft Computing, 99*, 106859.

Gupta, S., & Roy, S. (2019). Medav filter—filter for removal of image noise with the combination of median and average filters. In *Recent Trends in Signal and Image Processing* (pp. 11–19). Springer. doi:10.1007/978-981-10-8863-6_2

Guttikonda, G., Katamaneni, M., & Pandala, M. (2019). Diabetes Data Prediction Using Spark and Analysis in Hue Over Big Data. *2019 3rd International Conference on Computing Methodologies and Communication (ICCMC)*, 1112-1117.

Hall, P. (2018). *On the art and science of machine learning explanations.* arXiv preprint arXiv:1810.02909.

Han & Kamber. (2012). *Data Mining: Concepts and Techniques.* Academic Press.

Hasan, N., & Bao, Y. (2021). Comparing different feature selection algorithms for cardiovascular disease prediction. *Health and Technology, 11*(1), 49–62. doi:10.100712553-020-00499-2

Hashem, I. A. T., Ezugwu, A. E., Al-Garadi, M. A., Abdullahi, I. N., Otegbeye, O., Ahman, Q. O., . . . Chiroma, H. (2020). *A machine learning solution framework for combatting covid-19 in smart cities from multiple dimensions.* doi:. 05.18.20105577 doi:10.1101/2020

Hassantabar, S., Ahmadi, M., & Sharifi, A. (2020). Diagnosis and detection of infected tissue of COVID-19 patients based on lung x-ray image using convolution neural network approaches. *Chaos, Solitons and Fractals-Nonlinear Science, and Non-equilibrium and Complex Phenomena, 140*, 110170. PMID:32834651

Heidari, A. A., Faris, H., Aljarah, I., & Mirjalili, S. (2018). An Efficient Hybrid Multilayer Perceptron Neural Network with Grasshopper Optimization. *Soft Computing*, *2018*. Advance online publication. doi:10.100700500-018-3424-2

Heinrichs, B., & Eickhoff, S. B. (2020). Your evidence? Machine learning algorithms for medical diagnosis and prediction. *Human Brain Mapping*, *41*(6), 1435–1444.

Hengstler, M., Enkel, E., & Duelli, S. (2016). Applied artificial intelligence and trust—The case of autonomous vehicles and medical assistance devices. *Technological Forecasting and Social Change*, *105*, 105–120. doi:10.1016/j.techfore.2015.12.014

Ho, D. (2020). Addressing COVID-19 drug development with artificial intelligence. *Advanced Intelligent Systems*, *2*(5), 2000070. doi:10.1002/aisy.202000070 PMID:32838299

Hofman, J. M., Watts, D. J., Athey, S., Garip, F., Griffiths, T. L., Kleinberg, J., ... Yarkoni, T. (2021). Integrating explanation and prediction in computational social science. *Nature*, *595*(7866), 181–188.

Holzinger, A., Biemann, C., Pattichis, C. S., & Kell, D. B. (2017). *What do we need to build explainable AI systems for the medical domain?* arXiv preprint arXiv:1712.09923.

Holzinger, A. (2014). *Biomedical informatics: discovering knowledge in big data*. Springer.

Holzinger, A., Kieseberg, P., Weippl, E., & Tjoa, A. M. (2018, August). Current advances, trends and challenges of machine learning and knowledge extraction: from machine learning to explainable AI. In *International Cross-Domain Conference for Machine Learning and Knowledge Extraction* (pp. 1-8). Springer.

Hosny, A., Parmar, C., Quackenbush, J., Schwartz, L. H., & Aerts, H. J. (2018). Artificial intelligence in radiology. *Nature Reviews. Cancer*, *18*(8), 500–510. doi:10.103841568-018-0016-5 PMID:29777175

Hossain, M. M., McKyer, E. L. J., & Ma, P. (2020). Applications of artificial intelligence technologies on mental health research during COVID-19. doi:10.31235/osf.io/w6c9bosf.io/w6c9b

Hu, C., Liu, Z., Jiang, Y., Zhang, X., Shi, O., Xu, K., . . . Chen, X. (2020). Early prediction of mortality risk among severe COVID-19 patients using machine learning. MedRxiv. doi:10.1101/2020.04.13.20064329

Hua, K. L., Hsu, C. H., Hidayati, S. C., Cheng, W. H., & Chen, Y. J. (2015). Computer-aided classification of lung nodules on computed tomography images via deep learning technique. *OncoTargets and Therapy*, *8*.

Huang, Q., Yamada, M., Tian, Y., Singh, D., Yin, D., & Chang, Y. (2020). *Graphlime: Local interpretable model explanations for graph neural networks*. arXiv preprint arXiv:2001.06216.

Huang, Y., Shao, L., & Frangi, A. F. (2019). *Simultaneous super-resolution and cross-modality synthesis in magnetic resonance imaging Deep Learning and Convolutional Neural Networks for Medical Imaging and Clinical Informatics*. Springer.

Compilation of References

Hughes, J.P. (2011). *Principles of early drug discovery*. Doi:10.1111/j.1476-5381.2010.01127.x

Hui, D. S., Azhar, E. I., Madani, T. A., Ntoumi, F., Kock, R., Dar, O., ... Petersen, E. (2020). The continuing 2019-nCoV epidemic threat of novel coronaviruses to global health—The latest 2019 novel coronavirus outbreak in Wuhan, China. *International Journal of Infectious Diseases, 91*, 264–266. doi:10.1016/j.ijid.2020.01.009 PMID:31953166

Hu, R. (2011). Medical Data Mining Based on Decision Tree Algorithm. *Medical Data Mining Based on Decision Tree Algorithm., 4*(5), 14–19. doi:10.5539/cis.v4n5p14

Hwang, E. J., Park, S., Jin, K. N., Im Kim, J., Choi, S. Y., Lee, J. H., ... Park, C. M. (2019). Development and validation of a deep learning–based automated detection algorithm for major thoracic diseases on chest radiographs. *JAMA Network Open, 2*(3), e191095–e191095.

Ibarguren, I., Pérez, J. M., Muguerza, J., Arbelaitz, O., & Yera, A. (2022). PCTBagging: From inner ensembles to ensembles. A trade-off between discriminating capacity and interpretability. *Information Sciences, 583*, 219–238.

Ijaz, M. F., Attique, M., & Son, Y. (2020). Data-driven cervical cancer prediction model with outlier detection and over-sampling methods. *Sensors (Basel), 20*(10), 2809. doi:10.339020102809 PMID:32429090

Ijaz, M., Alfian, G., Syafrudin, M., & Rhee, J. (2018). Hybrid Prediction Model for Type 2 Diabetes and Hypertension Using DBSCAN-Based Outlier Detection, Synthetic Minority Over Sampling Technique (SMOTE), and Random Forest. *Applied Sciences (Basel, Switzerland), 8*(8), 1325. doi:10.3390/app8081325

Immorlica, N., Singla, S., & Waggoner, B. (2020, July). Prophet inequalities with linear correlations and augmentations. In *Proceedings of the 21st ACM Conference on Economics and Computation* (pp. 159-185). 10.1145/3391403.3399452

Imran, A., Posokhova, I., Qureshi, H. N., Masood, U., Riaz, M. S., Ali, K., John, C. N., Hussain, M. D. I., & Nabeel, M. (2020). AI4COVID-19: AI enabled preliminary diagnosis for COVID-19 from cough samples via an app. *Informatics in Medicine Unlocked, 20*, 100378. doi:10.1016/j.imu.2020.100378 PMID:32839734

Inam, R., Terra, A., Mujumdar, A., Fersman, E., & Feljan, A. V. (2021, April). *Explainable AI: How humans can trust Artificial Intelligence*. Ericsson White Paper. https://www.ericsson.com/en/reports-and-papers/white-papers/explainable-ai--how-humans-can-trust-ai

Inbaraj, L. R., George, C. E., & Chandrasingh, S. (2021). Seroprevalence of COVID-19 infection in a rural district of South India: A population-based seroepidemiological study. *PLoS One, 16*(3), e0249247.

Iqbal, H. T., Majeed, B., Khan, U., & Bin Altaf, M. A. (2019). An Infrared High classification Accuracy Hand-held Machine Learning based Breast-Cancer Detection System. *2019 IEEE Biomedical Circuits and Systems Conference (BioCAS)*, 1-4. 10.1109/BIOCAS.2019.8918687

Iwendi, C., Bashir, A. K., Peshkar, A., Sujatha, R., Chatterjee, J. M., Pasupuleti, S., Mishra, R., Pillai, S., & Jo, O. (2020). COVID-19 patient health prediction using boosted random forest algorithm. *Frontiers in Public Health*, 8, 357. doi:10.3389/fpubh.2020.00357 PMID:32719767

Jacovi, A., Marasović, A., Miller, T., & Goldberg, Y. (2021, March). Formalizing trust in artificial intelligence: Prerequisites, causes and goals of human trust in AI. In *Proceedings of the 2021 ACM conference on fairness, accountability, and transparency* (pp. 624-635). ACM.

Jagtap, V. S., More, P., & Jha, U. (2020). *A review of the 2019 novel coronavirus (COVID-19) based on current evidence.* . doi:10.1016/j.ijantimicag.2020.105948

Jha, I. P., Awasthi, R., Kumar, A., Kumar, V., & Sethi, T. (2020). *Explainable-machine-learning to discover drivers and to predict mental illness during covid-19.* . doi:10.2196/25097

Ji, D., Zhang, D., Xu, J., Chen, Z., Yang, T., Zhao, P., ... Qin, E. (2020). Prediction for progression risk in patients with COVID-19 pneumonia: The CALL score. *Clinical Infectious Diseases*, 71(6), 1393–1399.

Jimenez-Luna, J. (2020). *Drug Discovery with explainable artificial intelligence.* Nature Machine Language. doi:10.103842256-020-00236-4

Jiménez-Luna, J., Skalic, M., Weskamp, N., & Schneider, G. (2021). Coloring molecules with explainable artificial intelligence for preclinical relevance assessment. *Journal of Chemical Information and Modeling*, 61(3), 1083–1094.

Johnstone, S. (2020). *A viral warning for change. COVID-19 versus the red cross: Better solutions via blockchain and artificial intelligence. COVID-19 Versus the Red Cross: Better Solutions Via Blockchain and Artificial Intelligence.* University of Hong Kong Faculty of Law Research Paper, (2020/005). doi:10.2139/ssrn.3530756

Joshi, N. (2020). *5 Artificial intelligence implementation challenges in healthcare* [Blog]. Retrieved from https://www.bbntimes.com/technology/5-artificial-intelligence-implementation-challenges-in-healthcare

Joshi, S., Szweda, P., Szweda, P., Bichara, D., & Iggidr, A. (2011). *Expert Systems with Applications.* https://www.tandfonline.com/doi/full/10.1080/23737867.2016.1211495%0A

Kajala, A., & Jain, V. K. (2020). Diagnosis of Breast Cancer using Machine Learning Algorithms-A Review. *2020 International Conference on Emerging Trends in Communication, Control and Computing (ICONC3), Lakshmangarh, Sikar, India*, 1-5. 10.1109/ICONC345789.2020.9117320

Kamnitsas, K., Ferrante, E., Parisot, S., Ledig, C., Nori, A. V., Criminisi, A., ... Glocker, B. (2016, October). DeepMedic for brain tumor segmentation. In *International workshop on Brainlesion: Glioma, multiple sclerosis, stroke and traumatic brain injuries* (pp. 138-149). Springer.

Karakaya. (2020). LSTM: Understanding Output Types. *Deep Learning Tutorials with Keras.*

Kathirvel, S., & Thakur Rapporteurs, J. (2018). Sustainable development goals and non-communicable diseases: Roadmap till 2030 – A plenary session of world noncommunicable diseases Congress 2017. *International Journal of Noncommunicable Diseases*, *3*(1), 3. doi:10.4103/jncd.jncd_1_18

Kavakiotis, I., Tsave, O., Salifoglou, A., Maglaveras, N., Vlahavas, I., & Chouvarda, I. (2017). Machine learning and data mining methods in diabetes research. *Computational and Structural Biotechnology Journal*, *15*, 104–116. doi:10.1016/j.csbj.2016.12.005 PMID:28138367

Kavila, S. D., Muddana, M. K., Bharath, N., Sai Teja, N. K. S., Kumar, N. T., & Swaroop, L. J. (2021). *Explainable Artificial Intelligence to Predict Cardiovascular Diseases*. International Journal of Emerging Technologies and Innovative Research , 8.

Ke, Y. Y., Peng, T. T., Yeh, T. K., Huang, W. Z., Chang, S. E., Wu, S. H., Hung, H.-C., Hsu, T.-A., Lee, S.-J., Song, J.-S., Lin, W.-H., Chiang, T.-J., Lin, J.-H., Sytwu, H.-K., & Chen, C. T. (2020). Artificial intelligence approach fighting COVID-19 with repurposing drugs. *Biomedical Journal*, *43*(4), 355–362. doi:10.1016/j.bj.2020.05.001 PMID:32426387

Keys, R. (1981). *Cubic convolution interpolation for digital image processing*. Academic Press.

Khan, F. M., & Gupta, R. (2020). ARIMA and NAR based prediction model for time series analysis of COVID-19 cases in India. *Journal of Safety Science and Resilience*, *1*(1), 12–18. doi:10.1016/j.jnlssr.2020.06.007

Khatami, A., Khosravi, A., Nguyen, T., Lim, C. P., & Nahavandi, S. (2017). Medical image analysis using wavelet transform and deep belief networks. *Expert Systems with Applications*, *86*, 190–198. doi:10.1016/j.eswa.2017.05.073

Khattar, A., Jain, P. R., & Quadri, S. M. K. (2020, May). Effects of the disastrous pandemic COVID 19 on learning styles, activities and mental health of young Indian students-a machine learning approach. In *2020 4th International Conference on Intelligent Computing and Control Systems (ICICCS)* (pp. 1190-1195). IEEE. 10.1109/ICICCS48265.2020.9120955

Khuriwal, N., & Mishra, N. (2018). Breast cancer diagnosis using adaptive voting ensemble machine learning algorithm. *2018 IEEMA Engineer Infinite Conference (eTechNxT)*, 1-5. 10.1109/ETECHNXT.2018.8385355

Kim, J., Lee, J. K., & Lee, K. M. (2016). Accurate image super-resolution using very deep convolutional networks. *Proceedings of the IEEE conference on computer vision and pattern recognition*. 10.1109/CVPR.2016.182

Klosowski, J., & Frahm, J. (2017). Image denoising for real-time MRI. *Magnetic Resonance in Medicine*, *77*(3), 1340–1352. doi:10.1002/mrm.26205 PMID:27079944

Kolozsvari, L. R., Bérczes, T., Hajdu, A., Gesztelyi, R., Tiba, A., Varga, I., . . . Zsuga, J. (2021). Predicting the epidemic curve of the coronavirus (SARS-CoV-2) disease (COVID-19) using artificial intelligence. MedRxiv, 2020-04. doi:10.1101/2020.04.17.20069666

Krishna & Rao. (2018). Prediction Of Breast Cancer Using Machine Learning Techniques. *International Journal of Management, Technology And Engineering, 8*(12).

Krishna. (2019). *An Efficient Mixture Model Approach in Brain-Machine Interface Systems for Extracting the Psychological Status of Mentally Impaired Persons Using EEG Signals.* IEEE Access.

Krishna, N. (2013). Inferring the Human Emotional State of Mind using Asymetric Distrubution. *International Journal of Advanced Computer Science and Applications*, 116–118.

Krishna, N. M., Devi, J. S., & Yarramalle, S. (2017). A Novel Approach for Effective Emotion Recognition Using Double Truncated Gaussian Mixture Model and EEG. *I.J. Intelligent Systems and Applications, 6*(6), 33–42. doi:10.5815/ijisa.2017.06.04

Kumar, P., Kalita, H., Patairiya, S., Sharma, Y. D., Nanda, C., Rani, M., . . . Bhagavathula, A. S. (2020). Forecasting the dynamics of COVID-19 pandemic in top 15 countries in April 2020: ARIMA model with machine learning approach. MedRxiv. doi:10.1101/2020.03.30.20046227

Kumar, S. U., Kumar, D. T., Christopher, B. P., & Doss, C. (2020). The rise and impact of COVID-19 in India. *Frontiers in Medicine, 7*, 250.

Kundu, S., Elhalawani, H., Gichoya, J. W., & Kahn, C. E. Jr. (2020). How might AI and chest imaging help unravel COVID-19's mysteries? *Radiology. Artificial Intelligence, 2*(3), e200053. doi:10.1148/ryai.2020200053 PMID:33928254

Ladha, G. G., & Pippal, R. K. S. (2018, October). A computation analysis to predict diabetes based on data mining: a review. In *2018 3rd international conference on communication and electronics systems (ICCES)* (pp. 6-10). IEEE.

Laghmati, S., Tmiri, A., & Cherradi, B. (2019). Machine Learning based System for Prediction of Breast Cancer Severity. *2019 International Conference on Wireless Networks and Mobile Communications (WINCOM)*, 1-5. 10.1109/WINCOM47513.2019.8942575

Lai, W.-S., Huang, J.-B., Ahuja, N., & Yang, M.-H. (2017). Deep laplacian pyramid networks for fast and accurate super-resolution. *Proceedings of the IEEE conference on computer vision and pattern recognition*. 10.1109/CVPR.2017.618

Lakkaraju, H. (2017). Interpretable & Explorable Approximations of Black Box Models. *Workshop on Fairness, Accountability and Transparency in Machine Learning*.

Lalmuanawma, S., Hussain, J., & Chhakchhuak, L. (2020). Applications of machine learning and artificial intelligence for Covid-19 (SARS-CoV-2) pandemic: A review. *Chaos, Solitons, and Fractals, 139*, 110059. doi:10.1016/j.chaos.2020.110059 PMID:32834612

Landman, B. A., Huang, A. J., Gifford, A., Vikram, D. S., Lim, I. A. L., Farrell, J. A., . . . Jarso, S. (2011). *Multi-parametric neuroimaging reproducibility: a 3-T resource study*. Academic Press.

Lansdowne, L. E. (2020). *Exploring the Drug Development*. Technology Networks Drug Discovery.

Lauritsen, S. M., Kristensen, M., Olsen, M. V., Larsen, M. S., Lauritsen, K. M., Jørgensen, M. J., Lange, J., & Thiesson, B. (2020). undefined. *Nature Communications*, *11*(1). Advance online publication. doi:10.103841467-020-17431-x PMID:32737308

Lee, S. W., Jung, H., Ko, S., Kim, S., Kim, H., Doh, K., . . . Ha, J. W. (2020). *Carecall: a call-based active monitoring dialog agent for managing covid-19 pandemic.* doi:10.1016%2Fj.chaos.2020.110338

Li, X., & Orchard, M. (2001). *New edge-directed interpolation.* Academic Press.

Li, H. C., Yang, G., Yang, W., Du, Q., & Emery, W. J. (2020). Deep nonsmooth nonnegative matrix factorization network with semi-supervised learning for SAR image change detection. *ISPRS Journal of Photogrammetry and Remote Sensing*, *160*, 167–179. doi:10.1016/j.isprsjprs.2019.12.002

Li, J., Cheng, K., Wang, S., Morstatter, F., Trevino, R. P., Tang, J., & Liu, H. (2017). Feature selection: A data perspective. *ACM Computing Surveys*, *50*(6), 1–45. doi:10.1145/3136625

Li, Q., Wu, X., Xu, L., Chen, K., Yao, L., & Li, R. (2017). Multi-modal discriminative dictionary learning for Alzheimer's disease and mild cognitive impairment. *Computer Methods and Programs in Biomedicine*, *150*, 1–8. doi:10.1016/j.cmpb.2017.07.003 PMID:28859825

Li, S., Wang, Y., Xue, J., Zhao, N., & Zhu, T. (2020). The impact of COVID-19 epidemic declaration on psychological consequences: A study on active Weibo users. *International Journal of Environmental Research and Public Health*, *17*(6), 2032. doi:10.3390/ijerph17062032 PMID:32204411

Liu, M., Zhang, D., Shen, D., & Initiative, A. D. N. (2012). Ensemble sparse classification of Alzheimer's disease. *NeuroImage*, *60*(2), 1106–1116. doi:10.1016/j.neuroimage.2012.01.055 PMID:22270352

Liu, T., Fan, W., & Wu, C. (2019). A hybrid machine learning approach to cerebral stroke prediction based on imbalanced medical dataset. *Artificial Intelligence in Medicine*, *101*, 101723. doi:10.1016/j.artmed.2019.101723 PMID:31813482

Li, W. T., Ma, J., Shende, N., Castaneda, G., Chakladar, J., Tsai, J. C., Apostol, L., Honda, C. O., Xu, J., Wong, L. M., Zhang, T., Lee, A., Gnanasekar, A., Honda, T. K., Kuo, S. Z., Yu, M. A., Chang, E. Y., Rajasekaran, M. R., & Ongkeko, W. M. (2020). Using machine learning of clinical data to diagnose COVID-19: A systematic review and meta-analysis. *BMC Medical Informatics and Decision Making*, *20*(1), 1–13. doi:10.118612911-020-01266-z PMID:32993652

London, A. J. (2019). Artificial intelligence and black-box medical decisions: Accuracy versus explainability. *The Hastings Center Report*, *49*(1), 15–21. doi:10.1002/hast.973 PMID:30790315

Lui, A., & Lamb, G. W. (2018). Artificial intelligence and augmented intelligence collaboration: Regaining trust and confidence in the financial sector. *Information & Communications Technology Law*, *27*(3), 267–283. doi:10.1080/13600834.2018.1488659

Lundberg, S. M., & Lee, S. I. (2017, December 4). *A unified approach to interpreting model predictions*. ACM DigitalLibrary. https://dl.acm.org/doi/abs/10.5555/3295222.3295230

Lundberg, S. M., & Lee, S.-I. (2017). A unified approach to interpreting model predictions. *Advances in Neural Information Processing Systems*, *30*, 4765–4774.

Luo, S., & Cheng, B. (2010). *Diagnosing Breast Masses in Digital Mammography Using Feature Selection and Ensemble Methods*. doi:10.1007/s10916-010-9518-8

Luz, C. F., Vollmer, M., Decruyenaere, J., Nijsten, M. W., Glasner, C., & Sinha, B. (2020). Machine learning in infection management using routine electronic health records: Tools, techniques, and reporting of future technologies. *Clinical Microbiology and Infection*, *26*(10), 1291–1299. doi:10.1016/j.cmi.2020.02.003 PMID:32061798

Mahbooba, B., Timilsina, M., Sahal, R., & Serrano, M. (2021). Explainable artificial intelligence (xai) to enhance trust management in intrusion detection systems using decision tree model. *Complexity*.

Maher, A., Majdalawieh, M., & Nizamuddin, N. (2021). Modeling and forecasting of COVID-19 using a hybrid dynamic model based on SEIRD with ARIMA corrections. *Infectious Disease Modelling*, *6*, 98–111.

Mahjabeen Mirza Beg, M. J. (2012). An Analysis of the Methods Employed for Breast Cancer Diagnosis. *International Journal of Research in Computer Science*, *2*(3), 25–29. doi:10.7815/ijorcs.23.2012.025

Mak, K. K., & Pichika, M. R. (2019). Artificial intelligence in drug development: Present status and future prospects. *Drug Discovery Today*, *24*(3), 773–780. doi:10.1016/j.drudis.2018.11.014 PMID:30472429

Maldonado, S., Weber, R., & Famili, F. (2014). Feature selection for high-dimensional class-imbalanced data sets using Support Vector Machines. *Information Sciences*, *286*, 228–246. doi:10.1016/j.ins.2014.07.015

Maleki, M., & Arellano-Valle, R. B. (2017). Maximum a-posteriori estimation of autoregressive processes based on finite mixtures of scale-mixtures of skew-normal distributions. *Journal of Statistical Computation and Simulation*, *87*(6), 1061–1083.

Mandal, M. (2021). *Introduction to Convolutional Neural Networks (CNN)*. The Startup Medium.

Mandal, M., Singh, P., Ijaz, M., Shafi, J., & Sarkar, R. (2021). A Tri-Stage Wrapper-Filter Feature Selection Framework for Disease Classification. *Sensors (Basel)*, *21*(16), 5571. doi:10.339021165571 PMID:34451013

Martin Drance, A. (2021). Neuro symbolic XAI for computational Drug Repurposing. *Proceedings of the International Joint Conference on Knowledge Discovery, Knowledge Engineering and Knowledge Management (IC3K 2021)*, *2*, 220-225. Doi: 10.5220/0010714100003064

Maruhashi, K., Todoriki, M., Ohwa, T., Goto, K., Hasegawa, Y., Inakoshi, H., & Anai, H. (2018, April). Learning multi-way relations via tensor decomposition with neural networks. *Proceedings of the AAAI Conference on Artificial Intelligence*, *32*(1).

Mashamba-Thompson, T. P., & Crayton, E. D. (2020). Blockchain and artificial intelligence technology for novel coronavirus disease 2019 self-testing. *Diagnostics (Basel)*, *10*(4), 198. doi:10.3390/diagnostics10040198 PMID:32244841

Massie, A. B., Boyarsky, B. J., Werbel, W. A., Bae, S., Chow, E. K., Avery, R. K., Durand, C. M., Desai, N., Brennan, D., Garonzik-Wang, J. M., & Segev, D. L. (2020). Identifying scenarios of benefit or harm from kidney transplantation during the COVID-19 pandemic: A stochastic simulation and machine learning study. *American Journal of Transplantation*, *20*(11), 2997–3007. doi:10.1111/ajt.16117 PMID:32515544

Mathews, S. M. (2019, July). Explainable artificial intelligence applications in NLP, biomedical, and malware classification: a literature review. In *Intelligent computing-proceedings of the computing conference* (pp. 1269–1292). Springer.

Matuchansky, C. (2019). Deep medicine, artificial intelligence, and the practicing clinician. *Lancet*, *394*(10200), 736.

Mayr, A. (2018). *Large-scale comparison of machine learning methods for drug target prediction on ChEMBL*. Royal Society of Chemistry. doi:10.1039/C8SC00148K

Mayr, A., Klambauer, G., Unterthiner, T., & Hochreiter, S. (2016). DeepTox: Toxicity prediction using deep learning. *Frontiers in Environmental Science*, *3*. Advance online publication. doi:10.3389/fenvs.2015.00080

Mekha, P., & Teeyasuksaet, N. (2019). Deep Learning Algorithms for Predicting Breast Cancer Based on Tumor Cells. *2019 Joint International Conference on Digital Arts, Media and Technology with ECTI Northern Section Conference on Electrical, Electronics, Computer and Telecommunications Engineering (ECTI DAMT-NCON)*, 343-346. 10.1109/ECTI-NCON.2019.8692297

Metsky, H. C., Freije, C. A., Kosoko-Thoroddsen, T. S. F., Sabeti, P. C., & Myhrvold, C. (2020). CRISPR-based COVID-19 surveillance using a genomically-comprehensive machine learning approach. BioRxiv. doi:10.1101/2020.02.26.967026

Metz, C. (2015). *Google just open sourced tensorflow, its artificial intelligence engine*. Academic Press.

Miller, T. (2019). Explanation in artificial intelligence: Insights from the social sciences. *Artificial Intelligence*, *267*, 1–38.

Moftakhar, L., Mozhgan, S. E. I. F., & Safe, M. S. (2020). Exponentially increasing trend of infected patients with COVID-19 in Iran: a comparison of neural network and ARIMA forecasting models. *Iranian Journal of Public Health, 49*(Suppl 1), 92. 10.18502%2Fijph.v49iS1.3675

Mohanty, S., Rashid, M. H. A., Mridul, M., Mohanty, C., & Swayamsiddha, S. (2020). Application of Artificial Intelligence in COVID-19 drug repurposing. *Diabetes & Metabolic Syndrome*, *14*(5), 1027–1031. doi:10.1016/j.dsx.2020.06.068 PMID:32634717

Mohs, R. C., & Greig, N. H. (2017). Drug discovery and development: Role of basic biological research. *Alzheimer's & Dementia: Translational Research & Clinical Interventions*, *3*(4), 651–657. doi:10.1016/j.trci.2017.10.005 PMID:29255791

Mojrian, S. (2020). Hybrid Machine Learning Model of Extreme Learning Machine Radial basis function for Breast Cancer Detection and Diagnosis; a Multilayer Fuzzy Expert System. *2020 RIVF International Conference on Computing and Communication Technologies (RIVF)*, 1-7. 10.1109/RIVF48685.2020.9140744

Monaghan, C., Larkin, J. W., Chaudhuri, S., Han, H., Jiao, Y., Bermudez, K. M., . . . Maddux, F. W. (2020). Artificial intelligence for covid-19 risk classification in kidney disease: can technology unmask an unseen disease? medRxiv. doi:10.1101/2020.06.15.20131680

Muhammad, L. J., Algehyne, E. A., Usman, S. S., Ahmad, A., Chakraborty, C., & Mohammed, I. A. (2021). Supervised Machine Learning Models for Prediction of COVID-19 Infection using Epidemiology Dataset. *SN Computer Science*, *2*, 11.

Mustafa, A., & Azghadi, M.R. (2021). *Automated Machine Learning for Healthcare and Clinical Analysis*. Academic Press.

Naga Srinivasu, P., & Balas, V. E. (2021). Performance Measurement of Various Hybridized Kernels for Noise Normalization and Enhancement in High-Resolution MR Images. In Bio-inspired Neurocomputing. Studies in Computational Intelligence (vol. 903). Springer. doi:10.1007/978-981-15-5495-7_1

Naga Srinivasu, P., Ahmed, S., Alhumam, A., Bhoi Kumar, A., & Fazal Ijaz, M. (2021). An AW-HARIS Based Automated Segmentation of Human Liver Using CT Images. *Computers. Materials & Continua*, *69*(3), 3303–3319. doi:10.32604/cmc.2021.018472

Naga Srinivasu, P., Srinivasa Rao, T., Dicu, A. M., Mnerie, C. A., & Olariu, I. (2020). A comparative review of optimisation techniques in segmentation of brain MR images. *Journal of Intelligent & Fuzzy Systems*, *38*(5), 6031–6043. doi:10.3233/JIFS-179688

Naga Srinivasu, P., Srinivasa Rao, T., Srinivas, G., & Prasad Reddy, P. V. G. D. (2020). A computationally efficient skull scraping approach for brain MR image. *Recent Adv Comput Sci Commun*, *13*(5), 833–844. doi:10.2174/2213275912666190809111928

Nagaratnam, K., Harston, G., Flossmann, E., Canavan, C., Geraldes, R. C., & Edwards, C. (2020). Innovative use of artificial intelligence and digital communication in acute stroke pathway in response to COVID-19. *Future Healthcare Journal*, *7*(2), 169–173. doi:10.7861/fhj.2020-0034 PMID:32550287

Naga, S. P., Rao, T., & Dicu, A. (2020). Mihaela & Mnerie, Corina & Olariu, Iustin: A comparative review of optimisation techniques in segmentation of brain MR images. *Journal of Intelligent & Fuzzy Systems*, *38*, 1–12.

Nakasone, A. (2005). Emotion Recognition from Electromyography and Skin Conductance. *The Fifth International Workshop on Biosignal Interpretation*.

Nápoles, G., Grau, I., Bello, R., & Grau, R. (2014). Two-steps learning of Fuzzy Cognitive Maps for prediction and knowledge discovery on the HIV-1 drug resistance. *Expert Systems with Applications*, *41*(3), 821–830. doi:10.1016/j.eswa.2013.08.012

Natarajan, M., & Sathiamoorthy, S. (2018). *A Novel Pre-Processing Approach for the Denoising of Alzheimer Disease Image Dataset*. Academic Press.

Nawaz, N., Gomes, A. M., & Saldeen, M. A. (2020). Artificial intelligence (AI) applications for library services and resources in COVID-19 pandemic. *Artificial Intelligence (AI)*, *7*(18), 1951-1955. . doi:10.1016/j.dsx.2020.04.012

Naz, H., & Ahuja, S. (2020). Deep learning approach for diabetes prediction using PIMA Indian dataset. *Journal of Diabetes and Metabolic Disorders*, *19*, 391–403.

Nazir, T., Irtaza, A., Shabbir, Z., Javed, A., Akram, U., & Mahmood, M. T. (2019). Diabetic retinopathy detection through novel tetragonal local octa patterns and extreme learning machines. *Artificial Intelligence in Medicine*, *99*, 101695. doi:10.1016/j.artmed.2019.07.003 PMID:31606114

Nemati, M., Ansary, J., & Nemati, N. (2020). Machine-learning approaches in COVID-19 survival analysis and discharge-time likelihood prediction using clinical data. *Patterns*, *1*(5), 100074. doi:10.1016/j.patter.2020.100074 PMID:32835314

Neri, E., Miele, V., Coppola, F., & Grassi, R. (2020). Use of CT and artificial intelligence in suspected or COVID-19 positive patients: Statement of the Italian Society of Medical and Interventional Radiology. *La Radiologia Medica*, *125*(5), 505–508. doi:10.100711547-020-01197-9 PMID:32350794

Newman, S. J., & Furbank, R. T. (2021). Explainable machine learning models of major crop traits from satellite-monitored continent-wide field trial data. *Nature Plants*, *7*(10), 1354–1363.

Ngo, H. X., Garneau-Tsodikova, S., & Green, K. D. (2016). A complex game of hide and seek: The search for new antifungals. *MedChemComm*, *7*(7), 1285–1306. doi:10.1039/C6MD00222F PMID:27766140

Niţică, Ş., Czibula, G., & Tomescu, V. (2020). A comparative study on using unsupervised learning based data analysis techniques for breast cancer detection. *2020 IEEE 14th International Symposium on Applied Computational Intelligence and Informatics (SACI)*, 99-104. 10.1109/SACI49304.2020.9118783

Noncommunicable diseases country profiles 2018. (n.d.). https://apps.who.int/iris/handle/10665/274512

Noncommunicable diseases progress monitor 2017. (2017, September 1). *World Health Organization*. https://www.who.int/publications/i/item/9789241513029

Norouzi, N., de Rubens, G. Z., Choupanpiesheh, S., & Enevoldsen, P. (2020). When pandemics impact economies and climate change: Exploring the impacts of COVID-19 on oil and electricity demand in China. *Energy Research & Social Science, 68*, 101654. doi:10.1016/j.erss.2020.101654 PMID:32839693

Obinata, H., Ruan, P., Mori, H., Zhu, W., Sasaki, H., Tatsuya, K., . . . Yokobori, S. (2020). Can artificial intelligence predict the need for oxygen therapy in early stage COVID-19 pneumonia? doi:10.21203/rs.3.rs-33150/v1

Ofli, F., Chaudhry, R., Kurillo, G., Vidal, R., & Bajcsy, R. (2013). *Berkeley mhad: A comprehensive multimodal human action database*. Paper presented at the 2013 IEEE Workshop on Applications of Computer Vision (WACV). 10.1109/WACV.2013.6474999

Oladipo, I. D., AbdulRaheem, M., Awotunde, J. B., Bhoi, A. K., Adeniyi, E. A., & Abiodun, M. K. (2022). Machine Learning and Deep Learning Algorithms for Smart Cities: A Start-of-the-Art Review. *IoT and IoE Driven Smart Cities*, 143-162.

Onder, G., Rezza, G., & Brusaferro, S. (2020). Case-fatality rate and characteristics of patients dying in relation to COVID-19 in Italy. *Journal of the American Medical Association, 323*(18), 1775–1776. doi:10.1001/jama.2020.4683 PMID:32203977

Osborne, M. J., & Rubinstein, A. (1994). *A course in game theory*. MIT Press.

Othman, M. F. Bin, & Yau, T. M. S. (2007). Comparison of different classification techniques using WEKA for breast cancer. *3rd Kuala Lumpur International Conference on Biomedical Engineering 2006*, 520–523. 10.1007/978-3-540-68017-8_131

Ou, S., He, X., Ji, W., Chen, W., Sui, L., Gan, Y., Lu, Z., Lin, Z., Deng, S., Przesmitzki, S., & Bouchard, J. (2020). Machine learning model to project the impact of COVID-19 on US motor gasoline demand. *Nature Energy, 5*(9), 666–673. doi:10.103841560-020-0662-1 PMID:33052987

Pandey, R., Gautam, V., Pal, R., Bandhey, H., Dhingra, L. S., Misra, V., Sharma, H., Jain, C., Bhagat, K., Arushi, Patel, L., Agarwal, M., Agrawal, S., Jalan, R., Wadhwa, A., Garg, A., Agrawal, Y., Rana, B., Kumaraguru, P., & Sethi, T. (2022). A machine learning application for raising wash awareness in the times of covid-19 pandemic. *Scientific Reports, 12*(1), 1–10. doi:10.103841598-021-03869-6 PMID:35039533

Panigrahi, R., Borah, S., Bhoi, A. K., Ijaz, M. F., Pramanik, M., Jhaveri, R. H., & Chowdhary, C. L. (2021). Performance assessment of supervised classifiers for designing intrusion detection systems: A comprehensive review and recommendations for future research. *Mathematics, 9*(6), 690. doi:10.3390/math9060690

Panthong, R., & Srivihok, A. (2015). Wrapper Feature Subset Selection for Dimension Reduction Based on Ensemble Learning Algorithm. *Procedia Computer Science, 72*, 162–169. doi:10.1016/j.procs.2015.12.117

Parab, S., Rathod, P., Patil, D., & Chikkareddi, V. (2020). A Multilayer Hybrid Machine Learning Model for Diabetes Detection. In *ITM Web of Conferences* (Vol. 32). EDP Sciences.

Park. (2003). *Emotion Recognition and Acoustic Analysis from Speech Signal.* Academic Press.

Parte, R. S., Patil, A., Kad, A., & Kharat, S. (2019). Non-invasive method for diabetes detection using CNN and SVM classifier. *International Journal of Research in Engineering, Science and Management, 2*, 659-661.

Pasha, S. N., Ramesh, D., Mohmmad, S., Harshavardhan, A., & Shabana. (2020, December). Cardiovascular disease prediction using deep learning techniques. *IOP Conference Series. Materials Science and Engineering, 981*(2), 022006. doi:10.1088/1757-899X/981/2/022006

Paszke, A., Gross, S., Chintala, S., Chanan, G., Yang, E., DeVito, Z., Lerer, A. (2017). *Automatic differentiation in pytorch.* Academic Press.

Patankar, S. (2020). Deep learning-based computational drug discovery to inhibit the RNA Dependent RNA Polymerase: application to SARS-CoV and COVID-19. doi:10.31219/osf.io/6kpbgosf.io/6kpbg

Patel, P. (2021). EEG-based human emotion recognition using entropy as a feature extraction measure. Springer.

Patil, R., Majumder, L., Jain, M., & Patil, V. (2020). Diabetes Disease Prediction Using Machine Learning. International Journal of Research in Engineering, Science and Management, 3(6), 292-295.

Patil, T. R., & Sherekar, S. S. (2013). *Performance Analysis of Naive Bayes and J48 Classification Algorithm for Data Classification.* Academic Press.

Paulheim, H. (2017). Knowledge graph refinement: A survey of approaches and evaluation methods. *Semantic Web, 8*(3), 489–508.

Pauline-Graf, D., Mandel, S. E., Allen, H. W., & Devnew, L. E. (2021). Assumption Validation Process for the Assessment of Technology-Enhanced Learning. *Contemporary Educational Technology, 13*(4).

Paul, S. M., Mytelka, D. S., Dunwiddie, C. T., Persinger, C. C., Munos, B. H., Lindborg, S. R., & Schacht, A. L. (2010). How to improve R&D productivity: The pharmaceutical industry's grand challenge. *Nature Reviews. Drug Discovery, 9*(3), 203–214. doi:10.1038/nrd3078 PMID:20168317

Pawar, U., O'Shea, D., Rea, S., & O'Reilly, R. (2020). Explainable AI in Healthcare. *2020 International Conference on Cyber Situational Awareness, Data Analytics and Assessment (CyberSA)*, 1-2. 10.1109/CyberSA49311.2020.9139655

Peiffer-Smadja, N., Maatoug, R., Lescure, F. X., D'ortenzio, E., Pineau, J., & King, J. R. (2020). Machine learning for COVID-19 needs global collaboration and data-sharing. *Nature Machine Intelligence, 2*(6), 293–294. doi:10.103842256-020-0181-6

Peng, M., Yang, J., Shi, Q., Ying, L., Zhu, H., Zhu, G., ... Li, J. (2020). *Artificial intelligence application in COVID-19 diagnosis and prediction*. Academic Press.

Phillips, P. J., Hahn, C. A., Fontana, P. C., Broniatowski, D. A., & Przybocki, M. A. (2020). Four principles of explainable artificial intelligence. Academic Press.

Phillips-Wren, G., & Ichalkaranje, N. (Eds.). (2008). *Intelligent decision making: An AI-based approach* (Vol. 97). Springer Science & Business Media. doi:10.1007/978-3-540-76829-6

Piccolomini, E. L., & Zama, F. (2020). Monitoring Italian COVID-19 spread by a forced SEIRD model. *PLOS One, Global Health*. doi:10.1371/journal.pone.0237417

Pierce, R. (2019). *AI in Healthcare: Solutions, Challenges, and Dilemmas in Medical Decision-Making. SSRN Electronic Journal*. doi:10.2139srn.3806767

Pitsikalis. (2003). Some Advances on Speech Analysis using Generalized Dimensions. *ITRW on Non-Linear Speech Processing (NOLISP 03)*.

Pokkuluri, K. S., & Nedunuri, S. U. D. (2020). A novel cellular automata classifier for covid-19 prediction. *Journal of Health Sciences*, *10*(1), 34–38. doi:10.17532/jhsci.2020.907

Polyzos, S., Samitas, A., & Spyridou, A. E. (2021). Tourism demand and the COVID-19 pandemic: An LSTM approach. *Tourism Recreation Research*, *46*(2), 175–187. doi:10.1080/0 2508281.2020.1777053

Porto, R., Molina, J. M., Berlanga, A., & Patricio, M. A. (2021). Minimum Relevant Features to Obtain Explainable Systems for Predicting Cardiovascular Disease Using the Statlog Data Set. *Applied Sciences (Basel, Switzerland)*, *11*(3), 1285. doi:10.3390/app11031285

Pourhomayoun, M., & Shakibi, M. (2020). Predicting mortality risk in patients with COVID-19 using artificial intelligence to help medical decision-making. MedRxiv. doi:10.1101/2020.03.30.20047308

Prabhu, A. J., Sengan, S., Kamalam, G. K., Vellingiri, J., Jagadeesh, G., Velayutham, P., & Subramaniyaswamy, V. (2020, October). Medical information retrieval systems for e-Health care records using fuzzy based machine learning model. *Microprocessors and Microsystems*, *17*, 103344.

Prajapati, V. K. (2020). *AI in drug discovery and development: A brief commentary*. Pharma Tutor. https://www.pharmatutor.org/articles/ai-in-drug-discovery-and-development-a-brief-commentary

Preetha, S., Chandan, N., Darshan, N. K., & Gowrav, P. B. (2020). Diabetes Disease Prediction Using Machine Learning. *International Journal of Recent Trends in Engineering & Research*, *5*(6), 37–43.

Press, W. H., Teukolsky, S. A., Flannery, B. P., & Vetterling, W. T. (1992). Numerical recipes in Fortran 77: volume 1, volume 1 of Fortran numerical recipes: The art of scientific computing. Cambridge University Press.

Pu, X., Chen, K., Liu, J., Wen, J., Zhneng, S., & Li, H. (2020). Machine learning-based method for interpreting the guidelines of the diagnosis and treatment of COVID-19. *Sheng Wu Yi Xue Gong Cheng Xue Za Zhi= Journal of Biomedical Engineering= Shengwu Yixue Gongchengxue Zazhi, 37*(3), 365-372. . doi:10.7507/1001-5515.202003045

Puiutta, E., & Veith, E. (2020, August). Explainable reinforcement learning: A survey. In *International cross-domain conference for machine learning and knowledge extraction* (pp. 77-95). Springer.

Purushotham, S., Meng, C., Chea, Z., & Liua, Y. (2018). Benchmarking deep learning models on large healthcare datasets. *Journal of Biomedical Informatics, 83*, 112–134.

Pyzer-Knapp, E. O. (2020). *Using bayesian optimization to accelerate virtual screening for the discovery of therapeutics appropriate for repurposing for covid-19.* arXiv preprint arXiv:2005.07121.

Qiu, D., Cheng, Y., Wang, X., & Zhang, X. (2021). Multi-window back-projection residual networks for reconstructing COVID-19 CT super-resolution images. *Computer Methods and Programs in Biomedicine, 200*, 105934. doi:10.1016/j.cmpb.2021.105934 PMID:33454574

Qiu, D., Zheng, L., Zhu, J., & Huang, D. (2021). Multiple improved residual networks for medical image super-resolution. *Future Generation Computer Systems, 116*, 200–208. doi:10.1016/j.future.2020.11.001

Qureshi, K. N., Din, S., Jeon, G., & Piccialli, F. (2020). An accurate and dynamic predictive model for a smart M-Health system using machine learning. *Information Sciences, 538*, 486–502. doi:10.1016/j.ins.2020.06.025

Rahimi, I., Chen, F., & Gandomi, A. H. (2021). A review on COVID-19 forecasting models. *Neural Computing & Applications*, 1–11. PMID:33564213

Rahman, R. M., & Afroz, F. (2013). *Comparison of Various Classification Techniques Using Different Data Mining Tools for Diabetes Diagnosis.* Academic Press.

Rahman, S. A., AlRashed, R. A., AlZunaytan, D. N., AlHarbi, N. J., AlThubaiti, S. A., & AlHejeelan, M. K. (2020). Chronic Diseases System Based on Machine Learning Techniques. *Int. J. Data.Science, 1*(1), 18–36.

Rahul, B., & Kulkarni, P. (2018). Analysis of Classifiers for Prediction of Type II Diabetes Mellitus. *2018 Fourth International Conference on Computing Communication Control and Automation (ICCUBEA)*, 1-6. 10.1109/ICCUBEA.2018.8697856

Rathi, S. (2019). *Generating counterfactual and contrastive explanations using SHAP.* arXiv preprint arXiv:1906.09293.

Raza, K., & Singh, N. K. (2021). A tour of unsupervised deep learning for medical image analysis. *Current Medical Imaging, 17*(9), 1059–1077. doi:10.2174/1573405617666621012715 4257 PMID:33504314

Ribeiro, M. T., Singh, S., & Guestrin, C. (2016). "Why should i trust you?": Explaining the predictions of any classifier. In *Proceedings of the 22nd ACM SIGKDD International Conference on Knowledge Discovery and Data Mining, KDD '16* (pp. 1135–1144). ACM. doi: .293977810.1145/2939672

Ribeiro, M. T., Singh, S., & Guestrin, C. (2016). why should I trust you?: Explaining the predictions of any classifier. *Proceedings of the 22nd ACM SIGKDD International Conference on Knowledge Discovery and Data Mining*, 1135–1144. https://github.com/marcotcr/lime

Roberts, D. M. (2019). *How Artificial Intelligence is Transforming Drug Design*. Drug Discovery World.

Rodin, A. S., Litvinenko, A., Klos, K., Morrison, A. C., Woodage, T., Coresh, J., & Boerwinkle, E. (2009). Use of Wrapper Algorithms Coupled with a Random Forests Classifier for Variable Selection in Large-Scale Genomic Association Studies. *Journal of Computational Biology*, *16*(12), 1705–1718. doi:10.1089/cmb.2008.0037 PMID:20047492

Rodriguez, M. D., Ahmed, J., & Shah, M. (2008). *Action mach a spatio-temporal maximum average correlation height filter for action recognition*. Paper presented at the 2008 IEEE conference on computer vision and pattern recognition. 10.1109/CVPR.2008.4587727

Rohitha, E. P. (2019, December 13). *Explainability of AI: The challenges and possible workarounds*. https://medium.com/@rohithaelsa/explainability-of-ai-the-challenges-and-possible-workarounds-14d8389d2515

Rolain, J. M., Colson, P., & Raoult, D. (2007). Recycling of chloroquine and its hydroxyl analogue to face bacterial, fungal and viral infections in the 21st century. *International Journal of Antimicrobial Agents*, *30*(4), 297–308. doi:10.1016/j.ijantimicag.2007.05.015 PMID:17629679

Roosa, K., Lee, Y., Luo, R., Kirpich, A., Rothenberg, R., Hyman, J. M., ... Chowell, G. (2020). Real-time forecasts of the COVID-19 epidemic in China from February 5th to February 24th, 2020. *Infectious Disease Modelling*, *5*, 256–263.

Rubinstein, A., Wang, J. Z., & Weinberg, S. M. (2019). *Optimal single-choice prophet inequalities from samples*. arXiv preprint arXiv:1911.07945.

Rudin, C. (2019). Stop explaining black box machine learning models for high stakes decisions and use interpretable models instead. *Nature Machine Intelligence*, *1*(5), 206–215.

Ruiz EstradaM. A. (2020). *The uses of drones in case of massive epidemics contagious diseases relief humanitarian aid: Wuhan-COVID-19 crisis*. doi:10.2139/ssrn.3546547

S. (2020). Predicting community mortality risk due to CoVID-19 using machine learning and development of a prediction tool. medRxiv. doi:10.1101/2020.04.27.20081794

Sahiner, B., Pezeshk, A., Hadjiiski, L. M., Wang, X., Drukker, K., & Cha, K. H. (2019). Deep learning in medical imaging and radiation therapy. *Medical Physics*, *6*(1), 36.

Sahoo, A. K., Pradhan, C., & Das, H. (2020). *Performance Evaluation of Different Machine Learning Methods and Deep-Learning Based Convolutional Neural Network for Health Decision Making* (Vol. 871). Nature Inspired Computing for Data Science - Studies in Computational Intelligence.

Samanta, K., Avleen, M., Rohit, S., & Kary, F. (2020). Explainable Artificial Intelligence for Human Decision-Support System in Medical Domain. *Medical Physics*, *46*(1), 336.

Sarkar. (2019). *Google's New Explainable AI (XAI) Service, towards Data Science*. Academic Press.

Saru, S., & Subashree, S. (2019). Analysis and Prediction of Diabetes Using Machine Learning. *International Journal of Emerging Technology and Innovative Engineering*, *5*(4).

Sarwar, M. A., Kamal, N., Hamid, W., & Shah, M. A. (2018, September). Prediction of diabetes using machine learning algorithms in healthcare. In *2018 24th international conference on automation and computing (ICAC)* (pp. 1-6). IEEE.

Sarwinda, D., & Arymurthy, A. M. (2013). Feature selection using kernel PCA for Alzheimer's disease detection with 3D MR Images of brain. *2013 International Conference on Advanced Computer Science and Information Systems (ICACSIS)*, 329–333. 10.1109/ICACSIS.2013.6761597

Satrio, C. B. A., Darmawan, W., Nadia, B. U., & Hanafiah, N. (2021). Time series analysis and forecasting of coronavirus disease in Indonesia using ARIMA model and PROPHET. *Procedia Computer Science*, *179*, 524–532.

Saxena, S., & Gyanchandani, M. (2020). Machine learning methods for computer-aided breast cancer diagnosis using histopathology: A narrative review. *Journal of Medical Imaging and Radiation Sciences*, *51*(1), 182–193. doi:10.1016/j.jmir.2019.11.001 PMID:31884065

Schultz, M. B., Vera, D., & Sinclair, D. A. (2020). Can artificial intelligence identify effective COVID-19 therapies? *EMBO Molecular Medicine*, *12*(8), e12817. doi:10.15252/emmm.202012817 PMID:32569446

Sehanobish, A., Ravindra, N. G., & van Dijk, D. (2020). *Gaining insight into sars-cov-2 infection and covid-19 severity using self-supervised edge features and graph neural networks*. arXiv preprint arXiv:2006.12971. doi:10.1016%2Fj.chaos.2020.110338

Senoner, J., Netland, T., & Feuerriegel, S. (2021). Using explainable artificial intelligence to improve process quality: Evidence from semiconductor manufacturing. *Management Science*.

Shang, R., Qi, L., Jiao, L., Stolkin, R., & Li, Y. (2014). Change detection in SAR images by artificial immune multi-objective clustering. *Engineering Applications of Artificial Intelligence*, *31*, 53–67. doi:10.1016/j.engappai.2014.02.004

Shao, L., & Zhao, M. (2007). *Order statistic filters for image interpolation*. Paper presented at the 2007 IEEE International Conference on Multimedia and Expo. 10.1109/ICME.2007.4284684

Sharma & Nair. (2019). Efficient Breast Cancer Prediction Using Ensemble Machine Learning Models. *2019 4th International Conference on Recent Trends on Electronics, Information, Communication & Technology (RTEICT)*, 100-104. 10.1109/RTEICT46194.2019.9016968

Sharma, S. (2020). *Drawing Insights from COVID-19 Infected Patients With no Past Medical History Using CT Scan Images and Machine Learning Techniques: A Study on 200 Patients.* . doi:10.3390/ijerph17103437

Sharma, P., Choudhary, K., Gupta, K., Chawla, R., Gupta, D., & Sharma, A. (2020). Artificial plant optimization algorithm to detect heart rate & presence of heart disease using machine learning. *Artificial Intelligence in Medicine, 102*, 101752. doi:10.1016/j.artmed.2019.101752 PMID:31980091

Sheshadri, H. S., Shree, S. R. B., & Krishna, M. (2015). Diagnosis of Alzheimer's disease employing neuropsychological and classification techniques. *2015 5th International Conference on IT Convergence and Security (ICITCS)*, 1–6.

Shi, F., Cheng, J., Wang, L., Yap, P.-T., & Shen, D. (2015). *LRTV: MR image super-resolution with low-rank and total variation regularizations.* Academic Press.

Shi, Y., Zu, C., Hong, M., Zhou, L., Wang, L., Wu, X., & Zhou, J. (2020). ASMFS: Adaptive-Similarity-based Multi-modality Feature Selection for Classification of Alzheimer's Disease. *Computer Vision and Pattern Recognition*, 1–27.

Sh, K. F. (2021). Advantages of Magnetic Resonance Computer Tomography in the Diagnosis of Thyroid Cancer. *Pindus Journal of Culture, Literature, and ELT, 9*, 80–84.

Shortliffe, E. H. (1976). Books: Computer-Based Medical Consultations: MYCIN. *Journal of Clinical Engineering, 1*(1), 69. doi:10.1097/00004669-197610000-00011

Shrikumar, A., Greenside, P., & Kundaje, A. (2019). *Learning Important Features Through Propagating Activation Differences.* Opgehaal van. https://arxiv.org/abs/1704.02685

Singhal, S., & Jena, M. (2013). A Study on WEKA Tool for Data Preprocessing. *Classification and Clustering., 6*, 250–253.

Singh, V., & Aswani, D. (2018). Face detection in hybrid color space using HBF-KNN. *Proceedings of International Conference on Recent Advancement on Computer and Communication*, 489–498. 10.1007/978-981-10-8198-9_52

Sivapriya, J., Aravind Kumar, V., Siddarth Sai, S., & Sriram, S. (2019). Breast Cancer Prediction using Machine Learning. *International Journal of Recent Technology and Engineering, 8*(4).

Sneha, J., & Borse, M. (2016). Detection and Prediction of Diabetes Mellitus Using Back-Propagation Neural Network. *2016 International Conference on Micro-Electronics and Telecommunication Engineering (ICMETE)*, 110-113. 10.1109/ICMETE.2016.11

Sokol, K., & Flach, P. (2020, January). Explainability fact sheets: a framework for systematic assessment of explainable approaches. In *Proceedings of the 2020 Conference on Fairness, Accountability, and Transparency* (pp. 56-67). Academic Press.

Song, Z., Zhao, X., Hui, Y., & Jiang, H. (2021). Progressive back-projection network for COVID-CT super-resolution. *Computer Methods and Programs in Biomedicine*, *208*, 106193. doi:10.1016/j.cmpb.2021.106193 PMID:34107373

Soni, A. N. (2020). *Diabetes Mellitus Prediction Using Ensemble Machine Learning Techniques.* Available at SSRN 3642877..

Soni, J., Ansari, U., Sharma, D., & Soni, S. (2011). Predictive data mining for medical diagnosis: An overview of heart disease prediction. *International Journal of Computers and Applications*, *17*(8), 43–48. doi:10.5120/2237-2860

Sonntag, D. (2020). AI in Medicine, Covid-19 and Springer Nature's Open Access Agreement. *KI-Künstliche Intelligenz*, *34*(2), 123–125. doi:10.100713218-020-00661-y PMID:32518472

Sosa, A. L., Albanese, E., Prince, M., Acosta, D., Ferri, C. P., Guerra, M., Huang, Y., Jacob, K. S., de Rodriguez, J. L., Salas, A., Yang, F., Gaona, C., Joteeshwaran, A., Rodriguez, G., de la Torre, G. R., Williams, J. D., & Stewart, R. (2009). Population normative data for the 10/66 Dementia Research Group cognitive test battery from Latin America, India and China: A cross-sectional survey. *BMC Neurology*, *9*(1), 48. doi:10.1186/1471-2377-9-48 PMID:19709405

Srinivasan, S., Batra, R., Chan, H., Kamath, G., Cherukara, M. J., & Sankaranarayanan, S. K. (2021). Artificial intelligence-guided De novo molecular design targeting COVID-19. *ACS Omega*, *6*(19), 12557–12566. doi:10.1021/acsomega.1c00477 PMID:34056406

Srinivasu, P. N., Rao, T. S., & Balas, V. E. (2020). Volumetric estimation of the damaged area in the human brain from 2D MR image. *International Journal of Information System Modeling and Design*, *11*(1), 74–92. doi:10.4018/IJISMD.2020010105

Sriram, T. V. S., Rao, M. V., Narayana, G. S., Kaladhar, D., & Vital, T. P. R. (2013). Intelligent Parkinson disease prediction using machine learning algorithms. *Int. J. Eng. Innov. Technol*, *3*, 212–215.

Suhaimi, N. S., Mountstephens, J., & Teo, J. (2020). EEG-Based Emotion Recognition: A State-of-the-Art Review of Current Trends and Opportunities. *Computational Intelligence and Neuroscience*, *2020*, 1–19. doi:10.1155/2020/8875426 PMID:33014031

Su, J., Vargas, D. V., & Sakurai, K. (2019). One pixel attack for fooling deep neural networks. *IEEE Transactions on Evolutionary Computation*, *23*(5), 828–841.

Sultana, J., Sadaf, K., Jilani, A. K., & Alabdan, R. (2019). Diagnosing Breast Cancer using Support Vector Machine and Multi-Classifiers. *2019 International Conference on Computational Intelligence and Knowledge Economy (ICCIKE)*, 449-451. 10.1109/ICCIKE47802.2019.9004356

Suresh, K., Obulesu, O., & Ramudu, B. V. (2020). Diabetes Prediction using Machine Learning Techniques. Helix-The Scientific Explorer| Peer Reviewed Bimonthly. *International Journal (Toronto, Ont.)*, *10*(02), 136–142.

Sustersic, T., Blagojevic, A., Cvetkovic, D., Cvetkovic, A., Lorencin, I., Segota, S. B., Milovanovic, D., Baskic, D., Car, Z., & Filipovic, N. (2021, October). Epidemiological Predictive Modeling of COVID-19 Infection: Development, Testing, and Implementation on the Population of the Benelux Union. *Frontiers in Public Health, 28*, 727274. Advance online publication. doi:10.3389/fpubh.2021.727274 PMID:34778171

Szczepański, M., Choraś, M., Pawlicki, M., & Pawlicka, A. (2021, June). The methods and approaches of explainable artificial intelligence. In *International Conference on Computational Science* (pp. 3-17). Springer.

Tayarani-N, M. H., Yao, X., & Xu, H. (2014). Meta-heuristic algorithms in car engine design: A literature survey. *IEEE Transactions on Evolutionary Computation, 19*(5), 609–629. doi:10.1109/TEVC.2014.2355174

Taylor, J. E. T., & Taylor, G. W. (2021). Artificial cognition: How experimental psychology can help generate explainable artificial intelligence. *Psychonomic Bulletin & Review, 28*(2), 454–475.

Teixeira, F., Montenegro, J. L. Z., da Costa, C. A., & da Rosa Righi, R. (2019). An Analysis of Machine Learning Classifiers in Breast Cancer Diagnosis. *2019 XLV Latin American Computing Conference (CLEI)*, 1-10. 10.1109/CLEI47609.2019.235094

The big causes of death from noncommunicable diseases. (2016). Bulletin of the World Health Organization. doi:10.2471/BLT.16.030616

Thomas, M. (2021). *Machine Learning in Healthcare*. https://builtin.com/artificial-intelligence/machine-learning-healthcare

Thomas, T., Pradhan, N., & Dhaka, V. S. (2020). Comparative Analysis to Predict Breast Cancer using Machine Learning Algorithms: A Survey. *2020 International Conference on Inventive Computation Technologies (ICICT)*, 192-196. 10.1109/ICICT48043.2020.9112464

Thorsen-Meyer, H. C., Nielsen, A. B., Nielsen, A. P., Kaas-Hansen, B. S., Toft, P., Schierbeck, J., Strøm, T., Chmura, P. J., Heimann, M., Dybdahl, L., Spangsege, L., Hulsen, P., Belling, K., Brunak, S., & Perner, A. (2020). Dynamic and explainable machine learning prediction of mortality in patients in the intensive care unit: A retrospective study of high-frequency data in electronic patient records. *The Lancet. Digital Health, 2*(4), e179–e191. doi:10.1016/S2589-7500(20)30018-2 PMID:33328078

Tigga, N. P., & Garg, S. (2020). Prediction of type 2 diabetes using machine learning classification methods. *Procedia Computer Science, 167*, 706–716.

Tiwari, V., Deyal, N., & Bish, T. N. S. (2020). Mathematical Modeling Based Study and Prediction of COVID-19 Epidemic Dissemination Under the Impact of Lockdown in India. *Frontiers Physics*. doi:10.3389/fphy.2020.586899

Tiwari, A. (2020). Modeling and analysis of COVID-19 epidemic in India. *Journal of Safety Science and Resilience, 1*(2), 135–140. doi:10.1016/j.jnlssr.2020.11.005

Tjoa, E., & Guan, C. (2020). A survey on explainable artificial intelligence (xai): Toward medical xai. *IEEE Transactions on Neural Networks and Learning Systems*, *32*(11), 4793–4813. doi:10.1109/TNNLS.2020.3027314 PMID:33079674

Toğaçar, M., Ergen, B., & Cömert, Z. (2020). COVID-19 detection using deep learning models to exploit Social Mimic Optimization and structured chest X-ray images using fuzzy color and stacking approaches. *Computers in Biology and Medicine*, *121*, 103805. doi:10.1016/j.compbiomed.2020.103805 PMID:32568679

Trambaiolli, L. R., Spolaôr, N., Lorena, A. C., Anghinah, R., & Sato, J. R. (2017). Feature selection before EEG classification supports the diagnosis of Alzheimer's disease. *Clinical Neurophysiology*, *128*(10), 2058–2067. doi:10.1016/j.clinph.2017.06.251 PMID:28866471

Tran, D., & Sorokin, A. (2008). *Human activity recognition with metric learning*. Paper presented at the European conference on computer vision.

Tyler, N. S., Mosquera-Lopez, C. M., & Wilson, L. M. (2020). An artificial intelligence decision support system for the management of type 1 diabetes. Nat Metab, 2, 612–619.

Vaid, A., Somani, S., Russak, A. J., De Freitas, J. K., Chaudhry, F. F., Paranjpe, I., . . . Glicksberg, B. S. (2020). Machine learning to predict mortality and critical events in covid-19 positive new york city patients. medRxiv. doi:10.1101/2020.04.26.20073411

Vaka, A. R., Soni, B., & Reddy, S. (2020). Breast cancer detection by leveraging Machine Learning. *ICT Express*, *6*(4), 320–324. doi:10.1016/j.icte.2020.04.009

van der Waa, J., Nieuwburg, E., Cremers, A., & Neerincx, M. (2021). Evaluating XAI: A comparison of rule-based and example-based explanations. *Artificial Intelligence*, *291*, 103404.

Van Ouwerkerk, J. (2006). *Image super-resolution survey*. Academic Press.

Venkatramanana, S., Lewis, B., Chen, J., Higdon, D., Vullikanti, A., & Marathe, M. (2018). Using data-driven agent-based models for forecasting emerging infectious diseases. *Epidemics*, *22*, 43–49.

Verma, G., & Verma, H. (2020). A Multilayer Perceptron Neural Network Model For Predicting Diabetes. *International Journal of Grid and Distributed Computing*, *13*, 1018–1025.

Ververidis. (2006). *Emotional speech recognition: Resources, features, and methods*. Academic Press.

Vickers, N. J. (2017). Animal communication: When i'm calling you, will you answer too? *Current Biology*, *27*(14), R713–R715. doi:10.1016/j.cub.2017.05.064 PMID:28743020

Vilone, G., & Longo, L. (2021). Notions of explainability and evaluation approaches for explainable artificial intelligence. *Information Fusion*, *76*, 89–106.

Virani, S. S., Alonso, A., Aparicio, H. J., Benjamin, E. J., Bittencourt, M. S., Callaway, C. W., Carson, A. P., Chamberlain, A. M., Cheng, S., Delling, F. N., Elkind, M. S. V., Evenson, K. R., Ferguson, J. F., Gupta, D. K., Khan, S. S., Kissela, B. M., Knutson, K. L., Lee, C. D., Lewis, T. T., ... Tsao, C. W. (2021). Heart disease and stroke statistics—2021 update: A report from the American Heart Association. *Circulation*, *143*(8), e254–e743. doi:10.1161/CIR.0000000000000950 PMID:33501848

Wang, X., Zhou, D., Zeng, N., Yu, X., Hu, S. (2018). *Super-resolution image reconstruction using surface fitting with hierarchical structure*. Academic Press.

Wang, C., Zhu, X., Hong, J. C., & Zheng, D. (2019). Artificial intelligence in radiotherapy treatment planning: Present and future. *Technology in Cancer Research & Treatment*, *18*, 1533033819873922. doi:10.1177/1533033819873922 PMID:31495281

Wang, D., Yang, Q., Abdul, A., & Lim, B. Y. (2019, May). Designing theory-driven user-centric explainable AI. *Proceedings of the 2019 CHI conference on human factors in computing systems*, 1-15.

Wang, L., Zhu, H., He, Z., Jia, Y., & Du, J. (2022). Adjacent slices feature transformer network for single anisotropic 3D brain MRI image super-resolution. *Biomedical Signal Processing and Control*, *72*, 103339. doi:10.1016/j.bspc.2021.103339

Wang, Y., Lei, B., Elazab, A., Tan, E.-L., Wang, W., Huang, F., Gong, X., & Wang, T. (2020). Breast Cancer Image Classification via Multi-Network Features and Dual-Network Orthogonal Low-Rank Learning. *IEEE Access: Practical Innovations, Open Solutions*, *8*, 27779–27792. doi:10.1109/ACCESS.2020.2964276

Wan, X., Zou, Y., Wang, J., & Wang, W. (2021, August). Prediction of shale oil production based on Prophet algorithm. *Journal of Physics: Conference Series*, *2009*(1), 012056. doi:10.1088/1742-6596/2009/1/012056

Wei, L. (2009). Emotion-induced Higher Wavelet Entropy in the EEG with Depression during a Cognitive Task. *International Conference of the IEEE EMBS*, *22*, 5018-5021.

Wei, P., Zhao, Y., Zheng, N., & Zhu, S.-C. (2013). Modeling 4d human-object interactions for event and object recognition. *Proceedings of the IEEE International Conference on Computer Vision*. 10.1109/ICCV.2013.406

Weld, D. S., & Bansal, G. (2019). The challenge of crafting intelligible intelligence. *Communications of the ACM*, *62*(6), 70–79. doi:10.1145/3282486

Westerlund, A. M., Hawe, J. S., Heinig, M., & Schunkert, H. (2021). Risk Prediction of Cardiovascular Events by Exploration of Molecular Data with Explainable Artificial Intelligence. *International Journal of Molecular Sciences*, *22*(19), 10291. doi:10.3390/ijms221910291 PMID:34638627

WHO. (2019). *WHO's Country Office in the People's Republic of China picked up a media statement by the Wuhan Municipal Health Commission from their website on cases of 'viral pneumonia' in Wuhan, People's Republic of China.* https://www.who.int/

Xia, L., Chen, C.-C., & Aggarwal, J. K. (2012). *View invariant human action recognition using histograms of 3d joints.* Paper presented at the 2012 IEEE computer society conference on computer vision and pattern recognition workshops. 10.1109/CVPRW.2012.6239233

Xue, H., Li, J., Xie, H., & Wang, Y. (2018). Review of drug repositioning approaches and resources. *International Journal of Biological Sciences*, *14*(10), 1232–1244. doi:10.7150/ijbs.24612 PMID:30123072

Xu, X., Jiang, X., Mac, C., Dud, P., Li, X., Lv, S., Yu, L., Ni, Q., Chen, Y., Su, J., Lang, G., Li, Y., Zhao, H., Liu, J., Xu, K., Ruan, L., Sheng, J., Qiu, Y., Wua, W., ... Li, L. (2020). A Deep Learning System to Screen Novel Coronavirus Disease 2019 Pneumonia. *Engineering*, *6*, 1122–1129.

Xu, Z., & Wang, Z. (2019). A Risk Prediction Model for Type 2 Diabetes Based on Weighted Feature Selection of Random Forest and XGBoost Ensemble Classifier. *2019 Eleventh International Conference on Advanced Computational Intelligence (ICACI)*, 278-283. DOI: 10.1109/ICACI.2019.8778622

Yan, L., Zhang, H. T., Xiao, Y., Wang, M., Sun, C., Liang, J., . . . Yuan, Y. (2020). Prediction of survival for severe Covid-19 patients with three clinical features: development of a machine learning-based prognostic model with clinical data in Wuhan. medRxiv. doi:10.1101/2020.10.09.20165431

Yang, S. (2010). ECG Pattern Recognition Based on Wavelet Transform and BP Neural Network. *Second International Symposium on Networking and Network Security*, 246-249.

Yang, G., Ye, Q., & Xia, J. (2022). Unbox the black-box for the medical explainable ai via multi-modal and multi-centre data fusion: A mini-review, two showcases and beyond. *Information Fusion*, *77*, 29–52.

Yang, S. C. H., Folke, T., & Shafto, P. (2021). Abstraction, validation, and generalization for explainable artificial intelligence. *Applied AI Letters*, *2*(4), e37.

Yao, Z., Zheng, X., Zheng, Z., Wu, K., & Zheng, J. (2021). Construction and validation of a machine learning-based nomogram: A tool to predict the risk of getting severe coronavirus disease 2019 (COVID-19). *Immunity, Inflammation and Disease*, *9*(2), 595–607. doi:10.1002/iid3.421 PMID:33713584

Yarabarla, M. S., Ravi, L. K., & Sivasangari, A. (2019). Breast Cancer Prediction via Machine Learning. *2019 3rd International Conference on Trends in Electronics and Informatics (ICOEI)*, 121-124. 10.1109/ICOEI.2019.8862533

Yasnitsky, L. N., Dumler, A. A., Poleshchuk, A. N., Bogdanov, C. V., & Cherepanov, F. M. (2015). Artificial neural networks for obtaining new medical knowledge: Diagnostics and prediction of cardiovascular disease progression. *Biology and Medicine (Aligarh)*, *7*(2), 95.

Yuvaraj, N., & SriPreethaa, K.R. (2019). Diabetes prediction in healthcare systems using machine learning algorithms on Hadoop cluster. *Cluster Computing, 22*, 1–9. doi:10.1007/s10586-017-1532-x

Zhang, L., & Wu, X. (2006). *An edge-guided image interpolation algorithm via directional filtering and data fusion.* Academic Press.

Zhang, S., Liang, G., Pan, S., & Zheng, L. (2018). *A fast medical image super resolution method based on deep learning network.* Academic Press.

Zhang, L., Tan, J., Han, D., & Zhu, H. (2017). From Machine learning to Deep learning: Progress in machine intelligence fir rational drug discovery. *Drug Discovery Today, 22*(11), 1680–1685. doi:10.1016/j.drudis.2017.08.010 PMID:28881183

Zhao, X., Zhang, Y., Zhang, T., & Zou, X. (2019). *Channel splitting network for single MR image super-resolution.* Academic Press.

Zheng, Y., Li, Z., Xin, J., & Zhou, G. (2020). *A spatial-temporal graph based hybrid infectious disease model with application to COVID-19.* arXiv preprint arXiv:2010.09077. doi:10.1101/2020.07.20.20158568

Zheng, B., Yoon, S. W., & Lam, S. S. (2014). Breast cancer diagnosis based on feature extraction using a hybrid of K-means and support vector machine algorithms. *Expert Systems with Applications, 41*(4, Part 1), 1476–1482. doi:10.1016/j.eswa.2013.08.044

Zhou, J., Gandomi, A. H., Chen, F., & Holzinger, A. (2021). Evaluating the Quality of Machine Learning Explanations: A Survey on Methods and Metrics. *Electronics (Basel), 10*(5), 593. https://doi.org/10.3390/electronics10050593

Zhou, Y., Hou, Y., Shen, J., Huang, Y., Martin, W., & Cheng, F. (2020). Network-based drug repurposing for novel coronavirus 2019-nCoV/SARS-CoV-2. *Cell Discovery, 6*(1), 1–18. doi:10.103841421-020-0153-3 PMID:32194980

Zhu, J., Deng, Y. Q., Wang, X., Li, X. F., Zhang, N. N., Liu, Z., . . . Xie, Z. (2020). An artificial intelligence system reveals liquiritin inhibits SARS-CoV-2 by mimicking type I interferon. BioRxiv. doi:10.1101/2020.05.02.074021

Zhu, J., Yang, G., & Lio, P. (2019). *How can we make gan perform better in single medical image super-resolution? A lesion focused multi-scale approach.* Paper presented at the 2019 IEEE 16th International Symposium on Biomedical Imaging (ISBI 2019). 10.1109/ISBI.2019.8759517

Zhu, C., Idemudia, C. U., & Feng, W. (2019). Improved logistic regression model for diabetes prediction by integrating PCA and K-means techniques. *Informatics in Medicine Unlocked, 17*, 100179.

Zhu, C., Idemudia, C., & Feng, W. (2019). Improved logistic regression model for diabetes prediction by integrating PCA and K-means techniques. *Informatics in Medicine Unlocked, 17*, 100179. Advance online publication. doi:10.1016/j.imu.2019.100179

Compilation of References

Zhu, D., & Qiu, D. (2021). Residual dense network for medical magnetic resonance images super-resolution. *Computer Methods and Programs in Biomedicine, 209*, 106330. doi:10.1016/j.cmpb.2021.106330 PMID:34388684

Zhu, J., Liapis, A., Risi, S., Bidarra, R., & Youngblood, G. M. (2018, August). Explainable AI for designers: A human-centered perspective on mixed-initiative co-creation. In *2018 IEEE Conference on Computational Intelligence and Games (CIG)* (pp. 1-8). IEEE.

Zhu, X., Suk, H.-I., & Shen, D. (2014). A novel matrix-similarity based loss function for joint regression and classification in Alzheimer's Disease diagnosis. *NeuroImage, 100*, 91–105. doi:10.1016/j.neuroimage.2014.05.078 PMID:24911377

Zintgraf, L. M., Cohen, T. S., Adel, T., & Welling, M. (2017). *Visualizing deep neural network decisions: Prediction difference analysis.* Academic Press.

Zoabi, Y., & Shomron, N. (2020). COVID-19 diagnosis prediction by symptoms of tested individuals: a machine learning approach. MedRxiv. doi:10.1101/2020.05.07.20093948

Zubatiuk, T., & Isayev, O. (2021). Development of multimodal machine learning potentials: Toward a physics-aware artificial intelligence. *Accounts of Chemical Research, 54*(7), 1575–1585.

About the Contributors

Victor Hugo C. de Albuquerque has a PhD in Mechanical Engineering with emphasis on Materials from the Federal University of Paraíba (2010), an MSc in Teleinformatics Engineering from the Federal University of Ceará (2007), and he graduated in Mechatronics Technology at the Federal Center of Technological Education of Ceará (2006). He is currently Assistant VI Professor of the Graduate Program in Applied Informatics at the University of Fortaleza (UNIFOR). He has experience in Computer Systems, mainly in the research fields of: Applied Computing, Intelligent Systems, Visualization and Interaction, with specific interest in Pattern Recognition, Artificial Intelligence, Image Processing and Analysis, as well as Automation with respect to biological signal/image processing, image segmentation, biomedical circuits and human/brain-machine interaction, NeuroBiofeedback, Neurorehabilitation, Visual Stimulation, including Augmented and Virtual Reality Simulation Modeling for animals and humans. Additionally, he has research at the microstructural characterization field through the combination of non-destructive techniques with signal/image processing and analysis, and pattern recognition.

P. Naga Srinivasu procured his bachelor degree in computer science engineering in the year 2011 from JNTUK and Masters in Computer Science Technology in 2013 from Gitam University, Visakhapatnam. He is currently a research scholar in Gitam University and his areas of research include Biomedical Imaging, Image Enhancement, Image Segmentation, Object Recognition, Image Encryption.

Akash Kumar Bhoi (B.Tech, M.Tech, Ph.D) is currently associated with KIET Group of Institutions, India as Adjunct Faculty and Directorate of Research, Sikkim Manipal University as Adjunct Research Faculty. He is appointed as the honorary title of "Adjunct Fellow" Institute for Sustainable Industries & Liveable Cities (ISILC), Victoria University, Melbourne, Australia for the period from 1 August 2021 to 31 July 2022. He is also working as a Research Associate at Wireless Networks (WN) Research Laboratory, Institute of Information Science and Technologies, National Research Council (ISTI-CRN) Pisa, Italy. He was the University Ph.D. Course

Coordinator for "Research & Publication Ethics (RPE) at SMU." He is the former Assistant Professor (SG) of Sikkim Manipal Institute of Technology and served about 10 years. He is a member of IEEE, ISEIS, and IAENG, an associate member of IEI, UACEE, and an editorial board member reviewer of Indian and International journals. He is also a regular reviewer of reputed journals, namely IEEE, Springer, Elsevier, Taylor and Francis, Inderscience, etc. His research areas are Biomedical Technologies, the Internet of Things, Computational Intelligence, Antenna, Renewable Energy. He has published several papers in national and international journals and conferences. He has 130+ documents registered in the Scopus database by the year 2021. He has also served on numerous organizing panels for international conferences and workshops. He is currently editing several books with Springer Nature, Elsevier, and Routledge & CRC Press. He is also serving as Guest editor for special issues of the journal like Springer Nature and Inderscience.

Alfonso González Briones holds a Ph.D. in Computer Engineering from the University of Salamanca since 2018, his thesis obtained the second place in the 1st SENSORS+CIRTI Award for the best national thesis in smart cities (CAEPIA 2018). At the same university, he obtained his Bachelor of Technical Engineer in Computer Engineering (2012), Degree in Computer Engineering (2013), and Masters in Intelligent Systems (2014). Alfonso was Project Manager of Industry 4.0 and IoT projects in the AIR Institute, Lecturer at the International University of La Rioja (UNIR), and also "Juan De La Cierva" Postdoc at University Complutense of Madrid. Currently, he is Assistant Professor at the University of Salamanca in the Department of Computer Science and Automatics. He has published more than 30 articles in journals, more than 60 articles in books and international congresses and has participated in 10 international research projects. He is also Member of the scientific committee of the Advances in Distributed Computing and Artificial Intelligence Journal (ADCAIJ) and British Journal of Applied Science & Technology (BJAST) and Reviewer of international journals (Supercomputing Journal, Journal of King Saud University, Energies, Sensors, Electronics or Applied Sciences, among others). He has participated as Chair and Member of the technical committee of prestigious international congresses (AIPES, HAIS, FODERTICS, PAAMS, KDIR).

* * *

Kavinya A. completed the Master of technology in the field of information technology in 2021 and bachelor of technology in the field of information technology in 2015 from Vivekanandha College of Engineering for Women, Namakkal. She has attended more than 2 conferences and published 2 papers and worked as an intern for 2 months under Prof.Pushpavanam Department of chemical Engineering, IITM. She has published 2 book chapters. Her areas of research include Machine learning.

Muyideen AbdulRaheem is a lecturer in the Department of Computer Science, University of Ilorin, Ilorin, Nigeria. He obtained a Bachelor of Technology Computer Science at the Prestigious Abubakar Tafawa Balewa University Bauchi, in 1997, Master of Science in Mathematics (Computer Option), and Ph.D. Computer Science at the University of Ilorin, Ilorin, Nigeria. He is the author of more than 20 articles and conference proceedings. He is a member of the International Computer Professional Registration Council of Nigeria (MCPN), and Nigeria Computer Society (MNCS). His research area is on computer security, grid computing security, data, and information security, information security, and cybersecurity.

Joseph Bamidele Awotunde received a B.Sc. degree in Mathematics/Computer Science from Federal University of Technology, Minna, Nigeria, in 2007. M.Sc. and Ph.D. degrees in Computer Science from the University of Ilorin, Ilorin, Nigeria, in 2014 and 2019 respectively. From 2012 to 2015, and in 2018, he was a Computer Science Instructor with the University School, University of Ilorin, Ilorin, Nigeria. From 2017 to 2018, he was a Lecturer II with the McPherson University, Ijebo, Seriki-Sotayo, Nigeria. Since 2019, he has been a Lecturer II with the Computer Science Department, University, of Ilorin, Ilorin, Nigeria. He is the author of more than 40 articles, and more than 15 Conference Proceedings. His research interests include Information Security, Cybersecurity, Bioinformatics Artificial Intelligence, Internet of Medical Things, Wireless Body Sensor Networks, Wireless Networks, Telemedicine, m-Health/e-health, Medical Imaging, Information Security, Software Engineering, and Biometrics. He is a member of International Association of Engineers and Computer Scientists (MIAENG), Computer Professional Registration Council of Nigeria (MCPN), and the Nigeria Computer Society (MNCS). Internet Society.

Iswarya B., MCA., M.Phil., Ph.D., is working as an Assistant Professor, Department of Computer Applications, Sri G.V.G Visalakshi College For Women(Autonomous), Accredited with A+ Grade by NAAC (4th Cycle) An ISO 9001:2015 certified Institution, Udumalpet, Tiruppur(Dt). She has 10 Years of Teaching Experience. Published 4 International Journals in UGC Care/Scopus/Web of Science. She has presented 5 papers in National, International Conferences and published 3 Book Chapters in International Publications & published one Book.

Rajesh Bandaru completed a B.Tech degree in Computer Science & Information Technology from AITAM, affiliated with JNTU Hyderabad, in 2005, M.Tech degree in Computer Science Technology with a Specialization in Computer Networks from Andhra University, Visakhapatnam, in the year 2010. He is pursuing PhD. from GITAM (Deemed to be University). He is currently working as an Assistant Professor in the Department of Computer Science and Engineering, GIT, GITAM (Deemed to be University) Visakhapatnam. He has 16 years of academic experience and published more than ten research papers in reputed international journals and conferences. His research areas include Machine Learning and Natural Language Processing.

Shamayita Basu received her MSc. Degree in medical biotechnology at Sikkim Manipal University. Currently pursuing PhD in Department of Microbiology at University of Kalyani, she has 3 years of teaching experience. She has published more than 8 research articles. She also got 1 patent. She has published two book chapters. She has delivered more than 20 guest lectures.

M. Farida Begam, Ph.D. in Computer Science and Engineering, is a strong academician and is currently working as a Professor and Head of the Department, Information Science and Engineering at CMR Institute of Technology. She received Master's Degree, M.Tech in Computer Science, from the National Institute of Technology, Trichy, and pursued her Bachelor Degree B.E in Computer Science and Engineering in Mookambigai College of Engineering, Bharathidasan University, Trichy. Dr. Farida has published Scopus indexed papers in reputed Journals and Conferences. She has presented papers in conferences held in Kuwait, Dubai and India. She is passionate in continuous teaching learning processes and involved in research related to Machine Learning, Deep Learning, NLP and student centric learning methodologies. She worked in University of Bolton, RAK, U.A.E as an Adjunct Professor. She worked as an Adjunct Faculty in Higher Colleges of Technology Dubai Women's College, Murdoch University, Dubai and as a Senior Lecturer in the Department of Engineering and Information Technology, Manipal University Dubai Campus and handled various IT related basic and advanced courses. She has 20 years of teaching experience in various domains of Information Technology and Computer Science and Engineering. She had worked in various engineering colleges in Tamil Nadu including National Institute of Technology, Trichy, India. She also has industry experience and worked as a Technical Evangelist in the Education and Research department in Infosys Technologies Ltd. India. She is a Cisco Certified Network associate (CCNA) and handled CCNA training courses in Manipal University Dubai Campus.

Zuhaibuddin Bhutto received a PhD in electronic engineering from Dong-A University, South Korea in 2019, he also received B.E. degree in software engineering and M.E. Degree in information technology from Mehran University of

Engineering and Technology, Pakistan, in 2009 and 2011, respectively. Currently, he is pursuing a Ph.D. Degree in electronics engineering from Dong-A University, South Korea. Since 2011, he has been an assistant professor at the Department of Computer System Engineering, Balochistan University of Engineering and Technology, Pakistan. His research interests include, image processing, MIMO technology; in particular, cooperative relaying, adaptive transmission techniques, energy optimization, machine learning, and deep learning.

Abirami D. is currently working as Assistant Professor in the Department of Zoology at Sri GVG Visalakshi College for Women (Autonomous), Udumalpet, Tiruppur Dt., Tamil Nadu, India has completed MSc., B.Ed., PGDCA, Ph.D. She has 10 years of teaching experience. She has published 14 articles in the reputed journals. She has presented more than 15 papers at National and International conferences.

Oladipo Dauda Idowu was born in Offa, Offa Local Government Area of Kwara State, Nigerian in 1968. He received his B.Sc.(Edu.) degree in Computer Science from Ekiti State University, Ado-Ekiti, Ekiti State, Nigeria in 2005. He earned his M.Sc. and Ph.D degree in Computer Science from University of Ilorin, Ilorin, Nigeria, in 2010 and 2018 respectively. Since 2019, he has been a Lecturer II with the Department of Computer Science, University of Ilorin, Ilorin, Nigeria. He is the author of more than 20 articles, and more than 10 conference Proceedings. His research interests include Software Engineering, Bioinformatics, Information Security, Artificial Intelligence, Cyber Security and Computer Education. He is a member of International Computer Professional Registration Council of Nigeria (MCPN) and Nigeria Computer Society (MNCS).

J. Sirisha Devi has 15 years of teaching experience. currently working as a Associate Professor, CSE at Institute of Aeronautical Engineering, Hyderabad. She has published more than 25 publications in national and international journals.

Ayush Dubey is a final year Undergraduate Student of Information Science and Engineering from CMR Institute of Technology, Bangalore, affiliated to Visvesvaraya Technological University. His areas of interest include the machine intelligence models and natural language processing.

Rajavikram Gandham has 14 years of teaching experience. currently working as a head of the department, CSE at VIGNAN Institute of Technology and Science Hyderabad. He has published more than 20 publications in national and international journals.

S. Geetha obtained her undergraduate, B.Tech (Information Technology) degree from Francis Xavier Engineering College (affiliated to Anna University, Chennai), Tirunelveli by means of a First Class with Distinction in 2005. She had completed her postgraduate, M.Tech (Information Technology) from Satyabama University, Chennai again by means of First Class with Distinction in 2009, and distinguished herself in the Toppers list too. She worked as a faculty in different engineering colleges affiliated under Anna University, Tamilnadu as well as Visvesvaraya Technological University, Karnataka. Thereafter, she completed PhD in the Department of Computer Science and Engineering at Kalasalingam Academy of Research and Education in 2019. She is currently working as an associate professor in Department of Information Science and Engineering at BNM Institute of Technology, Bangalore. Her research interest includes wireless sensor networks, Data Mining and warehousing and sensor cloud. She has published her research in many Journals and conferences. Her specializing in Wireless Sensor Networks, Block chain.is missing a biography.

Manoj Gupta received his Ph.D in the Computer Science from University of Rajasthan, Jaipur (India). He received his M.Tech in Digital Signal Processing from H.N.B Garhwal Central University, Uttarakhand, India and B.Tech degree in Electronics and Communication Engineering from Institute of Engineering & Technology, M.J.P.Rohilkhand University Campus, Bareilly (U.P) India. His Overall Experience is more than 15 years. He has published more than 50+ research papers in international journals and National/International conferences and book chapters. He is having one patent grant and published 5 Patents in his credit and currently having one Indian Copyright and filled another one Indian Copyright in his credit. He is the Editor in Chief (EiC) of the Book Series "Advances in Antenna, Microwave and Communication Engineering", Scrivener (John Wiley), USA and the book series editor in chief (EiC) of the book series "Advances in Antenna Design, Wireless Communication and Mobile Network Technology, CRC Press, Taylor and Francis (USA) and Editor in Chief (EiC) of the Book Series of "Advances in Digital Signal Processing and Image Processing for Industrial Applications", CRC Press, Taylor and Francis, USA and the book series editor in chief of the book series "AAP Book Series on Digital Signal Processing, Computer Vision and Image Processing", Apple Academic Press, USA. His research interests are in Antenna and Wireless Communications, Biomedical Image & Signal Processing, Soft Computing, Computational Intelligence, Biomedical Engineering, Artificial Intelligence and Neuroscience. He is a Member of many Professional Bodies such as IEEE, IACSIT, ISTE, IAENG and many more. He has served as Technical Programme Committee (TPC) Member and Reviewer in various International Conferences such as, ICCIA 2020, ICCIA 2019 ICSIP 2018, ICSIP 2017, ICSIP 2016, AIPR 2017, AIPR 2016, ICCIA 2018, ICCIA 2017, ICCIA 2016, ICNIT 2018 and many more. He was invited for Keynote

Speaker/Invited Speaker in 2017 2nd IEEE International Conference on Signal and Image Processing (ICSIP 2017), August 04-06, 2017 in Nanyang Executive Centre, Singapore and Invited for Keynote Speaker in 2017 International Conferences on Public Health and Medical Sciences (ICPHMS 2017), May 23-24, 2017 in Xi'an, China. He is Editors, Associate editor and Reviewer of many international Journals. His name has been listed in Marquis Who's Who in Science and Engineering® USA and Marquis Who's Who in the World® USA). He is the Lead Guest Editor of the Special Issue Journal titled "Advanced 5G Communication System for Transforming Healthcare" in the Journal CMC Computers, Materials and Continua (Q1, SCI, Scopus, Impact Factor: 4.89). Presently he is working as an Associate Professor in Department of Electronics and Communication Engineering, JECRC University, Jaipur (Rajasthan), India.

Hariprasath K. is currently a research scholar of Anna University doing research in Blockchain and its futuristic applications. He has completed M.E. degree in Computer Science and Engineering in 2012 from the Anna University, Chennai. Currently working as an Assistant Professor in Department of Information technology at Vivekanandha College of Engineering for Women, Namakkal, India. He has more than 8 years of teaching experience in variety of subjects. Formerly, he worked as a faculty member in the Department of Computer Science & Engineering in Muthayammal College of Engineering, Namakkal. He had organized and participated various seminars and workshops. He has published over 10 papers in international, national journals, conference proceedings and 3 book chapters. His areas of research include IOT, Machine Learning, Blockchain, Image Processing, Wireless Sensor Networks and Network Security. He has delivered several special lectures in workshops and seminars.

Manimekalai K. is a Head & Assistant Professor in the Department of Computer Applications at Sri GVG Visalakshi College For Women(Autonomous), Udumalpet, Tiruppur Dt., She has completed MCA, M.Phil., In the year 2017, she passed the State Level Eligibility Test. She has 17 years of teaching experience. She has 13 international journal publications in Scopus, Web of Science, and UGC Care list. She has given 15 presentations at National and International conferences. She was a Session member as well as presenter at the International e-conference in CAPCDR in October 2021.She has published one book. She has published 5 book chapters in International publications.

Harikrishna Kamatham has 20 years of teaching experience. currently working as a principal, at AVN Institute of Engineering & Technology, Hyderabad. He has published more than 20 publications in national and international journals.

Selvani Deepthi Kavila received B.Tech degree in Computer Science & Information Technology from Al-Ameer College of Engineering, affiliated with JNTU Hyderabad, in 2005, M.Tech degree in Computer Science Technology with a Specialization in Artificial Intelligence & Robotics from Andhra University, Visakhapatnam, in the year of 2008. She has done a Ph.D. in computer science and Engineering from GITAM (Deemed to be University) in 2018. She is currently working as an Associate Professor in the Department of Computer Science and Engineering, ANITS, Visakhapatnam. She has a total of 16 years of teaching & research experience. She is a member of ACM, CSI, etc., and published more than 26 research papers in reputed international journals and conferences. She actively participated in reviewing research papers and book chapters and was a Program Committee member & Session chair of various Conferences. Her teaching and research interests include Artificial Intelligence, NLP, Machine Learning, and Deep Learning.

Namana Krishna, Professor & HOD, Department of CSE, AVN Institute of Engineering & Technology, Hyderabad, Telangana State, India, was awarded PhD, Computer Science and Engineering from GITAM University in the year 2014. He completed M.Tech., Computer Science and Technology from B.I.H.E.R in the year 2006. He has published more than 20 articles in reputed international journals and delivered guest lectures on different research topics like Human computer interaction, latest trends in signal processing, etc.

Wazir Laghari is currently working in Electrical Engineering Department, Balochistan University of Engineering and Technology (BUET) Khuzdar. He was received his doctoral degree from the Department of Electrical Engineering Chulalongkorn University Bangkok, Thailand in 2019. Previously he was obtained ME degree in the field of Communication Systems and Networks from Mehran University of Engineering and Technology, Jamshoro, Sindh, Pakistan respectively. His research interests lie in the areas of Electrical Engineering, Communication Systems, Neural Networks, and Machine Learning, specifically in Deep Learning image super-resolution.

Kaviyavarshini N. is doing research in Blockchain. Currently as Research Scholar of Anna University. She has completed M.Tech in the field of Information Technology at Vivekanandha College of Engineering for Women, Namakkal. She has attended more than 2 conferences and published 3 journal papers. She has published 2 book chapters. She also worked as an intern for 1 month under Mr. T. Vigneshwaran, Chief Executive Officer, Nandha Infotech, Coimbatore. Her area of research include Swarm Intelligence, Deep Learning, Machine Learning and Blockchain.

Saravana N. M. received his Ph.D. Degree in Information and Communication Engineering and M.E in Computer Science and Engineering at Anna University, Chennai. Currently working as a Professor in Department of Computer Science and Engineering at M. Kumarasamy College of Engineering, Karur, India. He is recognized as a Research Supervisor for Ph.D. Programme (By Research) in Information and Communication Engineering for Anna University, Chennai. He has more than 20 Years of teaching experience. He has attended more than 40 International Conferences and published around 40 papers in various reputed International Journals including Springer, Inderscience and Elsevier and is an editor of a book and published 3 book chapters. He also got 2 patents. He is guiding 11 research scholars. He has conducted more than 20 workshops on various fields of Big Data Analytics, Network Security, Cyber Security and Hadoop. He acts as a reviewer of various International journals. He has been contributed as a Technical committee member and session chair in and outside India. His interests include Network Security, Wireless & Mobile Communication and Distributed Systems. He is life member of ISTE, IAENG and CSI.

Hemaraju Pollayi has done Post-Docs in Mechanical and Aerospace Engineering at Utah State University-USA and in Mechanical Engineering at IISc Bengaluru-India. He has completed PhD in Aerospace Engineering (Structures) at IISc, MTech in Civil Engineering (Structures) at IIT-Guwahati and BE in Civil Engineering at Osmania University Hyderabad. Now he is working as an Associate Professor in Civil Engineering Department at School of Technology, GITAM University-Hyderabad. His research interests are in the area of AI & ML, Intelligent Systems, SHM, Non-Linear Mechanics and Damage Mechanics. He has 4-years of post-doc research experience in Solid Mechanics and Structural Health Monitoring (SHM) and 7-years of teaching experience in Structural Dynamics. His research work has published in high-impact factor International Journals and reputed International Conferences such as International Journal of Non-Linear Mechanics, International Journal of Composite Structures and International Journal of Engineering Structures. He has assisted a MS(Engg.), MS Plan-B and PhD dissertation during his PhD and Post-Doc. He has guided 5-MTech students, 12-BTech projects. Currently, he is guiding 5-PhD students.

Praveena Rao is currently pursuing PhD in Civil Engineering at GITAM University, Hyderabad in the area of Artificial Intelligence and Machine Learning applications for seismic analysis of structures. She has completed M.Tech in the specialization of Structural Engineering from KIIT Deemed to be University, Bhubaneswar and has performed experimental investigations in the area of Composite action of RCC and brick masonry walls. She has completed B.Tech in Civil Engineering and worked on ArcGIS for Geospatial analysis as BTech project. She has 3 years teaching experience as Assistant Professor ratified by JNTU-Hyderabad and BPUT, Odisha also worked as teaching assistant for a tenure of two years during M.Tech. She has guided B.Tech projects, 2 M.Tech projects. She has research publications in International Journals; presented papers at International Conferences and Symposia at Institution of Engineers, Bhubaneswar Student Chapter. Her research interests are in the area of Artificial Intelligence and Machine Learning Techniques, Structural Dynamics, Seismic Analysis, Earthquake Resistant Design and IoT based Structural Health Monitoring of civil engineering structures.

Joshua Samuel Raj R. received the B.E. Degree in computer science and engineering and M.E. degree in computer science and engineering from Anna University, Chennai, India, in 2005 and 2007, respectively, the Ph.D. degree from the Faculty of Information Technology, Kalasalingam University, India, in 2015, and the M.B.A. and the M.A. (literature) through the Distance Education Program from Manonmaniam Sundaranar University, Tirunelveli, India. He is a Life Member of the Indian Society for Technical Education and The Indian Science Congress. He is currently serving as a Professor in the Department of Information Science and Engineering, CMR Institute of Technology, Bengaluru. He has held key positions such as the Vice Principal, the Principal, and the Director of engineering colleges. He has authored over 60 articles in refereed international and domestic journals and conferences, and holds eight patents. His areas of interests include Grid Computing, Cloud Computing, Data Mining, Machine Learning, Scheduling and Artificial Intelligence.

Tamilselvi S. received her Ph.D. Degree in Science at Anna University and M.Phil in Biochemistry at Bharathiyar University. Currently working as a Associate Professor in Department of Biotechnology at Bannari Amman Institute of Technology Sathyamangalam. She is recognized as a Research Supervisor for Ph.D. in Science and Humanities for Anna University, Chennai. She has more than 15 Years of teaching experience. She has published more than 25 journal papers. She also got 4 patents. She has published a book chapter. She acts as a life member in ISTE (Indian Society for Technical Education), APP (Association of Pharmacy Professionals) and BRSI (Biotech Research Society of India). She has delivered more than 10 guest lectures.

Shakirat A. Salihu is a lecturer at the Department of Computer Science, Faculty of Communication and Information Sciences, University of Ilorin, Ilorin, Nigeria. She received her B.Sc. in Computer Science in 2006 from the University of Ilorin, subsequently obtained her M. Sc and Ph.D. degrees from the same University in

2011 and 2022 respectively. Her academic career began at Federal Polytechnic, Mubi, Adamawa State, Nigeria as an Assistant Lecturer in 2010 and rose to the level of Lecturer III in 2013. She later joined the service of the University of Ilorin as a lecturer in the Department of Computer Science in 2014. Her area of expert includes Software Engineering, Information Retrieval, Data Mining, and Knowledge Management.

Ayush Sengar is a final year Undergraduate Student of Information Science and Engineering from CMR Institute Of Technology, Bangalore, affiliated to Visvesvaraya Technological University. His areas of interest include the healthcare engineering and biomedical imaging technologies.

Jana Shafi is affiliated with the Department of Computer Science, Prince Sattam bin Abdul Aziz University, KSA. She has more than eight years of teaching and research experience. She has published in numerous journals such as Sensors, IEEE Access, Diagnostics, Symmetry, Mathematics and Wireless Communications, and Mobile Computing. Her research interests include Online Social Networks, Wearable Technology, Artificial Intelligence, Machine Learning, Deep Learning, Smart Health, and IOMT.

Index

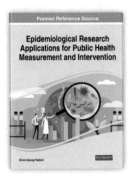
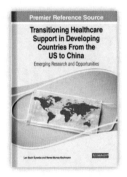
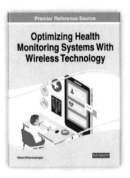
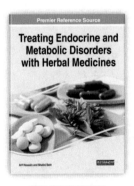
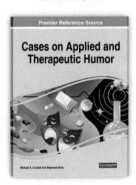
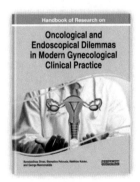
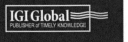

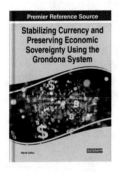
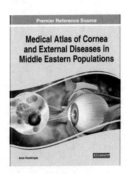
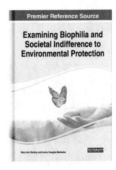
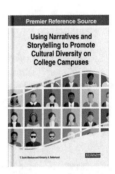

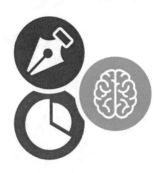
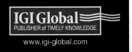

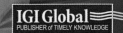

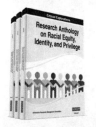
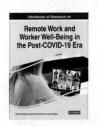
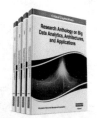
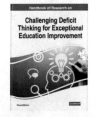

Have Your Work Published and Freely Accessible
Open Access Publishing

With the industry shifting from the more traditional publication models to an open access (OA) publication model, publishers are finding that OA publishing has many benefits that are awarded to authors and editors of published work.

Freely Share
Your Research

Higher Discoverability
& Citation Impact

Rigorous & Expedited
Publishing Process

Increased
Advancement &
Collaboration

Acquire & Open

When your library acquires an IGI Global e-Book and/or e-Journal Collection, your faculty's published work will be considered for immediate conversion to Open Access *(CC BY License)*, at no additional cost to the library or its faculty *(cost only applies to the e-Collection content being acquired)*, through our popular **Transformative Open Access (Read & Publish) Initiative**.

Provide Up To
100%
OA APC or
CPC Funding

Funding to
Convert or
Start a Journal to
**Platinum
OA**

Support for
Funding an
**OA
Reference
Book**

IGI Global publications are found in a number of prestigious indices, including Web of Science™, Scopus®, Compendex, and PsycINFO®. The selection criteria is very strict and to ensure that journals and books are accepted into the major indexes, IGI Global closely monitors publications against the criteria that the indexes provide to publishers.

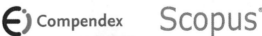

WEB OF SCIENCE™   Ⓔ Compendex   Scopus®

PsycINFO®   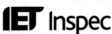 Inspec

---

**Learn More
Here:**

For Questions, Contact IGI Global's Open Access
Team at openaccessadmin@igi-global.com

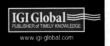
IGI Global
PUBLISHER of TIMELY KNOWLEDGE
www.igi-global.com

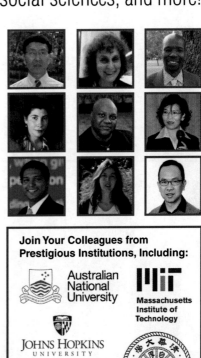

Printed in the United States
by Baker & Taylor Publisher Services